Passion

and

Purpose:

Black Female Surgeons

Stories and interviews to inspire and
motivate young women to follow their
dreams despite any obstacles.

By Dr. Praise Matemavi

Passion and Purpose: Black Female Surgeons

This is a work of non-fiction.

Text and Illustrations copyrighted

by Dr. Praise Matemavi ©2020

Library of Congress Control Number: 2020907376

Printed in the United States of America

A 2 Z Press LLC

PO Box 582

Deleon Springs, FL 32130

bestlittleonlinebookstore.com

sizemore3630@aol.com

440.241.3126

ISBN: 978-1-946908-35-3

DEDICATION

To every child and woman
who has a dream beyond
what they can see.

Introduction
About the Book

Passion and Purpose: Black Female Surgeons is a collection of stories and interviews of black women surgeons from 27 countries representing the United States of America, the United Kingdom, Europe, South America, the Caribbean, and Africa. These women were girls with visions who had the courage and fortitude to follow their dreams and embark on journeys that for most, no one who looked like them embarked on before. They set their sights on goals that were crystal clear in their minds even though at times no one else could see their vision. Surgical training is one of the most difficult of the training specialties in medicine and requires physical and mental stamina.

The contributors for this book overcame insurmountable odds. They are the definition of grit and resilience. They range in experience from intern to full professor. They are among the determined and fierce women featured in this book - The first African American female pediatric surgeon, the first female president of the Society of Black Academic Surgeons, the first African American Director of Member Services at the American College of Surgeons, the first female neurosurgeon in Uganda, the first female neurosurgeon in Rwanda, the first female urologist in Zambia, the first pediatric surgeon in Zambia, the only female breast cancer surgeon in Kenya, the first female cardio-thoracic surgeon in Nigeria and West Africa, the first female Zimbabwean orthopedic surgeon, and the first female pediatric and urological surgeon in Kenya. These and other phenomenal women share pearls of wisdom of how they achieved and thrive as women of color in a male-dominated field. All the surgical specialties are represented.

I was inspired to write this book when I finished my specialty training in multi-organ transplant and hepatobiliary (liver and gall bladder) surgery. As a child, I had the dream of becoming a doctor, but never had a frame of reference of a doctor that looked like me. This book has been a labor of love. I spent many nights and weekends contacting women via email and social media asking them if they would be part of this book. I remember wishing I had a book about women who looked like me doing what I wanted to do during my journey.

I read every book I could find about female surgeons. At the time, I only discovered two. I was motivated to collect stories about black female surgeons across the globe because we all have a unifying theme of grit, resilience, determination, perseverance, and experience of life in a way only those who look like us can relate to.

I hope all the brown-skinned girls everywhere in the world open this book and see women who look like them doing magnificent things in the field of surgery and become motivated to do whatever their hearts' desire. I hope girls and women are encouraged by these stories and interviews and will have the courage to take up space and flourish. This book is a celebration of those who have gone before us and the many men and women of different colors who have made it possible for us to reach our potential. We are certainly our ancestors' wildest dreams come true!

Dr. Praise Matemavi
Mississippi, USA

Table of Contents

CHAPTER NINE: Endocrine Surgery (surgery of the thyroids, parathyroids, and adrenals)

Dr. Aida Taye (Practicing in New York, USA)

CHAPTER TEN: Neurosurgery (surgery of the brain and spinal cord)

Dr. Juliet Sekabunga Nalwanga (Practicing in Uganda)

Dr. Claire Karekezi (Practicing in Rwanda)

Dr. J Nozipo Maraire (Practicing in Zimbabwe)

Dr. Coceka Mfundisi (Practicing in South Africa)

CHAPTER ELEVEN: Trauma and Critical Care Surgery (surgery for traumatic injuries and intensive care)

Dr. Violet Onkoba (Practicing in Michigan, USA)

Dr. Qaali Hussein (Practicing in Texas, USA)

Dr. Shuntaye Batson (Practicing in Mississippi, USA)

CHAPTER TWELVE: Obstetrics and Gynecologic Surgery (care of the pregnant patient and delivering babies, and surgery of female reproductive organs)

Dr. Keisha Bell Catchings (Practicing in Mississippi, USA)

Dr. Tosin Odunsi (Practicing in Washington State, USA)

Dr. Fatu Forna (Practicing in Georgia, USA)

Dr. Ruth Arumala (Practicing in Texas, USA)

CHAPTER THIRTEEN: Gynecologic Oncology (surgery for cancer of female reproductive organs – the ovaries and uterus)

Dr. Kemi Doll (Practicing in Washington State, USA)

Dr. Ebony Hoskins (Practicing in Washington D.C, USA)

CHAPTER FOURTEEN: Orthopedic Surgery (surgery of bones, ligaments, tendons, and muscles)

Dr. Samantha Z. Tross (Practicing in the UK)

Dr. Sonya Sloan (Practicing in Texas, USA)

Dr. Pamela Samoyo (Practicing in Zambia)

CHAPTER FIFTEEN: Cardio-thoracic Surgery (surgery of the heart and lungs)

Dr. Ogadinma Mgbajah (Practicing in Nigeria)

Dr. Lindiwe Sidali (Practicing in South Africa)

CHAPTER SIXTEEN: Vascular Surgery (surgery of the blood vessels)

Dr. Olamide Alabi (Practicing in Georgia, USA)

Fernanda Costa Sampaio Silva (Practicing in Brazil)

CHAPTER SEVENTEEN: Ophthalmology (surgery of the eyes)

Dr. Omofolasade Kosoko-Lasaki (Practicing in Nebraska, USA)

CHAPTER EIGHTEEN: Otolaryngologic Surgery (surgery of the ears, nose, throat, head, and neck

Dr. Gina Jefferson (Practicing in Mississippi, USA)

Dr. Barbara Grandison (Practicing in Montego Bay, Jamaica)

Dr. Tonia Farmer (Practicing in Ohio, USA)

CHAPTER NINETEEN: Plastics and Reconstructive Surgery & Cosmetic Surgery (surgery for the reconstruction of tissue and skin and hair transplant)

Dr. Metasebia Worku Abebe (Practicing in Addis Ababa, Ethiopia)

Dr. Sharone Jacobs (Practicing in Pennsylvania, USA)

Dr. Elizabeth Xoagus (Practicing in South Africa)

CHAPTER TWENTY: Surgical Oncology (surgery of cancers in the abdomen, breast, skin, and soft tissue)

Dr. Lori Wilson (Practicing in Washington D.C, USA)

CHAPTER TWENTY-ONE: Oral and Maxillofacial Surgery (surgery of the mouth and face)

Dr. Sandra Oyakhilome (Practicing in Cape Coast, Ghana)

CHAPTER ONE
Transplant Surgery

Transplant surgery is where an organ is replaced with an organ from a living donor or a deceased donor.

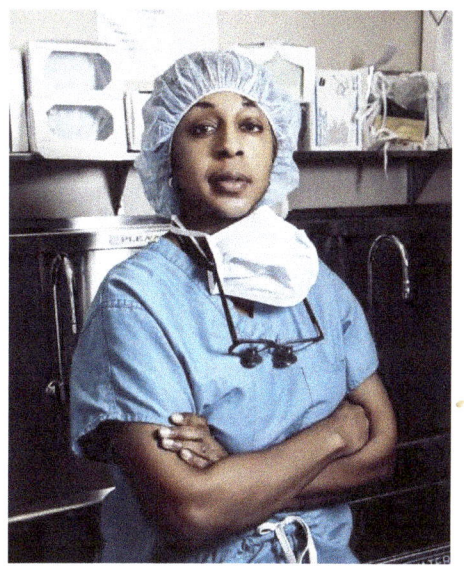

Dr. Sherilyn Gordon – Burroughs
(August 23, 1968 – March 19, 2017)

This book was created to inspire young women to dream big and know that, no matter what their dream is, nothing is impossible. It has also been created to honor the memory of one of the many talented and amazing female black surgeons in this book, transplant surgeon Dr. Sherilyn Gordon-Burroughs.

Dr. Sherilyn was a multi-organ transplant surgeon. Her parents migrated to Missouri, USA, from Jamaica in the 1960s. She was raised with strong family-oriented Jamaican influence. Her parents taught her the value and importance of an education at an early age. "Pray always, dream big, set goals, work hard, and enjoy your achievements," are the encouraging words her parents spoke into her life. These words were the driving force in her studies and work ethic.

Raised in a Seventh - day Adventist home, Dr. Sherilyn was a gifted child, and excelled academically. She began reading before her third birthday and, being the daughter of a father who was a microbiologist, she had the opportunity to tag along with him to work. This reinforced her love for science. From as far back as elementary school, she shared how several educators impacted her success. Educators throughout high school and medical school were also instrumental in encouraging her. And last, but not least, the people who trained her in general surgery and transplant surgery impacted her life dramatically. It cannot be overstated how the encouragement of educators give students entrusted to them a greater advantage when they invest positive influence and motivation. Teachers have the tremendous honor of finding something great in each student.

One high school science teacher, Mr. Scott, said, "I have never seen a more focused student." Dr. Sherilyn was awarded Science Student of the Year her junior year in high school.

Her focus extended into her undergraduate studies at Howard University in Washington, D.C., where Dr. Sherilyn was given a full academic scholarship and graduated *magna cum laude*. She attended medical school at Washington University in St Louis, Missouri, and returned to Howard University to complete her residency in general surgery.

During her residency, she completed an immunology research fellowship at the University of Pittsburgh in Pennsylvania. Finally, her long journey in education took her to the University of California, Los Angeles, where she completed her fellowship in multi-organ transplant surgery.

She had to be passionate about multi-organ transplant surgery because it is one of the most demanding subspecialty training programs of all the various specialties. Her parents agreed it was the most difficult time of her training, but she never complained.

After completing her fellowship, she was hired as faculty

at Dumont-UCLA Transplant Center, California, and worked for a few years before taking a job at the Methodist Hospital in Houston, Texas.

During interviews, Dr. Sherilyn shared about herself and her journey. When asked the secret to her personal and professional success and how she dealt with difficulties, she shared that it was her not taking herself too seriously. She felt this was the best advice she could tell herself. In fact, she said it served her well when dealing with both patients and colleagues as well as problems that arose. Dr. Sherilyn felt not taking herself too seriously was the most important thing because as she analyzed problems that came across her desk or issues that could inhibit her ability to deal with people, it helped to understand where they were coming from. She said, "Often, we get in our own way, and we do so by taking ourselves too seriously."

In addition to not taking herself too seriously, she shared that having a sense of humor went hand-in-hand with not taking herself too seriously. She claimed it was sometimes easy to mistake statements people made or offhanded comments as a slight. When she took the time to know people and where they were coming from, she found she was often surprised at how uncomfortable they were.

This never excused malicious things, but often in social or professional situations, people were just trying to walk a fine line that allowed them to say and be who they were while not necessarily being offensive. And, sometimes, it was just their way of embracing her. They did not always succeed, and this was okay. Dr. Sherilyn concluded that when she took herself too seriously and not having a sense of humor detracted from the ability to move forward in working relationships. So, she felt these two things go together.

She added a third secret to her personal and professional success. In the professional realm, what must trump all, is choosing to hold herself to the highest standard possible. In her own kind words, she said, "You can hold yourself to a high standard by reading and doing your homework and staying on top of your game. I also believe you should not make people feel you are the smartest person in the room or the person who knows the most who needs to be acknowledged for knowing."

She continued, "If you can balance this, I think it smooths things over nicely and work relations are built. Oftentimes in these social/professional situations people are just trying to walk a fine line that allows them to say and be who they are while not necessarily being offensive. And sometimes it's just a way of finding their way of embracing you."

Dr. Sherilyn aspired to become a Dean of Students and was passionate about the well-being and growth of medical students and residents. She was a gifted surgeon who absolutely loved her job. But the most important thing in her life was her daughter, Jasmine, whom she loved fiercely.

Despite all of Dr. Sherilyn's success, she unfortunately lost her life to domestic violence. She never complained about her home life and there were no outward signs she was in an abusive marriage. Domestic violence does not discriminate, it affects the most beautiful, the most successful, and the most amazing people. Though her death is tragic, it is not in vain. Her light continues to shine in all the lives she touched. She is greatly missed.

"Taking responsibility — practicing 100 percent responsibility every day — is about seeing ourselves not as right or wrong, but as an agent, chooser, problem solver, and learner in the complex interrelationships of our lives so that we can better integrate with the people and world around us. When we do this, we enjoy a better and more productive way to live and lead."
— Christopher Avery

Dr. Arika Hoffman

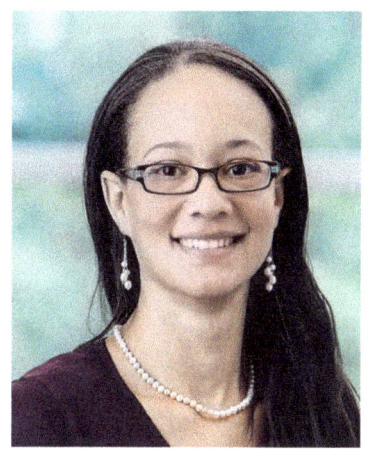

Dr. Arika Hoffman is an abdominal transplant surgeon at the University of Nebraska Medical Center in Omaha, Nebraska. She is a graduate of Dickinson College in Carlisle, Pennsylvania. She earned her degree in medicine from Wake Forest University, Winston Salem, North Carolina, and from there trained at Henry Ford Hospital, Detroit, Michigan, in general surgery. She completed an abdominal transplant surgery fellowship at the University of Alabama in Birmingham. Following her fellowship, she was recruited by the University of Nebraska where she currently specializes in adult and pediatric kidney transplantation.

Her clinical expertise is in living donor kidney transplant and pediatric transplantation. As one of only 10 African American female transplant surgeons in America, she carries her passion for education into research and mentorship. Her scientific interests include gender disparities in academia where she is nationally recognized for her work. She studies how gender differences in letters of recommendation for applicants entering surgical subspecialty fellowships provide insight into inherent gender bias and how this may influence candidate selection in these male-dominated fellowships. She hopes to make a difference for more young women applying for specialties.

Dr. Hoffman chose medicine because she believes it is a calling.

"I feel that if your purpose is to help people on a greater scale, this is the profession to pursue. I chose surgery because I love to operate," she explains. "I do not think you can pursue surgery unless you love to operate because you are going to do it when you are completely exhausted, stressed out, hungry and frustrated. And, if you do not love to operate, then these experiences will be horrible. If, however, you love to operate and you love surgery, then doing it when you feel like you can barely stand, when it is the middle of the night, actually feels more like a blessing."

What Dr. Hoffman has seen is that people who do not love surgery view it as a personal punishment during the tough times. For her, it has never been that way. She found herself trying to be in surgery as often as possible. When she realized surgery was where she preferred to be, she felt called to be a surgeon.

She shared some of the challenges she encountered in her journey. "I think of life in quotes. The saying, 'you cannot be what you cannot see' epitomizes the greatest challenge for me. For many of us, it is difficult to see something in yourself that you cannot see in someone else. I trained where there were very few female surgeons and even fewer black surgeons."

She sincerely added, "It is not that people did not believe in me, it was more so that people who did not look like me were more supported and it was as if the surgical community accepted them as surgeons before they accepted me. When you are surrounded by people who are afforded this privilege you realize that even though you are called to a specialty, it will be an uphill battle many days."

A few lessons Dr. Hoffman shared are to first find mentors and friends who are on a similar journey and path. She underestimated how important this is. Secondly, you are not a wave. You are part of an ocean. Your journey is part of a greater journey, so you recognize all the struggles of the people who have come before you. Many people have struggled for you in your place, so on your very worst day, if you can think how our ancestors paved the way, you can get through anything! And this is something she did not understand until she was further along in the process.

Thirdly, she feels you may love your position, your job, your residency, or fellowship, but your fellowship, your job, and your residency do not necessarily love you back. You must find value within yourself. If you are searching for value in a position, in a job, or in that place of employment, then you are doing it wrong. That employment or place believes you are dispensable and replaceable. You must find value in other things. You must remember that even if you love that position with everything you have it is not guaranteed that that position will love you back.

Dr. Hoffman's greatest accomplishment and proudest day was the day she walked into her office at the University of Nebraska Medical Center. It was then she realized she had made it! As she hung a picture on the wall – in *her* office – she realized, she was an academic surgeon and had arrived!

The advice she gives to every resident and fellow is never take a job on a promise because you may be disappointed. In other words, know exactly what job you are accepting in terms that are clear regarding responsibilities and expectations.

She is a mother of three young girls and juggles career and family well even though she realizes balance in life is not something she has found simple to achieve.

Dr. Hoffman candidly shared that if she was not a transplant surgeon, she would want to be a playwright. She was a playwright in college and wrote several plays she was never able to direct. She has many plays in her head just waiting to be developed.

If she could select three people to have dinner with, she would first pick Michelle Obama because she is simply amazing. Secondly, James Baldwin because he was ahead of his time. Dr. Hoffman feels she would love to see him and hear him now because everything that he said was going to happen has happened. And lastly, Ta-Nehisi Coates because he is so intelligent.

Dr. Hoffman hopes to inspire all young women by her story of courage and hard work.

Do your little bit of good where you are; it's those little bits of good put together that overwhelm the world." Desmond Tutu

Dr. Dinee Simpson

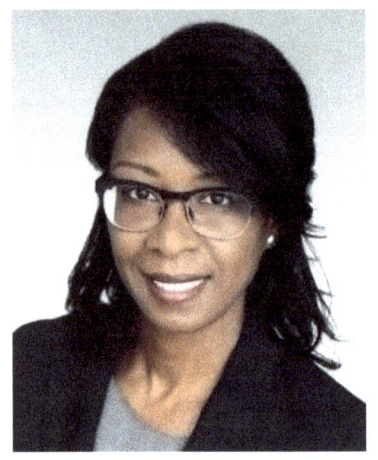

Dr. Dinee Simpson began her long journey in medicine at Colgate University in New York, where she received her bachelor's degree in chemistry. She was accepted to medical school at New York University, New York, New York.

After becoming a doctor, she attended Boston, Massachusetts's Brigham and Woman's Hospital, Harvard University Medical School and completed a post-doctoral fellowship. This is a fancy way of saying she finished additional study in research during her residency training in general surgery. She completed her general surgery residency at Brigham and Woman's Hospital before going to the University of Pennsylvania, Philadelphia, where she trained in liver and kidney transplant surgery.

After all her hard work, Dr. Simpson is now an assistant professor of surgery at Northwestern's Feinberg School of Medicine, Chicago, Illinois. Here, her academic focus is on disparities within the African American community regarding transplantation.

She is the founding director of Northwestern's African American Transplant Access Program, which aims to increase education about transplant, access to transplant, and help patients navigate through the evaluation and listing process. In addition to her many achievements, she also serves on the Board of Directors for the National Kidney Foundation of Illinois and the internal advisory board for Northwestern's George M. O'Brien Kidney Research Core Center (NUGoKidney).

When Dr. Simpson completed her bachelor's degree at Colgate University in New York, she majored in chemistry because she aspired to pursue a career discovering and researching new medications. During her junior year of college, she discovered a suspicious mass in her breast that required surgery.

She shared, "I was fearful because I did not know what to expect. When I awoke after surgery, the mass was gone, and this was a powerful experience for me. It was absolutely amazing to experience tangible results so quickly. It was at this time I knew I wanted to become a doctor, but it was too late to apply for medical school immediately following college because I was required to take the medical college admission test (MCAT) before I could apply."

So, while preparing for medical school, she worked at a tech startup in New York collecting data on how consumers searched for health care information online. A tech startup is a company that brings technology products or services to people to solve a problem where the solution is not obvious.

The company provided its data to drug manufacturers to help target marketing efforts. At that time, Dr. Simpson realized many of the commercials did not speak to either her or her family members. She feels healthcare needs to speak to peoples' culture.

This motivated her to use market research to consider how people from different cultures searched for healthcare information. She discovered there is a difference and presented her data to pharmaceutical clients. She used her data to create tailored commercials, depending on the target group. This was Dr. Simpson's first experience thinking about cultural competency when delivering a service.

During surgical residency training, she scrubbed into a living donor kidney transplant surgery and, when the blood flow was restored, the new kidney turned pink and began making urine immediately. She feels there is no better instant gratification than this. Even after completing several hundred transplants, it never gets old for Dr. Simpson. It is always as exciting as her first transplant!

Later that same day, she visited a kidney transplant evaluation clinic and saw six African American patients. She was overwhelmed and knew she wanted to be a transplant surgeon. The African American patients responded differently to Dr. Simpson than her colleagues who did not look like her. Some patients cried and some hugged her. Their reaction was incredible. It was simply because she looked like them. She was just a trainee at the time and did not have any special medical expertise or background, but this is what sealed her path and pushed her down this road.

Dr. Simpson's road has not been easy, but it has been worth it. Even when things were difficult, she pressed forward. One of the things motivating her was she wanted her sons to see that women can do anything they set their minds to do.

Her mission is to serve everybody but thinks there has been a disadvantage to African Americans because of social issues, genetic predispositions, and for many other reasons. She contends this cultural group needs assistance, and she recognizes she can provide some of this assistance just by looking the same way as they do.

"America has a dark history and it is remembered. Therefore, there is a mistrust of healthcare workers by the African American community," she says. "Patients have told me that they know transplant is experimental, and they know white people receive preference when it comes to time on the waiting list. Neither belief is true."

In some families, a deeply ingrained sense of betrayal is passed down through generations and can permeate doctor visits. It is a result of medical experiments widely performed on slaves in the mid-1800s, a result of the 40-year Tuskegee syphilis experiment that began in 1932 denying hundreds of black men a proper diagnosis or treatment for a debilitating disease.

The distrust and wrongful beliefs are also a result of quality medical care existing just out of geographic reach. This means that some poor do not have access to medical care and do not have the resources necessary for them to obtain adequate medical care. Dr. Simpson understands this and does everything possible to assuage this sense of betrayal, helping patients leave it in the past.

What she tries to help patients remember is, that is the past and we have come an awfully long way. She does not hide or minimize or sweep anything under the rug, but she educates patients on what the literature says about their disease and how she can help them.

Regardless of a patient's race, the transplant process is shrouded in mystery and misunderstanding. People worry that they will only recover a fraction of their former lives if they receive a new organ. Dr. Simpson tells them she wants them to return to where they were six months before they became ill, whether it relates to a liver or a kidney transplant.

To meet the rising need for living kidney transplant donors, Dr. Simpson shares, "Even though as a medical community we have found ways to make the risks minimal to donors, people are still fearful. Most of the time when we think about a living donor, we consider a family member. Many of our middle-aged and older parents would never ask a child to donate a kidney. But what I always tell my patients who voice this fear is that at the same time I am a mother, I am also a daughter. I would be upset with my parents if they did not allow me the opportunity to make the decision to be a donor for myself. I think this is an important message to relay and this is not just for the African American community. This is for everyone."

In addition to all her employment responsibilities, Dr. Simpson desires to be a mentor and motivate everyone. Every African American student or trainee who walks through her office door or into her operating room (OR) makes her think back to what she was like at that stage. She obtained mentorship from many different people for many different things during her career.

By far, the most important mentor she had was an African American surgeon who helped her on her darkest days realize she was not alone; she could make it through. He gave her countless hours of his time, and his only request for repayment was for her to pay it forward.

Dr. Dinee Simpson's heartfelt encouragement to every brown-skinned girl is, "Do not let anything hold you back. Even if you do not see someone who looks like you doing a particular thing, it does not mean it is not achievable."

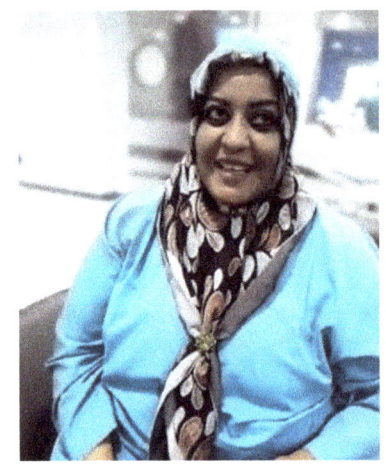

Dr. Manar Bushra Mohamed Abdalla

Dr. Manar Bushra Mohamed Abdalla is a general and kidney transplant surgeon. She is the head of the department of transplant surgery in the Ahmed Gasim Cardiac Surgery & Renal Transplantation Centre, Khartoum North, Sudan.

She is also the head of the department of surgery at Alban Jadeed Teaching Hospital and an associate professor of surgery at IBN Sina University in Khartoum, Sudan.

After finishing her fellowship in kidney transplantation in 2012 at Mansoura University in Egypt, she returned to her country where she is proud to be the only woman of the five transplant surgeons in Sudan.

Since she was a young girl, as young as five years old, Dr. Mohamed Abdalla always wanted to become a doctor. She loves to help people and finds great satisfaction in practicing medicine, especially surgery, because she enjoys using her hands for good. She likes that most of the time surgical recovery is rapid and patients' satisfaction is greater than in other medical specialties. Also, the population of patients is more diverse and disease profiles are more interesting and complex in surgical patients. Her greatest challenge in her journey to become a surgeon was as a female, not as a black woman, since she lives in Africa.

In 1999, she was the sixth woman to become a surgeon in Sudan and remained as such for at least another four years. Also, she was the second woman to work as the general director in a hospital from 1999 to 2004 at the Ahmed Gasim Cardiac & Renal Transplantation Center she established and supported in 1999 with the guidance of the Minister of Health in Khartoum State.

Sudan was one of the first countries in Africa to offer sophisticated cardiac care and kidney transplantation in 1974. Unfortunately, in 1985 this center closed due to unstable economic and political situations. It resumed functioning in 1999 when she became the director of the center.

As a 30-year-old young female general director, she faced many hardships giving instructions to young residents. Her peers and colleagues made it difficult for her to maintain a successfully functioning center.

Fortunately, she overcame these difficulties and is still the director. Through perseverance, patience, kindness, and being fair with her colleagues in the medical field, including paramedical staff, she was able to earn their respect. This was challenging because it was exhausting and sometimes extended into her personal life.

The lessons she learned are to be strong, confident, kind, and knowledgeable.

Dr. Mohamed Abdalla's greatest accomplishment and what she is proudest of, is the establishment of a cardiac center with all its functioning facilities, including an ICU, CCU, and cardiac catheterization unit.

She also established a hemodialysis and transplant center that has successfully competed with international centers in numbers of patients, positive survival outcomes, and success of transplants with neither major donor complication nor donor mortality.

Four days a week Dr. Mohamed Abdalla starts her day with two living-related kidney transplants where she participates in a donor nephrectomy, in which she surgically removes the donor organ, and then performs a kidney transplant into the recipient patient. The surgery takes anywhere from four to six hours. Afterwards, she completes surgical procedures on patients with kidney disease.

One procedure she performs is called an arteriovenous fistula. This procedure alters the patients' blood vessels by joining arteries and veins. Arteries carry oxygen-filled blood away from the heart to the body parts and veins carry carbon dioxide-filled blood away from the body parts to the heart. This type of fistula can be performed in blood vessels of the wrist, forearm, arm, or thigh.

This procedure allows patients with end-stage renal (kidney) disease to receive hemodialysis to clean his/her blood of toxins that accumulate in the body, the job of a healthy kidney.

Two of the four workdays end with Dr. Mohamed Abdalla working at her private surgical clinic which accepts patients from 7 p.m. to 11 p.m. The other two days, she is a teacher in a medical university and a consultant surgeon at a teaching hospital.

Her surgical team spends two days per week doing emergency practice-one day for the out-patient clinic, and one day for elective theater (operating room), which may include up to 15 operations ending by 6 p.m.

One of Dr. Mohamed Abdalla's kidney transplant days is fully dedicated to children at a pediatric nephrology center. Here she evaluates children for kidney transplantation and performs surgery for dialysis access so they can be dialyzed while they wait for their donor's kidney.

She finds balance with great difficulty because most of Dr. Mohamed Abdalla's work is government work. This means exceptionally low pay! It is not an easy job and keeping on track with her family and friends requires additional effort. She shared, "Honestly, sometimes I am not able to complete a day as it should be because of sheer fatigue and stress. Despite this, I would not trade doing surgery for anything else. It is just the way I am. Because I enjoy the nature of my work, this gives me an additional boost to keep going."

The best advice Dr. Mohamed Abdalla has received is to do her best and let her guide and leader be Prophet Muhammad.

Peace and prayers be upon Him and His Family.

Dr. Christie Gooden

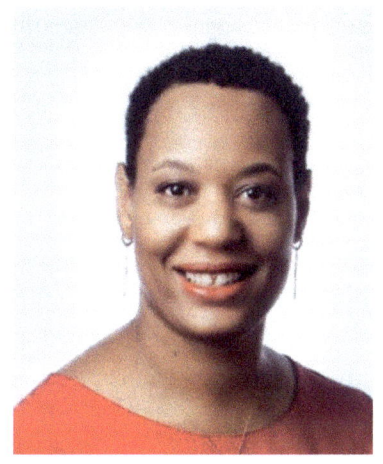

Two major events in Dr. Christie Gooden's life led her down the path to become a doctor. The first event was when she was a little girl and her father received a Ph.D. in physics and became the first Dr. Gooden. On his graduation day, almost all her family was in town for the celebration. They made jokes about different body parts hurting and needing him to examine them. After hearing her father remind them that he was not that kind of doctor, she told him that one day she would be the real Dr. Gooden. The second event was more traumatic and relates to her career choice.

Dr. Gooden remembered it as though it was yesterday. She went to the mall with her mother and everything was fine until her mother told her she was not feeling well. Shortly afterwards, her mother fainted. Dr. Gooden remembers feeling helpless because she did not know what to do.

Paramedics were called and came to evaluate her mother. When her mom was seen by a doctor, he discovered she had high blood pressure. This experience became a lifelong motivation for Dr. Gooden to have the education and tools to not only assist people in life-threatening situations but to also inform the community on preventative measures and healthy lifestyles. She loves being a surgeon but would rather people did not need surgery.

When Dr. Gooden was a teenager, she heard about Xavier University in Louisiana. She was told that African American students graduating from there had the highest rates of being accepted into medical school. So, it was a no-brainer for her to attend this school. To this day, she feels Xavier University is still number one, not only in being accepted to, but also graduating from medical school. Dr. Gooden claims earning her bachelor's at Xavier University was one of the best decisions of her life.

After graduating from Xavier University, she earned a four-year dual Medical Doctorate and Master of Public Health in Health Systems Management from Tulane University in New Orleans, Louisiana. She completed her general surgery residency training at the University of Alabama at Birmingham Medical Center (UAB), where she was also a National Institute of Health (NIH) scholar.

Dr. Gooden developed her love for transplant surgery during her general surgery residency. At UAB, she cared for many trauma patients, so she had the chance to help someone's life and add to the quantity of life but not necessarily the quality of life. This means that many trauma patients with injuries such as gunshot wounds, when treated, can have their lives prolonged, but many times they return to the same life they led before being shot.

What she saw with transplant surgery was the opportunity to immediately improve someone's quality of life as well as quantity. Dr. Gooden also appreciated that a team of medical professionals from different specialties worked together to accomplish patient-centered care. After deciding to change from heart surgery to transplant surgery, she completed her multi-organ transplant fellowship at the University of Michigan, Ann Arbor, Michigan.

Currently, Dr. Gooden is a multi-organ transplant surgeon at the Medical City Dallas Hospital in Dallas, Texas. Her special interests include liver, kidney, and pancreas transplantation as well as advanced laparoscopic and robotic surgery. This is surgery using a robot and keyhole surgery through small incisions.

She also performs dialysis access surgery such as creating arteriovenous fistulas (a procedure to connect an artery with a vein) for patients with kidney failure. This newly created special blood vessel is a way for patients to receive hemodialysis (cleaning toxins from the blood).

Any day she has a scalpel in her hand, and is in the operating room, is a great day. Other than being with her husband and two children, she is most at home in the operating room.

"I am blessed to be in the position that I am, living my dream, and living out my purpose. Along the way, I faced discrimination for being black and being a black female. Like many of us, I have been mistaken for the cleaning staff despite wearing a white coat. I have spent time with patients and their families, painstakingly reviewing all aspects of their case and the surgery recommended only to have them question who would be performing their surgery. Once I complete their surgery successfully and they are doing well, they are happy to introduce the black girl who did their surgery. The best thing to do in these circumstances is to not take the misunderstanding personally and strive to do your best every time. When it comes to discrimination, it is difficult to change the way people think. I allow my gift to speak for itself and continue to change the hearts of people by saving their lives. One heart at a time."

Dr. Gooden wants to encourage each reader to live his or her dream despite circumstances they may face. She hopes to inspire everyone to find their passion and work hard to walk in their purpose. She believes you go to medical school to have a career, not a job. A career is something you love. It is a part of you, sustains you, and defines who you are as much as it completes you.

A job is a paycheck and will never win passion or loyalty. Dr. Gooden urges everyone to ignore the myths about women in surgery. People will say you cannot be a wife or a mother and that you will have no personal life outside the hospital.

Her journey is evidence this is not true. She is happily married with two children (twins) and there are many others like her. Any success she has, she credits to her faith in God. In the transplant medical arena, surgeons are charged to turn tragedy into triumph. As she daily faces tragedy, Dr. Gooden is reminded of God's grace. It is an awesome responsibility and she is blessed

17

to be a part of every patient's story.

A few additional pearls of wisdom Dr. Gooden would like to share are, "Be fearless. You will hear "no" all the time. Do not let "no" keep you from believing in who you are meant to be. Nothing beats a cannot but a try! Never stop trying. Be an advocate. Advocate for your patients. If your patients come first, your decisions become easier. Advocate for yourself and others behind you. You earn respect when people know you are not concerned only about yourself. Respect is a currency that is difficult to come by. Pick your battles. A measured response is better than a response to everything. There are times you will need to swallow your pride and your tears. The key is keeping your head up and your mind on your goals, so you are not dragged down. Document everything because when it is time to battle, you want all your weapons ready."

Dr. Gooden credits her strength to achieve and her success to her faith and has developed mantras or little prayers, "Lord, Thank You for today. Thank You for yesterday because it's in the past and thank You for tomorrow if it is given, for I know it's not promised." If all else fails, her other go-to thought is, "They can't stop the clock," meaning no matter how difficult things become, they cannot stop time, so this too shall pass.

Dr. Gooden enjoys the benefits of music. So, when she is tired, certain songs play in her head like a soundtrack. From gospel to secular, she has go-to songs that speak to her.

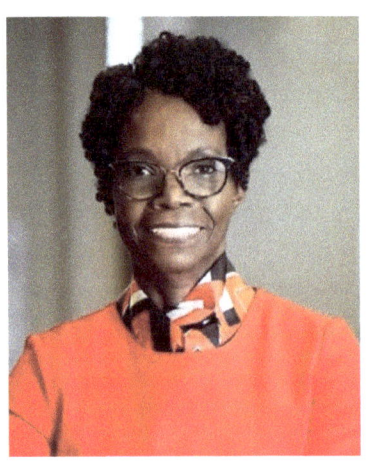

Dr. Velma Scantlebury

Dr. Velma P. Scantlebury is the associate director of the kidney transplant program at Christiana Care in Newark, Delaware. She accepted her position at Christiana Care after working at the University of South Alabama's Regional Transplant Center, Mobile. While there, she served as professor of surgery, assistant dean of community education, and director of transplantation. She has been named to both the "Best Doctors in America" and "Top Doctors in America" lists multiple times.

After earning her medical degree from Columbia University in New York City, Dr. Scantlebury completed her internship and residency in general surgery at Harlem Hospital Center in New York City. She finished her fellowship training in transplantation surgery at the University of Pittsburgh, Pennsylvania, and then joined the University of Pittsburgh School of Medicine as an assistant professor of surgery in 1989. She advanced to associate professor before her appointment at the University of Southern Alabama in Mobile, Alabama.

Dr. Scantlebury's special interests include researching the end results of donation and transplantation in African Americans, increasing organ donation in the African American community through education and awareness, increasing the incidence of living donor transplantation by education, and treating viral infections in kidneys.

She has been honored with the Woman of Spirit Award for inspiring others and the Gift of Life Award from the National Kidney Foundation. In addition to recognition by the Caribbean American Medical and Scientific Association, she received the Order of Barbados Gold Crown of Merit for her efforts to educate minorities about organ transplants. She has performed more than 2,000 transplants and published more than 85 peer-reviewed research papers, as well as 10 monographs and several book chapters. She is the best-selling author of her autobiography, *Beyond Every Wall: Becoming the 1st Black Female Transplant Surgeon.*

Dr. Scantlebury's amazing career began many years ago when her parents, her mother in particular, were passionate about education and knew she wanted to be a doctor. Her mother needed more for her children than Barbados had to offer, so she saw an opportunity and followed her heart. Some of Dr. Scantlebury's older brothers moved to England before Barbados gained independence, but her mother decided to move to New York.

Attending high school in Brooklyn was a tremendous culture shock! Dr. Scantlebury had few friends, was unfamiliar with the curriculum, and took multiple-choice tests. The testing in Barbados consisted more of problem-solving and essay-writing, with subjects such as English Literature, Latin, Scripture, and European history due to the British influence. In Brooklyn, she learned to stifle her desire to learn because if someone was timid like she was, they were beaten and forced to do other students' homework!

Despite this, once she was given an assignment to write an essay on, "My Career." Even at age 10, she wanted to help others and learn about what makes you sick. But, most importantly, she wanted to be her own boss. Her pediatrician was the only doctor she knew and he worked for himself. This is what she wanted to do.

Dr. Scantlebury's mother was her first mentor. Her mother pushed her to do what she knew she could do. Mom provided the opportunity to excel and constantly reminded her and her siblings about the hard work and responsibility that comes with success. As Dr. Scantlebury entered college, her biology teacher, Mr. Smith, provided advice and guidance and constantly encouraged her to strive for excellence.

She shared, "I think about the students in high school who, like me, were told not to consider going to college. This was an unacceptable option for my parents, who had high expectations for all of us, especially me. I was going to college if they made the rules. My high school counselors did not provide much encouragement and it seemed they had low expectations of many of the Black and Caribbean students. There were a few students of color who went on to college, but we did so without their help."

So, with little support, Dr. Scantlebury applied to two colleges in New York City that were close to home. She knew a little about loans but was aware her parents could not afford to pay for her college. As her mom always said, "God made a way!" Dr. Scantlebury was granted a full four-year scholarship to a nearby university. It was truly a blessing!

When Dr. Scantlebury attended medical school, there were only five black females and five black males in her class of 148 students. She was smitten with surgery the minute the class started studying gross anatomy the first year. Oh, what excitement it was to be able to do dissections, learn about the different muscles and nerves, and possess the ability to cure someone just with surgery. This was where she could be found late at night, in the anatomy laboratory, learning from her cadaver she named Suzy.

Also, while still in medical school, completing her rotations at Harlem Hospital Center, Dr. Scantlebury met the first female surgeon she ever knew. Her name is Dr. Barbara Barlow. She was chief of pediatric surgery. Dr. Scantlebury wanted to be just like her. Dr. Barlow maintained her femininity, poise, and demeanor in a way that conveyed confidence and trust, in and out of the operating room. Dr. Barlow became one of her mentors and taught her the fine skills of surgery. Later, when an opportunity arose to work with Dr. Hardy in transplant surgery, Dr. Barlow was instrumental in providing Dr. Scantlebury with her first research experience. It is always nice to have a friend and colleague.

During an interview for a research opportunity at the Children's Hospital of Pittsburgh, Dr. Scantlebury met Dr. Mark Ravitch. He suggested a two-year research fellowship in transplantation with Dr. Thomas Starzl. This gave her a competitive edge for acceptance into the pediatric fellowship program in Pittsburgh, Pennsylvania. Dr. Scantlebury arrived in Pittsburgh with plans of becoming a pediatric surgeon and became a transplant surgeon instead, completing her fellowship there in 1986, along with nine others that year.

Dr. Scantlebury was there because Dr. Ravitch spoke with Dr. Starzl regarding her need for more research in transplantation. At first, she did not give this fellowship in transplant much thought because it was meant to be a stepping-stone to her goal of becoming a pediatric surgeon. It was hard work, sleepless nights, and random midnight rounds with Dr. Starzl. As a fellow, you were either flying somewhere to retrieve organs or assisting in complicated transplant surgery with one of the senior attendings.

Dr. Scantlebury remembers, "In those days, some patients felt uncomfortable having a black female surgeon. I had to learn to not feel rejected because of their ignorance but embrace my skills and realize it was their loss not having me as their surgeon. On several occasions, the senior attending made it clear I would be the operating surgeon. Several of these patients stayed in touch for many years after their transplant. I won them over by saving their lives."

Some of the male surgeons in the group were supportive during Dr. Scantlebury's fellowship years but there were others who were not supportive to female fellows, therefore some female fellows gravitated to pediatric rotations at the Children's Hospital, where they spent most of their time. This kept them out of Dr. Starzl's path, their fearless leader who sought fellows at midnight for rounds on the numerous patients on the adult service. While it was an awesome opportunity to learn, it was grueling because they had to be up to date on all the patients' information and be ready with the answers, even at 1 a.m.

After her transplant training, an amazing doctor, Dr. Richard Simmons, then chair of the department of surgery, initiated a living donor kidney transplant program. As Dr. Scantlebury transitioned to an assistant professor of surgery, she worked with Dr. Ron Shapiro and focused less on liver transplants and more on kidney transplants. He was delightful to work with and treated her with respect as a colleague and a friend.

As she recalls, the department of surgery had no other female surgeons until Dr. Suzanne Ildstad joined the department as a pediatric surgeon in 1988. Women in surgery were few-and-far-between then. It was and still is a lonesome profession, especially for women and even more so for women of color.

It was not until Dr. Scantlebury's third year in Pittsburgh as a junior attending that word spread about her being the first black female transplant surgeon. Realizing there were no others before her was daunting. Many women paid the price for freedom, to get an education, to attend medical school, and even to become a surgeon. She was a transplant surgeon now, the first in her family to attend college, and the first black female transplant surgeon. Such status never meant much to her parents. She was just following God's plan for her life.

Dr. Scantlebury feels that in the past, African American patients faced disparities in access to kidney transplantation, either by late referrals or by not being referred at all for transplantation. Knowledge is power! With more education about treatment options for end-stage renal disease (ESRD) and understanding the advantages of early referral and listing, more patients of color have taken advantage of transplantation as a lifesaving option.

Despite this, more effort is necessary to educate the general population on the importance of organ donation and transplantation, including the advantages of living donation.

Dr. Scantlebury still sees patients who are diagnosed late with renal failure and need dialysis urgently. This is inadequate access or no access to appropriate healthcare and early diagnosis. She contends we still need to fix a much-needed healthcare system in a way that provides equal access for all, regardless of socioeconomic status.

Patients on dialysis who are listed for kidney transplantation encounter long waiting times and the increased risk of death on dialysis. This is unfortunate because we continue to struggle to increase the rates of organ donation. The continued challenge for all patients will be to stay healthy while on the waiting list and focus on finding a living donor that will provide them with the wonderful gift of life and excellent outcomes, thus avoiding increased morbidities on dialysis.

In addition to her challenging and busy career, Dr. Scantlebury has always had a love for teaching, and is aware of how important it is for someone in her position to reach back and bring others along. Her success is due in part to the many others who broke-down barriers and pushed ahead despite the obstacles they faced.

Dr. Scantlebury was told in medical school she would not make it as a surgeon, but today she is. She takes advantage of opportunities to volunteer in women's professional organizations, attends middle and high school career day sessions, and attends many invited sessions at various mentoring opportunities.

Her goal is to encourage, educate, and empower young women to aspire to achieve their goals and to seek positive reinforcement to help build self-esteem and the determination to succeed.

Dr. Scantlebury's advice to other transplant surgeons in training is to never doubt yourself or your capabilities. You have chosen this field because of your love for surgery and transplantation. While others may question the level of your surgical skills, know that women can make better surgeons, with equal or better talent and accomplishments.

Early in her career, Dr. Scantlebury was perceived as not being strong enough mentally or physically, but this has been proven to be incorrect. Women are resilient because they need to be. Women can carry this resilience capacity into a career as a surgeon.

The numbers of African American female transplant surgeons continue to increase each year, creating more role-models for young students aspiring to become transplant surgeons. Dr. Scantlebury's advice is to seek out mentors, perhaps more than one, and make connections through volunteer opportunities or professional groups. The more people you know, the more possibilities these connections will pay-off when needed.

Dr. Scantlebury is certainly balanced. She loves being a transplant surgeon, but when she gets home at the end of the day or night, she still has the responsibilities of being a wife, mother, sister, and now a caretaker for a young Sudanese student and her infant child. This is what she does. It is what she and her husband have always done. They are here for those in need.

She loves to cook, read, travel, and get massages. She treats herself to a monthly massage to relax and have someone else work on her body. It is heavenly. She thinks everyone should try it!

"I've missed more than 9000 shots in my career. I've lost almost 300 games. 26 times I've been trusted to take the game winning shot and missed. I've failed over and over and over again in my life. And that is why I succeed." – Michael Jordan

CHAPTER TWO
General Surgery

General surgery is a surgical specialty that focuses on abdominal contents, including the esophagus, stomach, small intestine, large intestine, liver, pancreas, gall bladder, appendix, bile ducts, and often, the thyroid gland. A general surgeon also deals with diseases involving the skin, breast, soft tissue, trauma, peripheral artery disease, and hernias as well as performs endoscopic procedures such as gastroscopy and colonoscopy.

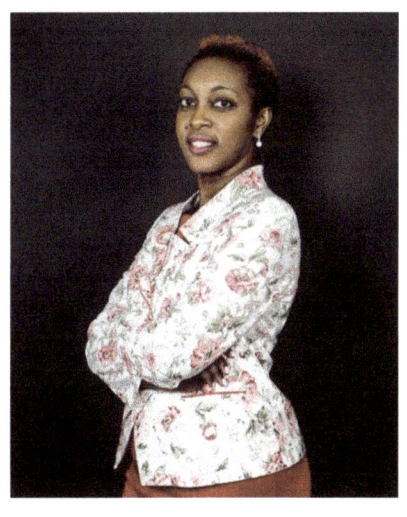

Dr. Faith Mugoha Odwaro

In some countries, students are required to earn a bachelor's degree (a four-year college degree) before they may apply to medical school. This is not the case in Africa and some European countries. Students with the goal of becoming a doctor apply to medical school after graduating from high school. This is what Dr. Faith Mugoha Odwaro did. After graduating from high school, she was accepted into and graduated from Odessa National Medical University, Ukraine in 2009.

She completed a one-year medical internship in her home country, Kenya, and worked as a medical officer at Mbagathi Hospital, in Nairobi, Kenya, after her internship. She returned to Odessa for general surgery training at the Department of General Surgery & Military Medicine, Odessa National Medical University, Ukraine.

Dr. Mugoha Odwaro is a general surgeon in Nairobi, Kenya. She and her husband are the creators and co-directors of the Mazira Foundation in Nairobi, founded in April 2006 in honor of her father, the late Reverend Hosea Mazira Odwaro. Her father battled acute leukemia for almost four years. During her hospital visits, both in Kenya and Canada, she was inspired to do what she now does with so much joy, serve her community and making a difference as a surgeon and community activist.

A community activist's responsibilities include assessing the health needs of their population and then enacting changes within the local communities, state, or federal government so that appropriate medical services may be accessed by people needing medical care in the community.

Dr. Mugoha Odwaro is an agent for change. She is passionate about health, leadership, and the empowerment of women. Her interest in global public health issues led her to work with communities to promote preventive medicine, giving her more than 13 years of practical experience working with the community through medical outreaches, health campaigns, and doing household visits with community health workers. As a surgeon, she works hard to ensure that those who otherwise do not have access to safe and timely surgical and medical care gain access to it. This is one of her motivations for building the Mazira Memorial Hospital which provides quality, affordable, and accessible health care services to the community to reduce the burden of diseases and enable communities to achieve better health.

Her long journey began when she was quite young. Growing up, she loved nursing the sick and wounded. This earned her the title of "Daktari" (meaning doctor in Swahili). When she was 15 years old, her experiences taking care of her ailing father in Kenya and Canada motivated her to join the fight against cancer. Being a doctor seemed like the best way to make an impact regarding health. Dr. Mugoha Odwaro would never have thought of surgery, however, when she worked with Dr. Nicholas Tinega, a senior consultant surgeon and mentor, he challenged her to pursue surgery. He is a phenomenal surgeon and teacher.

Dr. Mugoha Odwaro feels her greatest challenge while studying was proving she belonged at the big table with the senior surgeons and that her dreams to become a surgeon were valid as a woman. A second challenge was being considered to either be in the wrong place or being mistaken for a model, or anything but a doctor, let alone a surgeon.

She shared, "The most important thing is that you must believe in yourself enough to be taken seriously by senior surgeons. You must pursue surgery because you love it, knowing you will wake up each morning to save and transform lives. It is a huge responsibility for which you must be prepared."

Practicing in Kenya, Dr. Mugoha Odwaro claims her experience working with the community in Vihiga (a small county in Kenya, Africa, located on the eastern side of the Kakamega Forest, five kilometers from the equator) brought her to the realization of the inequalities affecting accessibility to quality and affordable healthcare. Kenya's health system is structured to deal with cases that come to the health facilities, which are sadly a small percentage of cases needing to be seen that receive care. Many times, people do not have transportation to come to health facilities. This results in patients dealing with their illnesses at home without access to care.

Doctors are constantly trying to treat preventable complications in an environment with insufficient resources such as medications or equipment. Doctors must deal with patients' personal as well as cultural beliefs that make them mistrust conventional medicine.

Prevention of complications of disease processes also includes providing medications necessary to treat conditions such as high blood pressure, diabetes, and others rather than waiting to treat patients when complications of the diseases arise. Potential complications may include stroke, diabetic foot ulcers, or end-stage renal (kidney) disease as well as other complications Dr. Mugoha Odwaro's passion is to change the present circumstance of non-accessible medical care to more accessible medical care and education.

Dr. Mugoha Odwaro's day starts at home with morning devotion with her loving husband followed by her arrival at the hospital for routine research and review of the patient procedures for the day.

Tuesdays and Thursdays are typically long hours in the theater (operating room). Mondays are major ward rounds days, including admission and review of patients scheduled for surgery. Ward rounds are when the team, including Dr. Mugoha Odwaro, surgical trainees, and nurses, visit each patient in the surgical ward who may need multi-disciplinary decisions about their care. Rounds also includes updates on patient illness, reviewing vital signs (blood pressure, heart and respiratory rates), laboratory results, medications, food and fluid intakes and outputs (urine, stool), and imaging tests that may have been completed such as X-rays or CAT scans. The doctors arrive at a plan of care for each patient which includes discharge plans and follow-up after they leave the hospital.

Wednesdays and Fridays are Dr. Mugoha Odwaro's days in the clinic where she sees patients on an outpatient basis.

She also has mentorship and mentee responsibilities. She is an alumna of the Emerging Leaders Foundation (ELF). This is an African youth-centered non-profit organization that provides practical values-based leadership development, mentorship, governance, and livelihoods training to young Africans so they can become positive agents of sustainable social, economic, and political transformation in society. Through the ELF, she has sessions with her mentor monthly where her mentor provides guidance and resources she may need to be a more effective leader in the foundation. Dr. Mugoha Odwaro is a mentor to other ELF mentees and several early career physicians. She also meets with them once a month and helps them formulate career goals and provides guidance as they work towards achieving their goals.

As mentioned earlier, Dr. Mugoha Odwaro and her husband created the Mazira Foundation. She tenderly shared, "I remember watching my mother, a young widow, cry herself to sleep, not sure how she would provide for our basic needs. A meal was difficult to come by and my education was often interrupted. She was my age when she became a widow, except she did not have higher education and was financially dependent on my late father. Because of this experience at a young age, I was passionate about finding solutions for the plight of widows. I devoted some time to working with the Solid Rock Widows in Kenya and provided monetary sponsorship through the Mazira Foundation. The foundation was birthed to advocate for accessible and affordable quality health services for people who are poor and disadvantaged and are unable to pay for services. It is also for those who can pay but cannot afford the expensive clinics and hospitals."

She added, "Women's health is a key determinant in reducing the disease burden, increasing productivity, and, therefore, alleviating poverty. We focus on the widow who is subjected to chronic stress which leads to metabolic syndrome with an exponential increase in hypertension (high blood pressure), diabetes (high blood sugars), obesity (being overweight) and cardiovascular (heart) diseases. When the widow is affected by stress and disease, everyone in her life is affected and predisposed to disease."

Dr. Mugoha Odwaro currently conducts public health programs including medical camps with an emphasis on preventive health through health education on nutrition, hygiene, first aid for home emergencies, screening and diagnostic testing, and early medical interventions. Also, she conducts health campaigns like the Adopt a Widow's Health program and the ongoing Own Your Health social media campaign. These programs have been instrumental in inspiring more than 10,000 people to own their health. They also encourage medical professionals to give back to the community by volunteering their professional time and resources.

In addition to all these wonderful endeavors Dr. Mugoha Odwaro is involved with, a few years ago she and others began the construction of a widow's center in Vihiga County in Kenya.

Seeing it stand and come to life and start operations makes her feel accomplished.

She believes she is the woman she is because her family believes in her, supports her initiatives, and understands her limitations. Her husband does not hesitate to step in to be the present parent when duty calls, and her mother always has her bags packed and is ready to house-sit on short notice. This allows her to attend international training events and conferences. Her family is her support system, propelling her to achieve greater heights. She remembers how her father told her to never be afraid to "Take the Road Less Traveled," quoting Robert Frost's famous poem.

There are times she is overwhelmed with her many responsibilities as a wife, mother, surgeon, and co-director of the Mazira Foundation, as well as her mentoring and teaching responsibilities. During these times, she leans on her support system and asks God to guide her and give her the strength to get through the day. Learning new skills and picking up new hobbies keeps her sane during stressful times. She loves gardening, homemaking, and baking and cooking for her family. What helps her find balance is the ability to engage with other women. She has taken up playing golf and loves to travel and engage in women leadership programs.

Dr. Elizabeth Mwachiro

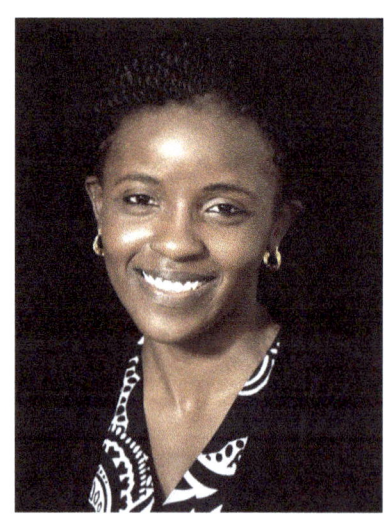

Dr. Elizabeth (Liz) Mwachiro completed her medical training at the University of Nairobi in Kenya. She was accepted for her medical internship at Tenwek Hospital, a faith-based institution in Bomet County, Kenya. After her internship, she relocated to

Kapenguria, north east of Kitale, where she worked in government hospitals as a medical officer. She returned to Tenwek Hospital to pursue her specialist training in general surgery through the Pan African Association of Christian Surgeons (PAACS) and the College of Surgeons of East, Central, and Southern Africa (COSECSA). She is a consultant general surgeon at Tenwek Hospital.

PAACS is a non-denominational, multinational service organization training African physicians to become surgeons who are willing to remain in Africa. This is to meet the growing need for surgeons to provide surgical care to the 56 million people in Africa. In many places in Africa, there is only one surgeon for a population of 250,000. In other areas, it is even more staggering. There may be only one surgeon for a population of 2.5 million people. The training through PAACS is offered at several well-established evangelical mission hospitals in Africa under the direction of experienced, board-certified missionary surgeons.

COSECSA is the largest surgical training institution in Sub-Saharan Africa. In 1996 it recognized that the quality and quantity of surgical services available to people within the region were inadequate. There was a fundamental need to formulate a common surgical training program that could be undertaken in designated training institutes in the region, all with a common exam and the award of an internationally recognized surgical qualification. COSECSA was established in 1999 to advance education, training, examination standards, research, and practice in surgical care by increasing the number of appropriately trained, well-qualified surgeons and surgically trained general medical officers.

In addition to her accomplishments as a physician, Dr. Mwachiro and her husband, a surgeon, researcher, and gastroenterologist, founded the Tenwek International School that currently provides early childhood education to 34 children.

Dr. Mwachiro's journey began when she was growing up. She remembers seeing her older brother dissecting lizards and sewing them back up. She was fascinated by his experiments.

After high school, she was selected to do a homeopathy program that allowed her to care for people who were ill. She realized she would love a career that allowed her to be close to patients and help them get well. As she rotated through the different medical specialties in medical school, Dr. Mwachiro was overly fascinated and enthralled with the operating room (OR) and the surgical procedures done there.

The first procedure she observed was the removal of a gallbladder via a laparoscopic cholecystectomy using a small scope and tiny incisions. The use of the small scope allows for faster recovery and avoids a large abdominal incision. She also observed bone surgery known as ORIF (open reduction and internal fixation) which means the surgeon opens the skin and uses pins or plates to fix a broken bone. This is an alternative to external fixation of broken bones, such as casting. She was fascinated and immediately knew she wanted to be a surgeon and her best rotation was surgery. As a medical intern, she felt drawn and called to pursue general surgery.

As a young African black woman, showing or proving she is equally as good, talented, or even better than her male colleagues has been especially challenging in Africa, where young female surgeons are viewed as less qualified.

Occasionally, she is referred to as a custodian or nurse or the physician assistant because she is female. She has appreciated and noted an increase in the number of women surgeons and chooses to be one of the female surgeons making the surgical field a more habitable arena for other female surgeons coming after her.

In addition to her family and work commitments, Dr. Mwachiro founded the Kenya Association of Women Surgeons (KAWS). This is an initiative and an organization working with the Surgical Society of Kenya that seeks to bring women together in training and in the surgical profession by allowing everyone to share their challenges and lift each other up.

As part of the KAWS initiative, Dr. Mwachiro and her team formed a KAWS Students group for the undergraduate and medical students interested in pursuing careers in surgery. They have sponsored several students interested in attending the KAWS meetings to motivate them and allow them to network with those in the surgical field. They also sponsor students to create scientific papers on case reports or outcomes research and submit them for surgical conferences, for oral presentations, and publications.

Through this group they are creating a mentorship task force to enhance mentor-mentee links and partnerships. Dr. Mwachiro and the team travel to high schools and talk about careers as surgeons throughout the country. This has made a positive impact in opening students' minds to the notion of females being surgeons.

Dr. Mwachiro is confident and attributes her confidence to hard-work and striving for excellence. As a woman surgeon there is tremendous pressure to be perfect. She never wants to be at fault for anything, but this is not realistic. Striving for excellence, but remembering she is human and fallible, is key. One must always be on their 'A' game. While training, Dr. Mwachiro surrounded herself with great mentors who guided her and showed her the right path and who continue to encourage her in her surgical career.

This is why Dr. Mwachiro is adamant that empowering those coming after her, guiding them, and supporting them, whether these are her junior peers, colleagues, or those in training should not only be her goal, but everyone's goal. As a mentor, another responsibility is to help make their journey better, lighter, and clearer. In Africa they say, it takes a whole village to raise a child. Dr. Mwachiro believes this is applicable and true in surgery. It takes a team of good and willing surgeons who have gone ahead to make the surgeons coming behind better surgeons. The goal is to provide the absolute best surgical and medical care for patients.

Dr. Mwachiro deals with failure and complications by accepting that they are part of growth and she learns from failure, especially in surgery. She participates in mortality and morbidity

(M&M) meetings with primary objectives to identify negative outcomes associated with medical error, to modify behavior and judgment based on previous experiences, and to prevent repetition of errors leading to complications. These conferences are non-punitive and focus on the goal to improve patient care. The proceedings are generally kept confidential by law. She now views these meetings as areas to learn and grow through failure and complications, digging deep into how everyone can improve.

Dr. Mwachiro's final words for the up-and-coming surgeons are, "The number one and most important thing is to love yourself and take care of yourself physically, emotionally, mentally, and spiritually. Keep your family and loved ones close, they need you and you need them. Know your tribe, friends, and colleagues, whether male or female, that will stand with you and walk with you through your journey; people who will hold you accountable and push you to your highest potential and beyond and encourage you when you feel drained. Do the same for them. As you pursue this surgical journey of training and establishing yourself in your field, seek to inspire those coming after you. Seek to empower, teach, and train the art of surgery. Strive to make the surgical field a better place for those coming after you. Seek to leave a legacy from where you are, wherever you are."

Leena Elsharief Elmokashfee Mohammed Ali

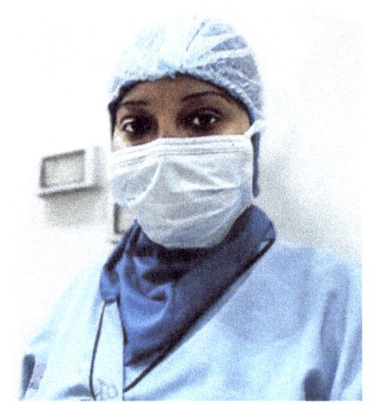

Dr. Leena Elsharief Elmokashfee Mohammed Ali received her medical degree from the University of Khartoum in Sudan. She completed a surgical internship at the Ministry of Health in Sudan as a house officer rotating through obstetrics and gynecology, ear, nose, and throat surgery, general surgery, orthopedic surgery, pediatrics, and medicine.

She finished her surgical residency in Sudan under the supervision of the Sudan Medical Specialization Board and is board certified by the Membership of the Royal Colleges of Surgeons, Edinburgh (MRCS Ed)). She is currently a general surgeon and an assistant professor of surgery at Nile University in Sudan and is pursuing a one-year breast surgical oncology fellowship in India.

This is what she would like to share.

My name, Leena, which means the palm tree that can grow tall, grow dates, and bear drought. My name teaches me to be patient, strong, and sweet despite the struggles I face. My life lessons are many.

Lesson 1: At a young age I learned the importance of finishing everything I started.

At nine years old, "*Leeeena, have you finished your project?*" My mother's words still ring in my ears. She urged me to finish everything I started. My first lesson for finishing projects was when I crocheted hats for my home economics class. I spent time after school working on my crocheting, and crocheted until my beautiful creations were completed. Through my mother's gentle guidance, I was able to learn to crochet, knit, needlepoint, and sew. I was small. I remember how she propped me up on a chair with pillows so I could reach the big sewing machine. I became proficient at sewing and it was one of my favorite things to do while growing up. I am convinced this helped me gain the surgical skill of suturing, which came naturally to me.

Lesson 2: With proper training and encouragement, you can achieve any goal you set for yourself. My confidence was built with each project I completed.

At 13 years old, "*Leena, I have a surprise for you.*" My father came home tired from working at the hospital and handed me a small bag. I opened the bag and inside was a surgical set. I was excited to have my own instruments and spent time imagining myself as a surgeon and using the instruments to help people who needed surgery.

Lesson 3: This surgical set sits on my desk and is a daily reminder of how far I have come from the little girl who never thought anything was impossible. Now I know you can achieve whatever you set your mind to do.

At 15 years old, the English woman teacher, Hibat Eltayeb, wrote a letter to my parents. "Thank Allah for giving you a unique daughter. Leena is a masterpiece that you must help grow to her full potential. I know that she will have a great future, whatever she chooses to do."

Lesson 4: Teachers have a powerful effect on their students which could be either negative or positive. Let us be inspiring teachers to those coming after us.

In high school, it was a typical evening in our neighborhood. The electricity was out, and we sat in the living room using candles to illuminate the room. My family waited for my secondary school exam results to arrive. As was the tradition during that time in Sudan, the highest-scoring students on the national secondary school exam we took at the end of high school were announced on the radio. We sat around our battery-powered small radio waiting. It was not long before my name was broadcast. My family was happy about my success and my brothers joked I had become famous. My brothers have been my source of support, unconditional love, and encouragement.

Lesson 5: Take care of your loved ones. They are your source of support as you strive to reach your goals.

My first year in medical school, "This is the best specimen that has been dissected in this lab, except for the small fact that you cut into the gut tube." This is what my zoology professor said about my dissected cockroach.

Lesson 6: It is important to find ways to criticize in a loving and constructive manner. I learned from experience that small faults do not spoil great efforts. Keep striving to be the best you can be and always do your best.

In my second year in medical school, there was a senior nurse in my first surgical rotation who assisted with surgeries. She taught me basic suturing. By the time I finished medical school, I had developed good suturing skills which made me a better and more efficient intern as I entered surgical training.

Lesson 7: We are all part of a team and we should work hard for the patient to win. We must work well together as a team and help each other to be the best we can be.

In my fourth year in medical school, I was in a general surgery rotation and our team was busy evaluating surgical patients in the emergency room and operating. We finally had some downtime in the middle of the night as we waited for another ready operating room. I chose to sleep on the carpet in the female doctors' restroom as I waited to assist with the next operation so our on-call registrar (resident) was able to enjoy an hour of good sleep on the bed. At times, teamwork means putting someone else above ourselves.

Lesson 8: Always be considerate of others who may need something more than you. Be empathetic to others.

At my medical school graduation, I was not surprised to graduate with distinction in surgery because I put my all into my rotations. Surgery is what I wanted to do so I spent as much time as I could in the operating room learning from the registrars (residents) and consultant surgeons.

Lesson 9: Pure honey cannot be taken without painful bee stings. This means that for any big dream, you must be willing to work hard to achieve it. Do not expect anything to be handed to you.

During my registrarship (residency), *"It is sometimes impossible to accomplish 100% perfection,"* Dr. Mohammed Eltayeb advised me during surgery. He is the mentor who guided me from a novice to an expert surgeon. Gently, efficiently, and knowledgeably, he took me through each step of many of the operations we performed together. He taught me many other life lessons by watching how he treated patients and other people. He is highly respected by his colleagues. He influenced my development as a surgeon.

Lesson 10: Whenever we share our knowledge generously, we will remain in the minds and hearts of those whose lives we touch.

During my Membership of the Royal Colleges of Surgeons (MRCS) preparation course, (the certifying examination for general surgery allowing a surgeon to practice independently in Sudan), one of the professors training us for the course said, "You are one of our best candidates throughout the world. Why don't you join training through the scholarships we provide to Sudanese candidates?" Before this, I did not know there were scholarship opportunities available for me to continue my training in breast oncology surgery.

Lesson 11: Work hard. Always do your best. Be excellent and doors will open for you.

My journey to become a surgeon has been filled with tears, obstacles, triumphs, and growth as a person and as a physician. I wanted to share snippets in my timeline to show the importance we each play in other's lives. I look back at these experiences and it rejuvenates my spirit and motivates me to continue working hard for my patients. Our lives are filled with difficulties, but each struggle is a rung on the ladder of success. Teamwork is the soul of success. We should continue to encourage each other along this journey.

"Every great dream begins with a dreamer. Always remember, you have within you the strength, the patience, and the passion to reach for the stars to change the world." – Harriet Tubman

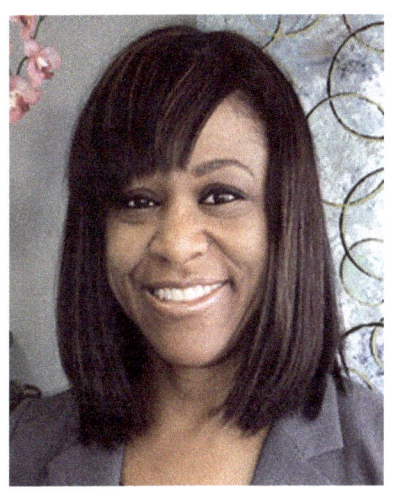

Dr. Carla Pugh

Dr. Carla Pugh is a professor of surgery at Stanford University School of Medicine, Stanford, California. She is also the director of the Technology Enabled Clinical Improvement (T.E.C.I.) Center, Stanford, California.

Her clinical area of expertise is acute care surgery. Prior to joining the faculty at Stanford, Dr. Pugh held the titles of vice chair of innovation and entrepreneurship and vice chair of education and patient safety at the University of Wisconsin, Madison, Wisconsin.

Dr. Pugh earned her undergraduate degree at the University of California, Berkeley in neurobiology and her medical degree at Howard University School of Medicine, Washington, D.C. After completing her surgical training at Howard University Hospital, she continued on to Stanford University and obtained a PhD in education. She is the first surgeon in the United States to obtain a PhD in education. This has allowed her to integrate the study of education and science with medicine.

Her research has led to new ways of using technologies, most notably simulations, to teach doctors how to best practice. This enables doctors to receive hands-on experience without putting patients at risk and it relies on the insights she gained as a doctoral student in education at Stanford. She does innovative work with sensors and human-computer interactions to help healthcare professionals learn how to practice medicine.

Over the last two decades, Dr. Pugh has developed at least 15 devices that provide medical students with life-like training experiences and enable instructors to capture measurable data to better assess their students' skills.

Dr. Pugh's research involves the use of simulation and advanced engineering technologies to develop new approaches for assessing and defining competency in clinical procedural skills. She holds three patents on the use of sensor and data acquisition technology to measure and characterize hands-on clinical skills.

Her pelvic examination simulator, for instance, is used in more than 200 medical and nursing schools. These simulators allow students to perform exams on the internal pelvic structures and when they do so, a computer verifies if they have done the exam correctly.

In addition, a dozen of her simulation-based clinical exam courses and accompanying teacher-training courses and curricula are used around the world. Dr. Pugh uses technology to change the face of medical and surgical education.

Her work has received numerous awards from medical and engineering organizations. In 2011 Dr. Pugh received the Presidential Early Career Award for scientists and engineers from President Barak Obama at The White House. She is considered a leading international expert on the use of sensors and motion tracking technology for performance measurement.

In 2014 she was invited to give a TEDMED talk on the potential uses of technology to transform how we measure clinical skills in medicine. In April 2018, Dr. Pugh was inducted into the American Institute for Medical and Biological Engineering.

Dr. Pugh knew she wanted to be a doctor at the age of five. She grew up in Berkeley, California. During childhood, she heard tales of both her mother's and father's family in the Deep South in the 1930s, where a family member delivered all the babies at home and tended to every medical need for both people and animals. They did not go to the hospital. They went to whoever was nearest to the farm who possessed the skills to help. Both her parents were born at home and delivered by their grandmother or great aunt who was the midwife, as well as the veterinarian for all the animals. She grew up thinking these women were superwomen. In her mind they were physicians who took care of people and animals and this was what she wanted to do with her life.

Dr. Pugh originally wanted to be a cranio-facial reconstructive surgeon when she was 14 years old. She was in an advanced science class in high school and had an amazing teacher who taught everyone how to dissect insects. As part of the class, the teacher showed a movie about Dr. Paul Tessier, a renowned cranio-surgical reconstruction surgeon. This experience helped her realize she could be creative and help people.

Fifteen years later, she had the opportunity to perform this same surgery with a surgeon who trained under Dr. Tessier when she was a surgical resident and described her experience as simply incredible.

As a young child, Dr. Pugh enjoyed taking things apart and recreating them. Other children in the neighborhood often brought their dolls for her to fix. Dr. Pugh loved to fix things and loved working with her hands and tools.

At the University of California, Berkley, none of the faculty in Dr. Pugh's STEM classes were African American. There was one black faculty member who taught social sciences. Dr. Pugh was very much the minority at the school and in a competitive pre-medicine program. She read about Howard University and applied there for medical school. She was accepted and had a wonderful experience.

It was the first time she was being taught by African Americans and seeing so many successful black people of various socioeconomic backgrounds.

As a medical student she was frustrated as she watched doctor's complete breast, prostate or pelvic exams because when she did her exams, she was unsure whether she was touching the right places or using the correct pressure. So, years later, she created the simulators to give medical students a better idea of the correct palpation techniques.

Her simulators are attached to sensors that are interpreted by computers that display a diagram of the anatomy. When a student practices performing an internal exam, lights, bells and whistles go off to show the instructor when the student has touched the correct area and applied the proper degree of pressure.

Dr. Pugh realized the best way to improve medical care was to improve how doctors are trained, and she decided the best way to train them was to learn about learning, about curriculum, and about assessment in a structured way.

As much as Dr. Pugh loves to create things and teach students and residents, she loves to operate and care for patients. She is a mentor and when asked what advice she would give to early career surgeons in academic surgery practice, she states, "One has to understand that it is a journey and it takes time to accomplish goals as an academic surgeon. It is important to have a realistic timeline for when you want to achieve your goals and to build a team of people to help you achieve these goals, understanding that the team may change in time as you grow in your profession. It is important to have set goals and to be flexible along the way and keep your eyes open to opportunities."

Remembering Sherilyn

"I knew Sherilyn Gordon-Burroughs well and looked forward to meeting her at annual meetings each year where a group of us girlfriends, who are surgeons, meet annually. I miss her very much. I miss her smile. The energy she had in her voice and her presence were inspiring. She was always remarkably upbeat and was the kind of person who would get anything done. She was an encourager, motivator, challenger, and a sister to keep you accountable. She was easy to talk with and a great friend.

Life Lesson: You must learn how to play the game whatever it is you decide you want to do in life. It is important that you understand the rules and play to win. You cannot criticize the game, you cannot fight it, you cannot take everything personal, and you have to understand who your team members are and how to promote them and how to have tolerance for different points of view and always work hard and play to win.

CHAPTER THREE

Minimally Invasive Surgery

A minimally invasive surgeon uses a laparoscope, a thin tube with a light and tiny video camera on the end, to see inside the body and makes tiny incisions and uses long tiny surgical instruments to do surgery. A bariatric surgeon does surgeries to help people who are overweight lose weight.

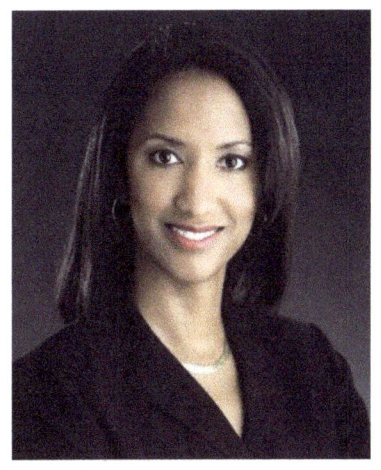

Dr. Patricia L. Turner

Dr. Patricia Turner earned her bachelor's degree at the University of Pennsylvania, Philadelphia, and her medical degree from the Bowman Gray School of Medicine at Wake Forest University in Winston-Salem, North Carolina. She continued her training as both an intern in surgery and a surgical resident at Howard University Hospital in Washington, D.C.

During her residency, she spent two years between her second and third years of residency completing a research fellowship at the National Institute of Health (NIH). Her work there focused on dysregulation of sodium transport in the kidney and nitric oxide's role in the changing abundance of nephron transporter proteins. This means she was working with problems associated with salt transport in the kidneys and how nitric oxide affects the transport of proteins in the kidney and their absorption.

She completed her fellowship training in minimally invasive (MIS) and bariatric surgery at the Mount Sinai School of Medicine, Weill-Cornell University School of Medicine, and

Columbia University School of Medicine in Manhattan, New York. This fellowship program rotated through and trained in all these hospitals at the same time.

Dr. Turner is board-certified in surgery and is a Fellow of the American College of Surgeons. The designation 'Fellow' is used to indicate that the surgeon's education and training, professional qualifications, surgical competence, and ethical conduct have passed a rigorous evaluation, and have been found to be consistent with the high standards established and demanded by American College of Surgeons (ACS).

After completing her fellowship training in New York, she became an associate professor of surgery at the University of Maryland, School of Medicine (UMMC), Baltimore, Maryland, where she was most recently the program director for the general surgery residency program in addition to her surgical practice. In this capacity, she was responsible for the education and credentialing of general surgery residents. During her employment there, she was the medical director of the UMMC Surgical Acute Care Unit where she provided guidance and leadership for the clinical staff on that unit.

She was also a member of the UMMC Medical Executive Committee. A medical executive committee acts as a representative of the medical staff. The committee proposes change and enacts policies, procedures, and other protocols to improve patient care and medical staff structure.

As a member of the UMMC Graduate Medical Education Committee, Dr. Turner was responsible for supporting all the residency and fellowship training programs in the institution. She was also Vice-Chair of the UMMC Credentialing Committee, responsible for developing monitoring and maintaining standards of education, training, and licensing of practitioners in the hospital.

Lastly, she was the chair of the UMMC Executive Infection Control Committee whose responsibility was to monitor infection control policies and implement them while also recommending corrective actions if there is an infection issue.

Her clinical expertise is in minimally invasive and laparoscopic gastrointestinal and endocrine surgery. Endocrine surgery is surgery of the different glands in the body, such as the thyroid gland, the adrenal gland, and all other glands.

Presently, Dr. Turner is director of the Division of Member Services at the American College of Surgeons and is a clinical associate professor of surgery at the University of Chicago in Chicago, Illinois. Additional leadership roles in national organizations include her current position as a director of the American Medical Association (AMA) Foundation whose mission is to bring together physicians and communities to improve the health of the nation. She was also an executive committee member of the Surgical Section of the National Medical Association, the largest and oldest national organization representing African American physicians and their patients in the United States. She is the first female president of the Society of Black Academic Surgeons whose mission is to improve health, advance science, and foster careers of African American and other underrepresented minority surgeons.

She has anchored and provided ongoing medical expertise and commentary for health-related segments on *Good Morning America* (GMA) and *GMA Health* and was featured in an issue of *Black Enterprise* magazine focusing on innovative physicians. Her opinions on the *State of Black Health in America* were featured in the November 2010 anniversary issue of *Ebony* magazine.

Dr. Turner's incredible journey began as a child raised in Washington, D.C. She never wanted to be anything but a surgeon since the first grade. She did not know any, nor had she ever met any surgeons. Her mother was a junior high school science teacher so this may have influenced her desire to be a doctor. She was proficient in math and science and her mother was encouraging and always told her she could do whatever she wanted to do.

Excelling in math and science was important because Dr. Turner was focused on being accepted into college when she was in high school. And after earning her undergraduate degree, she focused on being accepted into medical school.

There was a time in high school when she wanted to be a neurosurgeon, surgery of the brain and spinal cord, and a time in medical school she considered orthopedic surgery, bone surgery. But she realized during medical school that she loved gastrointestinal surgery, surgery on the stomach and intestines. She decided to complete her fellowship in minimally invasive surgery and bariatric surgery.

Despite being an exceptional student she faced challenges along the way. She feels, intersectionality (the interconnected nature of social categorizations such as race, class, and gender as they apply to a given individual or group, regarded as creating overlapping and interdependent systems of discrimination or disadvantage) was part of her experience.

She shares, "In general, it is difficult to discern why some people may make things difficult for you or may not care for you. Is it race, is it gender, is it where you are from? You cannot try to figure out why people do not care for you. I mainly focused on getting the work done to the best of my abilities and letting the work speak for me. You can spend a great deal of time and energy getting caught up in trying to figure out what people's biases are, and you may never understand them. At the end of the day it does not matter. I had many positive supporters and advocates of all races and genders. I did not have mentors that were all women or people of color. It is a much more complex situation that cannot be explained."

Dr. Turner feels the most important goal is for patient outcomes to be positive. This means that the patient has survived and is doing well. Everything else flows from this. At the end of the day, surgeons care for patients. This is the primary goal; this is the purpose. There may be research, or educational responsibilities, or professional societies that are responsibilities as well; but at the end of the day a surgeon's job is to provide exemplary care for patients, period! This must be a doctor's highest priority. Once a surgeon has passed the steep learning curve of practicing on his/her own, it is the same for everyone, no matter how fantastic they are or were as a chief resident or fellow. Then, one can start taking on more responsibilities in their hospital and national societies.

Doctors must rely on the excellent training they have received to help them during challenging situations, because many times there is no one near to assist or take over during a difficult surgery. Sometimes, one must make difficult decisions and rely on their instincts, training, and work ethic to achieve success. Doctors have partners they can call in case the difficulties require experienced help; this ensures that patients are safe because ultimately this is what matters.

In the first few years practicing on their own, a doctor needs to make certain their judgment is good, their outcomes are positive, and their patients do well. With positive and successful clinical outcomes as a foundation, one can then build on other things like leadership roles within your institution or national organizations, research, education, and mentoring. All of this must be built on a solid foundation of excellent patient care and great outcomes.

Even with great education and talent, complications are part of a surgeon's life. Everyone has heard the adage, "The only way to not have complications is to not operate." Dr. Turner thinks this is true because surgeons who do not have complications are the ones who are not being truthful when they claim they do not have complications or are the ones who do not operate.

Keeping this perspective in mind is helpful, but it does not make it easier. Every complication a doctor has as an attending is devastating. Dr. Turner does not think people can fully grasp how devastated surgeons are. Neither the patient nor the public knows. It is especially important to have colleagues and friends and non-judgmental advisers that a physician can rely on to help process complications and the devastating feelings caused by these complications.

Many doctors are privileged to know other surgeons they can call in their circle of friends that may not be at the same institution. Their non-surgeon support system can be loving and sympathetic and supportive, but they will not understand. Surgeons must lean on surgeon friends because they are the only people who can understand because they have personal experience.

It is important to have someone who has been down this road before, senior surgeon advisers who are at different institutions to call and talk to about the case and receive honest feedback. With someone looking from the outside-in who understands and can help navigate through the situation, they can help figure out what could have been done differently. At times, they will be there to say there was nothing they believe that could have been done differently. Because the truth is, sometimes everything can be done correctly and there will still be an unfortunate outcome. A doctor needs to talk about it so the event does not break his/her confidence.

Dr. Turner contends complications present a two-hit phenomenon. The first hit is when a complication happens and a doctor manages the patient and their family, working to have the patient thrive through the complication. The second hit is being judged by colleagues. By the time they are finished harshly judging and criticizing a doctor for complications, that doctor just wants to quit. Some departments are exceptionally good about the morbidity and mortality conference and using it as an educational tool rather than as a place where people are berated and humiliated.

For this and every other reason both mentorship and sponsorship cannot be overstated. Mentorship is crucial and it is critically important to have multiple mentors because no one person can fill all the mentorship needs for an individual. Dr. Turner feels you may have a mentor for clinical cases, someone for life and work balance, someone for promotion and tenure assistance, and someone at your institution to help navigate politics or someone who helps you with the business aspect of medicine. Mentors provide advice and counsel for these different areas of life.

The sponsorship and advocacy aspects of becoming and being a doctor are critically important and undervalued. Everyone needs a person who is willing to say nice things about them behind closed doors. At times, you may not know the person who is advocating for you. It could be someone on the program committee who mentions your name when the committee is looking for a moderator for a national conference. It could be someone mentioning you to someone looking for an author for a chapter in a textbook. It could also be the person who nominates you for an officer position in a professional society or someone who puts in a word for you in the search committee where you are looking for a job. These are examples of when you do not necessarily know who your advocate is or who is sponsoring you, but you sure do appreciate them.

A sponsor or advocate may also be someone that stands up for you if someone is disparaging or saying negative things about you. They may advocate for you and dispel a rumor that is not true. These are meaningful relationships and may be more subtle and sporadic, but important in terms of advancing in a career. In Dr. Turner's experience, she is certain she would not be where she is today without the many wonderful people who were sponsors and advocates for her. They are extraordinary leaders who always took interest in her and advised her and have allowed her to speak with them in confidence about delicate situations and have given great advice. For this, she is forever grateful.

Sponsors and advocates may not necessarily be older than you. They can be people in your brain trust, a group of experts who advise you, that are your age or younger than you. When Dr. Sherilyn Gordon-Burroughs was with us, Dr. Turner talked with her as well as other friends who helped her grow as a surgeon and leader. Sometimes others have good judgment to share or a different skill level or may have better communication skills, making it beneficial to share ideas with them. You can ask how they would approach and handle a specific situation. Sometimes this helps to learn and grow as a doctor and every physician is always learning and always growing as a professional their entire career. Dr. Turner feels it is her duty to advocate for others.

Finally, Dr. Turner shares these words, "Surgery is an amazing career and it is doable. You can be a surgeon if you desire. There is a whole community of us who are already surgeons and want to support you and help you because you are the future of the profession."

Dr. Turner honors Dr. Sherilyn Gordon-Burroughs: "There is so much to say, but she was truly inspirational. She was a surgeon's surgeon; very smart, accomplished, generous with her time, influential, extraordinarily savvy, and really took an interest in educating the younger generation. She was an incredible mother, daughter, and friend. An extraordinary surgeon and scholar and just an amazing human being. We are all much poorer for her no longer being with us."

Dr. Angeles Boleko Ribas

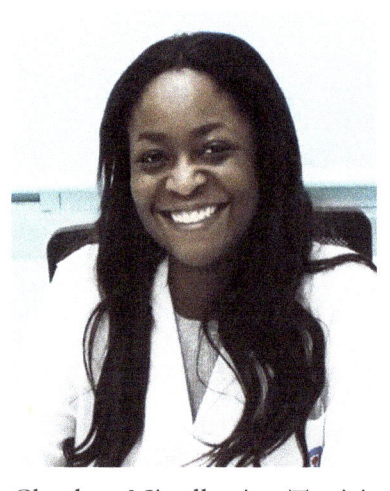

Dr. Angeles Boleko Ribas earned her medical degree from the University of Barcelona in Spain. She completed her general surgery residency at Vall d'Hebrón University Hospital, Spain. During her surgical residency, she rotated through various hospitals including Sao Joao University Hospital in Porto, Portugal, Charles Nicolle in Tunisia, and Charlotte Maxeke General Academic Hospital in Johannesburg, South Africa. During her rotations, she gained extensive experience in emergency surgery and polytrauma.

Dr. Boleko Ribas obtained Advanced Trauma Life Support (ATLS) and Definitive Surgical Trauma Care (DSTC) certificates during her rotation in Johannesburg. She earned a Master of Nutrition and Health Degree at the University Oberta de Catalunya in Barcelona, Spain, and completed a Bariatric

Surgery Fellowship in Barcelona. She also worked with Doctors Without Borders, doing humanitarian work. She is currently a specialist surgeon in Barcelona at the Hospital de Barcelona, Hospital Quiron El Pilar, and Hospital Quirón Dexeus. Spain, like many European countries, only has a handful of black surgeons.

Dr. Boleko Ribas was born 36 years ago in Barcelona. Both her parents are from Equatorial Guinea. They came to Spain when Guinea was part of a Spanish colony in the early '60s.

She chose medicine because whenever she visited her mother at the clinic where she worked as a nurse-midwife, she felt at home. Growing up, she religiously watched the television show ER and was fascinated by Eriq LaSalle's character, the amazing Dr. Peter Benton. Dr. Boleko Ribas dreamed of one day being like him, an amazing surgeon.

There were challenges along the way. Dr. Boleko Ribas discovered she had to show she could be a skilled surgeon despite not having mentors that resembled her. Also, during her first year of training she faced another challenge. A female surgeon made training difficult because she was not supportive and was extremely critical in a negative way during each encounter Dr. Boleko Ribas had with her. To overcome these challenges, Dr. Boleko Ribas worked hard in residency and stayed focused on her goal. Things have become easier for her since graduating from residency. With time, she has learned to not take it personally when she is underestimated.

Dr. Boleko Ribas shared her pearls of wisdom for young black females considering medicine and surgery, "Never give up. Set your goals and work extremely hard until you achieve them. Be a team player. There is no need to trample on others so you can shine. When you are great, your work and results speak for themselves. Life is more than work. Have a life outside of work."

Dr. Boleko Ribas is confident now, but has not always been so. During her residency training, she lacked confidence because she listened and internalized the criticism from people who judged her based on her skin color and gender without allowing her the chance to prove herself. By realizing how difficult it is to teach others, Dr. Boleko Ribas began putting more effort into teaching and, in turn, this helped her develop confidence as a surgeon and teacher.

She wakes early to go to the hospital for rounds with her team. They examine patients and formulate plans of care for them. Then, she either heads to the operating room if she has cases scheduled that day or sees patients in the office.

Dr. Boleko Ribas feels her greatest accomplishment is to know that all she has accomplished is due exclusively to her own efforts. Nobody has given her anything and she has not had to step on anyone to achieve her goals. Her proudest moments are when she took the exam to choose her specialty (in Spain it is called MIR, Medico Interno Residente). She was number 998 of more than 7000 exam takers. Another proud moment was when she realized she could perform surgery without assistance, trusting her instincts and knowledge. This was an amazing day. She is also immensely proud whenever she sees her patients for follow-up visits and they are thankful, happy, and well.

Dr. Boleko Ribas shares the best advice she has received, "One of my teachers in surgical residency said, 'Cirujano es el que opera,' meaning 'complications are part of our job description.' It is comforting when there is an unexpected outcome or complication to know this happens to even the absolute best surgeons. We as surgeons need to support each other during these times and help each other grow from these experiences to better serve our patients."

She feels that life goes beyond work. Though she loves her job, she believes life is much more than just being a surgeon. She enjoys spending time with her family and friends. She is currently reading Bromatology. In her spare time, she is studying to be a dietitian.

Dr. Boleko Ribas would love to meet her maternal and paternal grandmothers. They were both phenomenal women and she would love to learn about life from them. She would also like to have dinner with Chimamanda Ngozi Adichie because she is an amazing prolific Nigerian author of three novels, Purple Hibiscus (2003), Half of a Yellow Sun (2006), and Americanah (2013), and also a short story collection, The Thing around Your Neck (2009). Her TEDx talk, "We Should All Be Feminists," has garnered more than 5 million views.

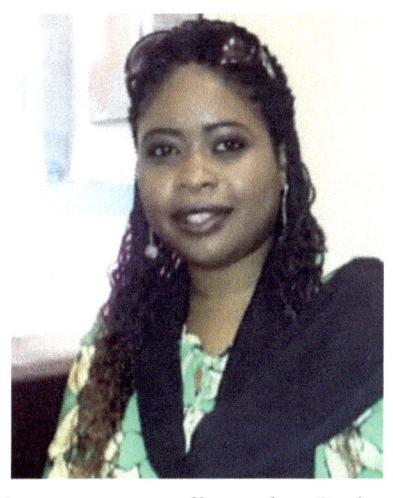

Dr. Sally Omer El-Goni

Dr. Sally Omer El-Goni is a specialist in general and laparoscopic surgery in Khartoum, Sudan. She is originally from South Sudan and is a member of the Women in Surgery Africa (WISA) where she won the She for She Award in 2019. She is also a member of the Sudan Association of Surgery, as well as the Sudanese Society of Gastroenterology (SSG) and the World Association of Minimally Invasive Surgery.

Dr. Omer El-Goni had a dream of becoming a cardiac (heart) surgeon since she was a child. She does not remember exactly how old she was or why this was her dream, but she thinks she was influenced by Egyptian movies. In one movie, a patient presented having a heart attack and was immediately taken to the operating theater (operating room). Then, within a short time, the patient recovered. She thought this was incredible. Dr. Omer El-Goni's family knew she wanted to be a doctor and encouraged her by calling her Dr. Sally from a young age.

When she was 11 years old, Dr. Omer El-Goni began reading about mummies and how they were made. She became so interested in mummies she began mummifying birds. She took dead birds, emptied their stomachs, and filled them with preservative material using natural ingredients from the kitchen, such as salt, lemon, and a special small stone from the Western Sudan Mountains. These mummified birds were used as decorations in her living room.

Dr. Omer El-Goni does not know exactly what surgery meant despite dreaming of being a surgeon until she enrolled in medical school. It was then that she understood what surgery entailed.

She excelled in anatomy because, at an early age, Dr. Omer El-Goni understood that to be a great surgeon, one must understand anatomy very well. She fell in love with dissecting cadavers. After graduating from medical school, she changed her goal from cardiac surgery to general surgery. Her mother and siblings were supportive from the beginning. Her father, however, was against her pursuing surgery because of the extreme stress that comes with being a surgeon as well as the sacrifices one must make compared to other disciplines in medicine. Once he realized how determined his daughter was, he also supported her career choice.

Initially, her friends felt it would be too difficult for her to be a surgeon. They worried she would be unable to have a family. Now, however, they are happy she is a surgeon and feel safe when she operates on their relatives. The love and support of family have had the greatest impact on Dr. Omer El-Goni's career in medicine and surgery. They are always understanding when she is on call and cannot make it to social events. For this, she is incredibly grateful.

The greatest challenge Dr. Omer El-Goni faces is the community because they are not familiar with female surgeons. It takes time to convince people who are not used to seeing a woman surgeon that she is as competent, at times more competent than men. It still seems to be a very male-dominated field.

The best advice Dr. Omer El-Goni received is "Come and work at Ibn Sina Hospital and you will see some amazing surgery!" stated Professor Abdel Majed Massad, professor of gastrointestinal and hepatobiliary surgery in Sudan. When Dr. Omer El-Goni joined his team, she realized she sincerely wanted to be a hepatobiliary surgeon someday. She grew professionally and refined her surgical skills and expanded her medical and surgical knowledge as she worked with him.

A typical day for Dr. Omer El-Goni is waking early in the morning, reading something inspirational, and then eating breakfast with a cup of coffee. She arrives at the hospital and depending on the day, reviews patients with her team before attending ward rounds where they make decisions regarding patient care and discharges. On days she has teaching responsibilities, Dr. Omer El-Goni trains medical students and surgical residents. On days she operates, she is in the OR (operating room).

Operating can be stressful, but she feels it is also extremely rewarding work because many times results are seen quickly. For instance, if a patient presents with an inflamed gallbladder and surgery is indicated to remove it, the patient feels better soon, if not immediately, after surgery. On a typical day, Dr. Omer El-Goni also sees patients in the outpatient clinic throughout the day.

Once work is completed at the hospital, she heads home to rest for a short while before cooking with her family. Sometimes, she watches television with the family before they all gather for prayer. Then, she prepares for the following day and, at times, if there is a critically ill patient in the hospital, she is required to make an evening or night visit.

Thursday is a special day for Dr. Omer El-Goni's family because they make a point of sitting together in the evening, around the tea tray, discussing the events of the week. Sometimes, there is a social activity she attends in the evening or on the weekend. She has great friends and most of them are doctors she met at different times in training. They plan times to get together, and she tries as much as possible to meet with them.

Dr. Omer El-Goni shares, "It is difficult to find balance with a medical career, especially when you are a surgeon. Your time is not completely yours. Your time also belongs to patients and their families. In a country like Sudan, you are always a doctor. Also, at social events, if people know you are a doctor, they ask for medical advice. They even expect you to write medicine prescriptions for them regardless of what type of doctor you are. Doctors only treat patients with disorders in their specific branch of medicine or surgery. I find it frustrating because many times I just want to enjoy the social event and not be a doctor for a while."

Three people Dr. Omer El-Goni would like to have dinner with and learn about are Sir Alfred Cuschieri, a Maltese-British academic surgeon most notable for his pioneering contribution to minimal access surgery, also known as key-hole surgery. She would love to pick his brain and learn as much as she can from him. Also, she would like to meet Dr. R.K. Mishra, a laparoscopic and robotic surgeon who is world renown and teaches surgeons from countries all over the world. Lastly, she would like to learn from and enhance her surgical skills from Dr. Sami Elderderi, a general and laparoscopic surgeon in Sudan.

Words of advice Dr. Omer El-Goni wants to share with others interested in becoming surgeons are to believe in yourself, to follow your dreams, and to be strong because you can do it.

Dr. Crystal Johnson-Mann

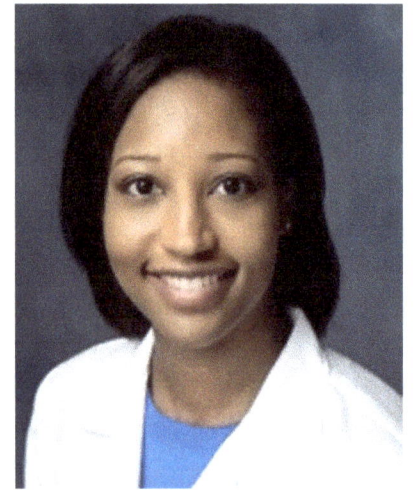

Dr. Crystal Johnson-Mann is currently an assistant professor and a minimally invasive and bariatric surgeon (MIS) within the division of gastrointestinal surgery at the University of Florida, College of Medicine, Gainesville, Florida, USA.

She earned her bachelor's degree at the University of South Carolina in Columbia, South Carolina. While there, she divided her time as a student-athlete with a major in biological sciences and as a member of the varsity volleyball team. She completed her medical education at the Medical University of South

Carolina (MUSC) in Charleston, South Carolina and completed her general surgery residency at the same institution. She finished a fellowship in minimally invasive surgery at the University of Virginia Health System, Charlottesville, and is board certified in general surgery by the American Board of Surgery.

Her clinical and research interests include bariatric surgery (weight loss surgery), anti-reflux surgery (surgery to relieve stomach reflux), minimally invasive hernia repair, fixing hernias (which are bulges that happen when an organ or fatty tissue squeeze through a weak spot in a surrounding muscle or tissue that holds it in place), and healthcare disparities. She is a member of the American College of Surgeons, Association for Women Surgeons, American Society for Metabolic and Bariatric Surgeons, National Medical Association, Society of American Gastrointestinal and Endoscopic Surgeons, and the Society of Black Academic Surgeons (SBAS).

Dr. Johnson-Mann grew up in a small town where her father was the first African American director of the emergency medical services (EMS) at their hospital. He did so after working his way for years from an orderly/ambulance attendant to an emergency medical technician (EMT) to a Paramedic, then becoming the director.

In addition to his day job, he taught EMT certification courses at night. Dr. Johnson-Mann tagged along during school breaks because she wanted to follow her dad everywhere. This set the foundation for her exposure to medicine; trailing behind her dad to his classes, flipping through his EMT textbooks in the ER when he left her with the nurses for an emergency call, and seeing him in action via simulation when she played the victim at the annual EMS Symposium.

Even with this exposure, however, she never considered medicine seriously until she elected to take honors biology during her sophomore year in high school. Until this time, Dr. Johnson-Mann avoided science classes, but this class was taught by Mr. Horton and, it was different. From this point forward, she was on the trajectory to pre-medicine in college.

In college, she was an athlete, playing volleyball at a well-known Division 1-A school. Unfortunately, she was unable to play her freshman year due to an injury to her shoulder that needed surgery. Sports always attracted her, and she initially thought she wanted to pursue orthopedic surgery as a career so she could focus on sports medicine.

While in medical school, Dr. Johnson-Mann carried this vision with her and actively sought exposure to the orthopedic surgery attending physicians. She became quite active in the leadership of the orthopedics student interest group. Halfway through her third year of medical school, on the GI (stomach and intestinal) surgery rotation, she met someone that ultimately changed her life, Dr. David B. Adams.

Because of him, she fell in love of general surgery, specifically the surgery of the foregut, the first part of the gastrointestinal tract from the mouth to the duodenum, (the section of the small intestine connected to the stomach), and includes the liver, gallbladder, pancreas, and spleen. As a resident at the same institution, on the GI surgery service with her bariatric attendings, she also fell in love with bariatric surgery (weight loss surgery). It is technically challenging but immensely gratifying as she helps her bariatric patients have a second shot at life. There is no greater reward.

The greatest challenge Dr. Johnson-Mann faced in training was the relative lack of other black women in medicine. Where she attended medical school, she was aware of a few black female attending physicians, but only one was still an attending when she was finishing her residency. Unfortunately, this attending was also on her way to another institution. There were no black female surgeons within her department during her residency. At the time, there were two black male surgical attending physicians who were both fantastic.

Lucky for her, there were a few black females in Dr. Johnson-Mann's residency program, so they became a support system for the minority female medical students interested in surgery and other disciplines through their involvement in campus organizations.

Fellowship experience was a hybrid, according to Dr. Johnson-Mann. She was a fellow and a junior attending physician. There were days she was the attending physician responsible for her personal cases and at the same time was scrubbing for surgical cases with the attending physicians teaching and overseeing her surgery fellowship training.

Most operating room days, she would wake by 6 a.m. to quickly shower, grab something to eat, make herself a cappuccino, let the dog out, and feed both the cat and dog. Then off to the hospital. Her husband was on pet duty when he was home.

Dr. Johnson-Mann talked to patients before surgery. Then, it was into the operating room. If she cared for inpatients in the hospital, she rounded and saw these patients on the surgical unit with one of the residents between other surgical cases. At the end of the day, she signed notes, and went home to hang out with her husband and pets. Things have changed since she became an attending physician and they have added a baby to their family.

To find balance in her fellowship, Dr. Johnson-Mann made sure to retain the activities she loved outside of medicine. She is still a huge sports fanatic but does not let herself play volleyball anymore for fear of injury. Her car radio station is set to ESPN. *Sports Center* is usually on when she has the television playing.

The best advice Dr. Johnson-Mann received was from Dr. David Adams who said, "Kick to the wall." It means, "Finish the race strong. Don't slow down."

Dr. Johnson-Mann would like to encourage every reader by saying, "Trust in yourself. You got here because you worked hard and deserve to be here. Self-doubt plagued me during my first couple years of residency. Ask for help if you need it. No one is perfect. Find a good mentor; ideally in your chosen specialty, but mentors can exist in other disciplines as well. I was lucky because I found one in medical school.

Dr. Rania Hassan Saad

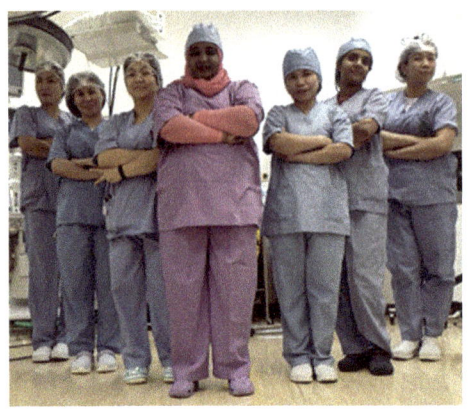

Dr. Rania Hassan Saad is a general surgeon in Sudan. She is a member of the Royal College of Surgeons-Edinburgh (MRCS, Ed), the Sudan Association of Surgeons, and a member of the World Association of Laparoscopic surgeons and Sudan Education Supporting Organization (SEDSO) and she is a Primarily Trauma Care (PTC) instructor.

Studying medicine provides the chance to deal with the most precious thing in life, health. When one is healthy, it is reflected in all other aspects of their life. Dr. Hassan Saad chose surgery because it is a dynamic job characterized by a unique relationship between patients and physicians. A patient relinquishes all control and puts their trust in his/her surgeon while they sleep, trusting their surgeon will do the absolute best for them. It is a great responsibility filled with great reward and satisfaction. A surgeon is constantly learning and with time and throughout training, develops knowledge, promptitude, confidence, and patience.

Dr. Hassan Saad did not know what a career in surgery entailed, but she was consumed by everything that had to do with surgery since she was a medical student; from taking care of patients in the emergency room to taking them into the operating room for their operations. She watched teachers as they examined each abdomen or threw each stitch while sewing bowel (intestines) together. Dr. Hassan Saad was a sponge, soaking it all in for a time when she would be the one to do it and teach others.

Each step of the way, she thirsted for more knowledge and wanted to learn more skills. During her internship, she was on the plastics, burn, and reconstructive surgery unit and loved taking care of these patients and watching them recover. She had such a positive attitude and genuinely enjoyed her work so much that this caught the attention of several specialists who advised her to take the surgical exam, which would allow her to start a surgical residency. Dr. Hassan Saad took the test and passed the first time. Thus, began her journey into the amazing, intricate world of surgery.

Challenges she faced along the way related to things like her being 154 cm (5ft 0.5in) tall and being in a discipline that she feels affords men preferential treatment in many respects, whether it is just the fact that patients are not accustomed to having a female surgeon or the equipment used by surgeons is made for large male hands.

Since she was the shortest physician in the group, and a woman, patients often sat in front of one of her junior residents for their physical exam and treatment. The patients often refused to be treated by Dr. Hassan Saad because they viewed her as inexperienced since she was short and a woman. The junior residents explained to patients that she was, in fact, the senior surgeon in the group.

Another huge challenge she faced during her journey was finding balance between standing up for herself so she received the same training opportunities as her male colleagues, and maintaining the respect and dignity of her colleagues who had different ideas of roles of women in surgery. She was challenged to stay feminine and avoid becoming like one of the men to fit in.

Dr. Hassan Saad's proudest moment was when she thought of quitting because surgical training is exceedingly difficult. She persevered and eventually passed her general surgery exam. Now, she is in a new era of finding herself again after years of rigorous training. She is in pursuit of establishing her name among the many great surgeons. She continues to work to improve her surgical skills and, one surgery at a time, she is carving her fingerprint in the vast world of surgery.

Also, Dr. Hassan Saad joined the Sudan Association of Surgeons and is one of its most active members. She participates in conferences as a presenter and organizes various surgical events. There are many female surgeons in her country and the numbers are continuing to grow. They probably have one of the largest groups of female surgeons in Africa. This motivated them to create the Sudanese Women in Surgery Society to provide support and mentorship to all female Sudanese surgeons in all stages of their training and careers. She is also interested in breast surgical oncology because she wants to be able to provide comprehensive management to female patients because often, religion is a barrier to seeking consultation from male surgeons.

Sudan is a predominantly Muslim country and female patients have a difficult time in the hospital system when they must be taken care of by male medical staff. This is because it is culturally unacceptable for them to be exposed when there is a man present who is not their family. Dr. Hassan Saad hopes to establish a specialized care hospital with an all-female staff someday, including the receptionists, custodial staff, food services, physicians, nurses, respiratory therapists, administration, and the CEO. This way, female patients can be cared for without experiencing the anxiety of being taken care of by men. She knows it is a huge goal and seems impossible, but she continues to work hard and keeps trying.

Three people Dr. Hassan Saad would like to have dinner with and learn from are Professor Sir Alfred Cuschieri, the pioneer in minimal access surgery. She met him in 2013. At this time, he was the main guest at the international conference organized by the Sudan Association of Surgeons and was the man that inspired her to overcome her anxieties about going into surgery as a woman. Her second choice is Professor Alla Illyinichna Levushkina, the oldest female surgeon currently 91-one-years-old. She said, "Being a doctor isn't just a profession, but a lifestyle. Why else would the surgeon live, if not to work?" She has clearly taught Dr.

Hassan Saad that nothing is impossible if you work hard and try your best at all times. The sky is the only limit. And finally, she would love to meet with her deceased father one more time and thank him for believing in her and for putting the seeds of human service in her soul. She would tell him that she will continue to strive to be the absolute best that she can until the day she dies.

The most precious advice Dr. Hassan Saad received was, "Your juniors are the future. Teach them well and show how proud you are of them when they do well because positive reinforcement is enormously powerful."

The most precious advice Dr. Hassan Saad received was, "Your juniors are the future. Teach them well and show how proud you are of them when they do well because positive reinforcement is enormously powerful."

Things she would like to share are, "Be knowledgeable and honest. Be confident. Keep working hard and do not give up."

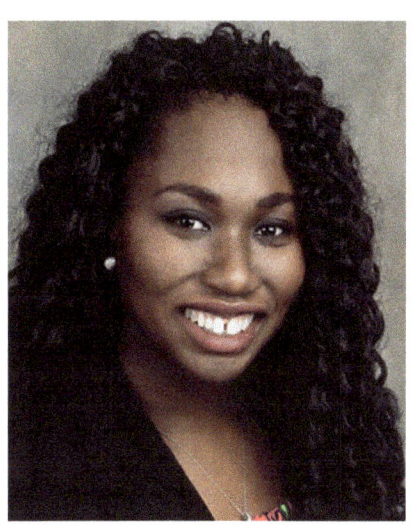

Dr. Iyore James

Dr. Iyore James earned her bachelor's degree in science at the University of Massachusetts in Boston, Massachusetts, and her medical degree from Tufts University School of Medicine also in Boston. She completed a general surgery residency at the Ohio State University Wexner Medical Center in Columbus, Ohio, where she also trained in an abdominal organ transplant surgery fellowship. She currently works as a general surgeon in Charlotte, South Carolina, and is interested in laparoscopic and robotic surgery.

Dr. James chose medicine during her pre-teen years

growing up in Nigeria because she saw the healthcare problems in her country. She wanted a career in medicine and policy because she thought that as a doctor, she would be able to help people who are sick and dying. At the time she considered infectious diseases as a specialty because infectious diseases were what were killing her people. She felt this was the major medical issue in Nigeria.

As a third-year medical student during her general surgery rotation, she enjoyed working in the operating room. It was satisfying to be able to see a problem and fix it. When she was completing a rotation at a community hospital, one of the chief residents on service with her, cheered her on to pursue surgery as a specialty.

During her journey to become a doctor, Dr. James feels developing relationships with mentors and peers was her greatest challenge. Also, her own internal drive of wanting to be the best was a challenge, but she learned to be kind to herself and not expect perfection.

Dr. James feels her greatest confidence builder was her father. He believed in her and encouraged her to always do her best. Her dad always told her that with hard work she can achieve anything and will be rewarded. She has found this to be true. Dr. James studied diligently and did excellent work. This built her confidence as she progressed in training.

Currently, she works in a private practice multi-surgical group and performs general surgery and minimally invasive surgery, laparoscopic, and robotic surgery. She mostly performs gastrointestinal (GI) surgeries, such as colon resections, hiatal hernias, stomach resections, and hernias. She has one full day of operating and then spends a half-day seeing clinic patients and half-day operating the other days of the week.

If she could only do one operation for the rest of her career, she would do a laparoscopic cholecystectomy, gallbladder removal surgery.

In addition to her private practice, Dr. James frequently joins others on mission trips. She has been back to Nigeria to provide care. She understands mission trips are not for long-term problem solving, but a means to help a few people at a time. Her hope and goal are to be able to help the local doctors and healthcare systems develop long-term care availability.

She partners with Dr. Obi Ekwanna, a urologist and transplant surgeon. They provide surgical care on mission trips. Their most recent trip lasted five days and they performed two kidney transplants.

The enthusiasm of the people motivates Dr. James to continue this work. Many things at our disposal in the United States are not available in Nigeria.

Experiencing healthcare conditions in both countries has had a tremendous impact on her career development. On one hand, Dr. James appreciates the abundance of resources and has learned to not be wasteful. On the other hand, she learned to improvise while getting the job done safely in an environment with limited resources.

One priority on the service trip is education. It is essential to educate and train because this strengthens the local capacity of the healthcare providers in Nigeria. It is not enough to do a procedure, there needs to be continuation of care. It has been a life-long dream of Dr. James to help her native country.

"Just before I left Nigeria, when I was 16 years old starting my college education, my father sat me down and told me that if I am good at what I do, this cannot be denied. Even if there are people that do not like me, ultimately my work speaks for itself! My dad is my hero. He has so much insight and has helped me look at things in different ways."

Dr. James would love to have dinner with and learn from Nelson Mandela. In the face of hatred and great injustice, he blessed his enemies and was driven by what was good and best for his people and not for himself. He sacrificed his freedom for what he believed in. Secondly, she always loves talking with her father who is still alive. They have disagreements at times, but they typically have fruitful conversations. They talk about everything from politics to how to deal with people. She loves her talks with her dad. Lastly, she would like to speak with Ruth Bader Ginsburg, Supreme Court Justice of the United States. She is a strong woman with a vision and goal. Dr. James would love to talk to her!

Dr. James wants every young lady with the desire to pursue a career in medicine to be true to themselves and be confident. She is convinced everyone continues to learn their entire careers and that no one arrives at a point where they have learned everything, so open your mind to keep learning. Even when there are failures, find lessons in them. Lastly, she feels that you must have support. Have champions in your corner to encourage you. Keep your relationships because they are important. It is stressful and you need to have a great support system. It is true that it takes a village for you to be successful.

Finally, when choosing a career path, your path may change along the way. It may be very different from what you originally thought you would choose. Dr. James's journey is a testament to the fact that direction changes depending on life circumstances.

When she was in general surgery residency, she considered pediatric surgery which required her to complete two years of research to be a competitive applicant for pediatric surgery. She, however, did not match into a pediatric fellowship so, instead of waiting another year and reapplying to a pediatric surgery fellowship, she considered transplant surgery and doing pediatric surgery as a transplant surgeon.

During her transplant surgery fellowship her plans changed again after she became pregnant with twins. She experienced another difficult pregnancy with complications that required her to revisit what she wanted to do with her career as her premature twins struggled for their lives.

Dr. James shares, "Life happens and decisions made during difficult times define who you are. Some people consider it a failure if you wanted to do one thing and then choose something else. It is alright to decide later what you want to do or to change your mind if circumstances change."

CHAPTER FOUR
Pediatric Surgery

Pediatric surgery is a subspecialty of surgery involving the surgery of fetuses, infants, children, adolescents, and young adults.

Dr. Andrea Hayes-Jordan

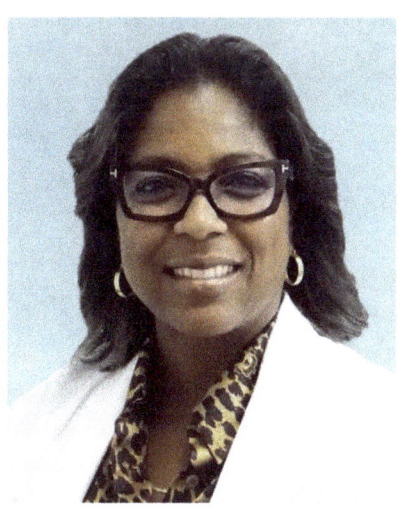

Dr. Andrea Hayes-Jordan is a professor of pediatric surgery and surgical oncology (cancer) at the University of North Carolina (UNC) Children's Hospital, Chapel Hill, North Carolina. She is the surgeon-in-chief of the UNC Children's Hospital and the division chief of pediatric surgery at UNC. Before becoming a surgeon-in-chief at UNC Children's Hospital, she was the director of pediatric surgical oncology and associate professor of surgical oncology and pediatrics at the University of Texas MD Anderson Cancer Center, Houston. She is the first African American pediatric surgeon.

Dr. Hayes-Jordan is originally from Los Angeles, California. Her mother told her that from her first words she knew she wanted to be a doctor. She started talking at 18 months, reading at age two, and her mother said no matter who asked her, she always answered, "I want to be a baby doctor." She does not remember ever wanting to be anything else.

She loves taking care of children, but she feels working in pediatrics is a calling. It can be emotionally draining to care for children because it takes more of your being. When she was in medical school, Dr. Hayes-Jordan thought she wanted to be a pediatrician. As she progressed through her training, she realized she wanted to be a surgeon. Then, a series of events happened where God led her to pediatric surgery.

In her fourth year of medical school at Dartmouth in Hanover, New Hampshire, Dr. Hayes-Jordan applied for a sub-internship at Stanford in California. This was before the internet and before cell phones, so all correspondence was done by mail. On her first day, she was told there was no room for medical students on the general surgery service because it was full. She moved to California from the east coast, so she was committed to making something work. She thought, "Well, I'm here. What are my choices?"

There happened to be openings in orthopedic surgery and pediatric surgery. Having already completed an orthopedic surgery rotation, she reluctantly chose pediatric surgery. Dr. Hayes-Jordan said, "My second day on the service, the first day I worked with patients, I fell in love. It was an eye-opening revelation on rounds to see the children and be part of treating their diseases. What I realized was when I help a child with any disease, I am not helping only one person, but I am also helping generations. This one child lives. They have children and their children have children and so on. So, it is easy to see how in pediatrics that one life is more than one life. This is what I love about it."

Before this, she received her undergraduate degree from Dartmouth. She majored in religion but completed all the required premedical courses. Dr. Hayes-Jordan spent 10 hours doing research in a leukemia lab, and this was the beginning of her development as a researcher. She attended medical school at Dartmouth and then completed her general surgery residency at the University of California, Davis. She completed a two-year fellowship in molecular biology at the University of California, San Francisco (UCSF) during her surgical residency.

After finishing her residency, she completed a melanoma and sarcoma fellowship (two types of cancers) at the University of Texas MD Anderson Cancer Center, Houston, and a pediatric surgical oncology fellowship at St Jude Children's Research Hospital, Memphis, Tennessee. She finalized her pediatric surgery fellowship at the Hospital for Sick Children in Toronto, Canada. After completing this fellowship, Dr. Hayes-Jordan discovered she was the first black female pediatric surgeon.

Dr. Hayes-Jordan experienced challenges along the way. When she applied for her pediatric surgery fellowship training, not a single institution accepted her. She tried again and again with the same results. At the time, there were only about 25 available opportunities for this training. Dr. Hayes-Jordan did not want to blame it on her race, but when she could not find another explanation, this is the only conclusion she felt she could make. She had done everything everyone who was accepted had done.

Her mentors made calls to find out why she was rejected. One surgeon at a southern hospital replied that bringing in the first black woman was too much of a risk for his program. Dr. Hayes-Jordan continued to affirm she knew this is what she was meant to do, and she refused to give up and choose another specialty! In 2000, she secured a fellowship in Canada at the University of Toronto Hospital for Sick Children.

While training at St. Jude's, she met a patient who had a disease called desmoplastic small round cell tumor. It was extensive and he had hundreds of tumors in his belly cavity. No one could help him. Dr. Hayes-Jordan was the one who told his mother that her son's tumor could not be operated on and that he was going to die.

This experience impressed upon her the importance of finding a cure for this disease. After reading about this type of tumor and studying the disease and the outcomes, it was clear to Dr. Hayes-Jordan that new therapy was needed. This changed her career path and what she does now. She is a pioneer for the development of hyperthermic, intraperitoneal chemotherapy that is delivered to patients with desmoplastic small round cell tumors. This procedure, abbreviated HIPEC, is what she has built her career on.

Desmoplastic small round cell tumors (DSRCT), a rare

sarcoma, spreads throughout the abdominal and chest cavities. Instead of one large tumor, there are hundreds of tiny malignant tumors everywhere in the abdominal cavity (malignant tumors are tumors that spread to other areas of the body and usually result in loss of the patient). Before Dr. Hayes-Jordan started treating this disease, it was considered hopeless. Many physicians would not offer treatment because it was considered inoperable. In her 15 years of research, Dr. Hayes-Jordan discovered that these tumors are treatable. These children can live longer, and some can even be cured.

Before, the survival rate for over five years was 15% to 30%. Now, the survival rate has improved to approximately 60% with aggressive surgery. The surgery is called a cytoreductive (which means we reduce the cells of the tumors) procedure and takes anywhere from 10 to 20 hours to remove every one of these tumors.

Once the removal is complete, the child is treated with hyperthermic, intraperitoneal chemotherapy (HIPEC). This means the abdominal cavity is washed with extremely hot chemotherapy. This prevents the tumors from returning. Five or 10 years ago, this procedure was considered experimental. Progress over the last 12 years has advanced and now it is part of the standard treatment for these patients.

Implementing research into practice takes a great deal of time; progress in medicine is slow. However, because Dr. Hayes-Jordan has a laboratory where she can study the genes and scientific parts of the cancer cells in these tumors, progress is quicker. She can see a specific problem in a patient, return to her laboratory, and then determine how to best fix that problem. She does so by figuring out how her discoveries affect the patient at the cellular level and then she creates a plan to halt the disease so the patient can live longer.

Dr. Hayes-Jordan's greatest satisfaction is being able to treat children from all over the world for a disease that, a few years ago, was considered hopeless. When she was completing her medical training, physicians were not treating this disease.

They were not operating on these patients, so there were no techniques available for removing these tumors; no solution to make certain they did not reappear. Dr. Hayes-Jordan knew there had to be a way to give these children a fighting chance for survival. Dr. Hayes-Jordan's greatest achievement has been perfecting the technique of removing 300 to 2000 tiny tumors inside a child's chest and abdominal cavity and then being able to treat them successfully with heated chemotherapy with very few side effects.

When asked what keeps her going, Dr. Hayes-Jordan states, "The one thing that gives me hope is knowing that God is in control and I am here doing the best I can, but ultimately, I am not in control of the world or the outcome of the patients. I think what gives me peace is knowing that God is in control. I spend a lot of time praying. God keeps me going. He keeps me strong." Her favorite motto is, "I can do all things through Christ who strengthens me." (Philippians 4.13)

The best advice she has ever received was from Dr. Claude Organ Junior, former president of the American College of Surgeons, who said "Hard work is no guarantee of success." She feels this is a difficult sentence to swallow because there are hundreds of thousands of people who are working hard who are not necessarily successful, but she believes surrounding yourself with a great team is the key to success.

Dr. Hayes-Jordan also agrees that mentorship is important because she realizes that, in her career, one of the reasons she has been successful is because of her mentors. Her mentors helped a great deal in her long journey which you really cannot do it without help. No matter how smart you are, no matter how persistent you are, no matter how great you are at what you do, you always need someone who has navigated the waters before you to guide you. Dr. Hayes-Jordan was appreciative to have had several mentors who were supportive of what she was doing. Some people were not supportive. But even if people are not supportive, a mentor can be there and let you know what you should or should not be doing and give their opinion, opinions based on caring. Dr. Hayes-Jordan feels a responsibility to give back because someone mentored her. She does not want another person to endure the same mistakes she did.

Her final words of encouragement are, "Do what you need to do to get where you need to be in life. Do not be concerned about the amount of time it will take to get there. Do not give up. Keep trying until you get where you want to be. Be confident. Exude confidence. Always do your best in whatever you are doing, no matter where you are because you never know who could be looking at you. In everything do your best and be confident and you will be successful."

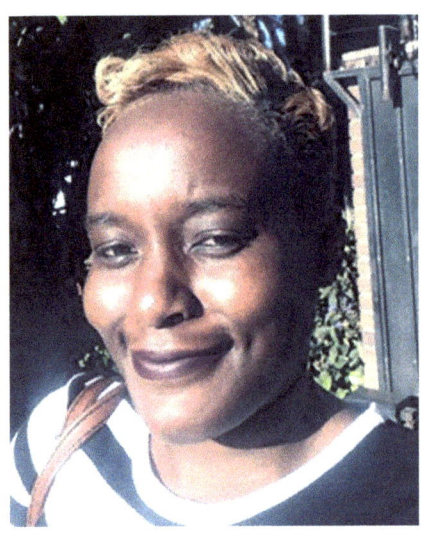

Dr. Kudzayi Sarah Munanzvi

Dr. Kudzayi Sarah Munanzvi is a pediatric surgeon in Zimbabwe. She completed her medical training at the University of Zimbabwe and developed an interest in surgery during her medical internship.

She spent several years working under the mentorship of a renowned pediatric surgeon, Dr. Bothwell Mbuwayesango, learning the art of surgery before beginning her surgical training. During this time, she was part of a team that successfully separated conjoined twins.

She recently completed her pediatric surgery fellowship training with the College of Surgeons of East Central and Southern Africa (COSECSA), Arusha, Tanzania. She was awarded the best pediatric surgery trainee in the region. Her areas of interest include minimal access surgery, surgery using small tiny incisions and a camera with small tiny instruments, and neonatal surgery, surgery in newborns less than 28 days old. She enjoys mentoring young people and encouraging them, not just to become surgeons, but to become leaders.

One of the most common conditions a pediatric surgeon must manage is a congenital abnormality, a birth-related disorder, known as gastroschisis. This is a condition in which the baby's bowels (intestines) are outside the abdominal cavity at birth. In developed countries, survival for babies born with this defect is about 95%. In developing countries, however, survival is anywhere between 0-33%. These children have poor odds of survival from birth.

There was one patient who left an indelible mark on Dr. Munanzvi. The infant was born with gastroschisis and was referred to Dr. Munanzvi's hospital from a hospital 250km (155 miles) away. The child's mother, age 24, had a thick accent typical of people native to the eastern part of the country. She was older than other mothers (mainly teenagers) who delivered babies with gastroschisis. Nevertheless, her age is not the only thing that distinguished her; she was always cheerful, always asking questions, always hopeful.

Her baby had a low birth weight. She weighed 2000grams (4 lbs. 4 oz.) whereas normal birth weight is between 3500g (5.5 lbs.) and 4500g (10 lbs.). She also presented with low body temperature. These findings cause doctors to worry because they indicate the baby is terribly ill and most likely will not survive.

Because the infant had exposed bowel, a plastic bag known as a silo was attached to the abdominal wall around the defect to temporarily contain the bowel. The bowel is then reduced (put back) slowly back into the abdomen over five-seven days. From the beginning, this patient developed every possible complication including infection, low blood sugar, inability for the medical team to gain intravenous access (a piece of plastic in a vein to allow the administration of medications and fluids for hydration), pneumonia, and many more complications. On three separate occasions, she was resuscitated after her heart stopped.

In addition to all these complications, the baby needed her silo replaced three times and had two failed attempts to close her abdomen. Time was running out for this baby. She was more than two weeks old, had not been feeding well, and had a severe systemic infection (infection in her bloodstream). Dr. Munanzvi was on call on a busy Saturday when she received the call that the baby's silo came off again. She was in the theater (operating room) at the time and was not able to help the baby until 10 p.m. Dr. Munanzvi attempted to close the abdomen once more, but things quickly went wrong.

The baby vomited and stopped breathing. Soon after, her heart stopped. Dr. Munanzvi resuscitated the baby (brought her back to life) by herself for 10 minutes before her pulse returned. Resuscitation should always be done with a team, but, with critical staff shortages in her country, it is not uncommon for a doctor or nurse to resuscitate a baby alone.

After this, Dr. Munanzvi proceeded to carefully and gently close the baby's abdomen using a permanent suture (a suture that does not dissolve) to attempt to contain the bowel. Her skin was extremely thin and friable after the many previously attempted procedures.

It was close to midnight when Dr. Munanzvi finished and left the baby breathing but barely holding on. The baby's mother was waiting for Dr. Munanzvi. Dr. Munanzvi's heart was in her shoes and she could not speak. She mumbled a few words and shook her head, Dr. Munanzvi feared if she said more, an unending torrent of tears would overwhelm her. Dr. Munanzvi choked back the tears and made a hasty exit.

For the next week, Dr. Munanzvi avoided the neonatal unit. When the team rounded there, she found work to do elsewhere. Her heart could not take it. When she finally made it there, she was astounded to find the little patient there, alive, hanging on! Several weeks and many more battles later, the baby and mother were sent home! When Dr. Munanzvi saw her last, she was 10 months old, growing, thriving, and achieving all her developmental milestones. The many scars across her abdomen are the only remnant of her victorious battle against the odds. It is patients such as these that make the work she does worthwhile.

Pediatric surgery was never Dr. Munanzvi's objective. She stumbled upon it quite serendipitously on her quest to becoming a surgeon. The person she chose to be her mentor, Dr. Bothwell Mbuwayesango, was a pediatric surgeon. She knew he was a natural teacher; approachable and always available. He welcomed her onto his team with open arms. Over the years she realized she made one of the best decisions of her life. Dr. Munanzvi was painstakingly groomed from a raw intern with no surgical skills, into a surgeon with a deliberate thought process and well-trained hands.

Whenever she was unsure, Dr. Mbuwayesango listened to her viewpoint and asked questions that pointed her in the correct direction without overshadowing her. Each time she reported a misstep, he delivered carefully weighted words enabling her to correct her mistake without belittling her. What Dr. Munanzvi learned from her mentor is that surgery is not only about operating but also about cultivating strong teams, respecting patients and their families, and making well-informed decisions. She thrived in the department. Along the way, Dr. Munanzvi had many other surgeons mentor her. Each laying a brick in the creation of the surgeon she became.

Mr. Zimunhu strove to teach her excellence. As a deliberate and meticulous surgeon, he pushed her out of her comfort zone and challenged her to be more than mediocre.

Mr. Chitsika insisted she think outside the box and not restrict her thinking. He taught her the art of critical thinking.

Mr. Matron Shaka always questioned her approach which made her continually renew her attitude and conduct as a leader. The environment Dr. Munanzvi was immersed in was ideal to nurture an aspiring surgeon.

Despite all this, it was years before Dr. Munanzvi enrolled in a formal surgical training program. She meandered for a long while, enjoying being a middle-level doctor and raising her children. Starting the process of an academic program was a challenge she eventually felt compelled to tackle. Soon, her mother's subtle hints at her pursuing her dream of becoming a pediatric surgeon became louder and could no longer be ignored. Her mother always said she would support her and help her with childcare so Dr. Munanzvi could realize her dream because her mother saw how passionate she was about it.

Then, Dr. Munanzvi realized, although she was not the sharpest tool in the shed, she made life immensely difficult for herself by not tackling the work using a learning method appropriate for her. She found it was easier to learn through teaching. Teaching medical students became her new passion. Dr. Munanzvi found their unique questions opened new avenues of thought for her while she challenged her students. The more she taught, the easier it was for her to retain the material she was learning herself.

As Dr. Munanzvi tackled studying and work, she thought she had all her ducks in a row until, quite suddenly, her world came crashing around her when her son was struck by illness. She said, "I was confused and helpless. Everyone at home expected me to be in control and have all the answers. The team at work closed ranks around me. I fell apart and no one judged me. I was given time off work, offers of help, and encouragement. When I returned to work, I was eased back into it gently."

She tenderly confirmed, "My path to becoming a surgeon was never the straight trajectory of a rising star, but all these experiences molded me into a better surgeon. In Africa, there is a saying, 'umuntu ngumuntu ngabantu' which literally translated means that a person is a person because of people. It rings true of my journey to become a surgeon."

"I learned that courage was not the absence of fear, but the triumph over it. The brave man is not he who does not feel afraid, but he who conquers that fear." – Nelson Mandela

Dr. Zaria Murrell

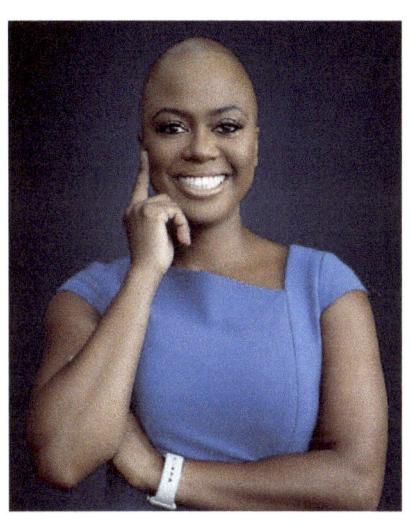

Dr. Zaria Murrell is a pediatric surgeon in Huntsville, Alabama. She completed her bachelor's degree at Howard University, Washington, D.C., and earned her medical degree from the University of Maryland Medical School, College Park, Maryland. She finished her general surgery residency at the State University of New York (SUNY) Health Science Center in Brooklyn, New York, before completing a fellowship in minimally invasive and bariatric surgery (surgery using tiny incisions and endoscope with tiny long instruments) at New York Medical College, Valhalla, New York.

She practiced for seven years as a minimally invasive and bariatric surgeon before completing a fellowship in fetal surgery and hemangioma and pediatric vascular malformations at the Cincinnati Children's Hospital Medical Center, Cincinnati, Ohio. Hemangiomas are noncancerous growths of the smallest blood vessels, called capillaries, and vascular malformations are abnormally formed blood vessels. Lastly, she completed a pediatric surgery fellowship at the University of Louisville, Kentucky.

Dr. Murrell is a native New Yorker, but her parents are from the Caribbean. Her mother is from a small island called Montserrat and her father is from the French side of St. Martin. She was born and raised in New York City with a strong Afro-Caribbean influence and spent summers in the Caribbean. Dr. Murrell does not know when she fell in love with medicine, she just remembers watching the 1976 Olympics and seeing Nadia Comaneci.

She was fascinated with athletics, so she initially went into medical school thinking she would pursue sports medicine. Dr. Murrell had a rude awakening, however, when she saw a broken bone being set and was sick to her stomach. For some reason seeing intestines and stool did not faze her one bit. Shortly after, she finished a pediatric surgery rotation and fell in love. Dr. Murrell has always loved fixing things, so a career in surgery is rewarding because she knows she has helped correct something that is wrong and is causing pain to patients. She is always excited about being used as an instrument to bring healing to a variety of patients with surgical issues.

Dr. Murrell has always loved the discipline of pediatric surgery and had every intention of pursuing it. She completed two years of research during her residency. She was also interested in the new technologies in surgery like laparoscopic and robotic surgery (surgery using tiny incisions and using the robot to help you with the surgery). Initially, Dr. Murrell chose a fellowship in minimally invasive (laparoscopic) surgery and after completing this fellowship, she worked as a laparoscopic and bariatric surgeon for seven years before deciding to pursue her true love. When she finished her fellowship in minimally invasive surgery, she was a new wife with an infant and shortly after, became a mother of two.

After putting a great deal of thought into seeking another specialty training and talking with multiple mentors who encouraged her to follow her passion, Dr. Murrell applied for a pediatric surgery fellowship. Unfortunately, she was not accepted into any program for pediatric surgery training, but God provided an opportunity for another fellowship with children. So, she took the position she was offered and became a fetal surgery fellow and then a pediatric vascular anomalies fellow at the Cincinnati Children's Hospital Medical Center (CCHMC).

These fellowships were not accredited by the board of pediatric surgery. This meant Dr. Murrell needed to find and complete an accredited pediatric surgery fellowship program. Once again, God provided! Two weeks after completing her vascular anomalies fellowship, while working on fetal research projects at CCHMC, she received an email about a sudden opening for an accredited pediatric surgery fellowship position in Louisville, Kentucky. She was accepted for the position and completed her two-year pediatric surgery fellowship at the University of Louisville, Kentucky.

A typical day in fellowship started by arriving at work at 5:45 a.m. to round on babies in the neonatal intensive care unit (NICU), then completing surgery rounds with residents from 6:30–7:30 a.m. and NICU teaching rounds from 7:30–8:00 a.m. Depending on which cases the residents and Dr. Murrell were assigned, she was in the operating room from 8:00 a.m.-4:00 p.m. In between operative cases, she saw new consults (patients needing their care) in the emergency room or NICU, discharged patients, and completed the necessary patient care. They were busy days, but fellowship went by fast!

Dr. Murrell shared, "This process is long; sometimes taking longer than five-seven years and, at times, nine, 10, 11, or even 12 years. If you not only focus on the endpoint, but also learn to enjoy the journey, you will thrive. Expect a significant amount of growth, the process is necessary. I cannot emphasize the importance of honesty, even in the little things. Do not say you examined the patient or any aspect of the body when you did not look. This is someone's life in your hands and giving inaccurate data can cause harm to a patient and make you untrustworthy to your superiors. Honesty is key. Thoroughness and dedication are also immensely important."

Dr. Murrell added, "For the undergraduate student, good study habits are a must. Being disciplined in college is beneficial for the remainder of your training. Study habits formed in college will impact your medical education. If possible, take a review course for the Medical College Admission Test (MCAT) and do as many practice questions as you possibly can. For the medical student, pray and ask God for guidance; realizing you must love surgery to choose such a demanding lifestyle. Communicate well with your team and read about every surgical case before going to the operating room. Do not be afraid to ask thoughtful questions. Ask yourself on your surgical rotation, 'Do I really love this, and can I live like this?'"

Dr. Murrell fell in love with academic surgery when she was in private practice. She feels everyone should have a goal of reassessing their life plans and life journey every five-ten years because to grow as individuals, changes must happen. As she reassessed her life goals in her late thirties, she realized that as much as she enjoyed and was content with adult general surgery, she had a longing for pediatric surgery. What crazy woman goes back and considers doing a pediatric surgery fellowship at age 40? She did.

After much prayer and fasting and conversations with her husband and the pediatric surgeon in town she worked with and admired, Dr. Murrell realized how much she missed being around residents and medical students and teaching. There were many things she learned in private practice that she has been able to teach residents she otherwise would not have known.

As much as she loved academic surgery, she returned to private practice for family reasons. Her mother was diagnosed with cancer and died within two months and her father was getting older with many medical issues associated with age. She is his primary caregiver. For Dr. Murrell, her family is most important. She also has young children and wanted to spend more time with them. Dr. Murrell chose to leave academic medicine to focus on her family's needs, knowing that academic medicine gladly received her before. She expects it will be there when the times comes that she is able to return.

Dr. Murrell confirms her journey has been challenging. She would not have been able to do anything without the support of her husband. He was always encouraging and willing to fill the gaps when she was away for long periods of time. Her mother was also always there. She herself was a mother of five and was Dr. Murrell's children's main care provider for their first few months of life; her son for nine months and her daughter for six months. Dr. Murrell was committed to spending a certain amount of time with her children, so she cared for them in the mornings and her husband cared for them in the evenings. It worked well. She loves spending time with family, running, international travel, medical missionary trips, and she plays the piano.

In addition to work in the USA, Dr. Murrell also participates in mission work. She has been traveling to Kenya since 2009. A nurse anesthetist she worked with when she was an adult surgeon has an organization called kenyarelief.org which is in a rural part of Kenya near the Tanzania border. He always asked her to go, but it was never the right time. Dr. Murrell's children were young, and she worried about traveling so far, leaving them behind.

One day, while working on a case together, he peeked over the drape and said, "We have all these young girls at the orphanage that have never seen a female surgeon who looks like them before." Dr. Murrell was sold, if for nothing else than for the sake of being a role model and mentor to these young girls. When she went the first time, she fell in love with Kenya. It reminded her of her Caribbean roots. She felt at home. Dr. Murrell has young ladies she sponsors and mentors, and considers it is such a wonderful experience to work with them.

The journey has never been smooth. Dr. Murrell strongly dislikes stereotypes. She contends it should not matter what she looks like on the outside. She has extensive training. She still dislikes it when some people first see her and ask, "Who's that black girl? Are you a nurse? (Not that there is anything wrong with being a nurse.) Are you cleaning up?" Some people look at her as though she is suspicious, as though to say, "Do you really know what you are doing?" And she has been asked, "How long have you been doing this? I googled you. I asked around." And she respects this because unfortunately, we live in a society where people are judged by their appearance, which is so unfair.

While she was in New York, Dr. Murrell was chief resident and clearly remembers when rounding and talking to a patient that the patient asked the intern, who happened to be a young white male, "What is going to happen next?" The young man looked at her, and said, "You're going to have to ask my chief. She is the one who really knows what's going on with you." This stumped the patient. Dr. Murrell does not remember the patient's race. It was just the fact that he addressed the white male in the group even though it was obvious in group rounds at the patients' bedsides that they reported to her. The patient was looking for authority from this young man. It is not that he did not have authority, but he realized where he was in the hierarchy. Dr. Murrell had six years more experience than he had.

Dr. Murrell's faith is part of every single aspect of her life as a surgeon. Being a surgeon is her vocation, it is not just a job. She loves what she does. It is what she is called to do. Dr. Murrell has seen God work time and time again in everything throughout her journey and in practice. For instance, she sees Him in how He orchestrated her being in Cincinnati for the fellowship she was accepted to.

Once, she was operating on a child in Kenya and was looking for a mesh to fix a hernia. Instead, she found a fistula anal plug (a plug used to treat an abnormal opening in the anal area of a child). She was disappointed she could not find what she wanted, but 24 hours later, a patient with a fistula-in-ano walked in and she had exactly what she needed to care for this child's problem. In all the times she was on mission trips to Kenya, she never saw a fistula-in-ano. She would not have known a plug was available if she had not been looking for something else for someone else. Every step of the way she sees God's hand in her life.

"I learned a variety of lessons, and one of the most important is this: You can't hit a target you can't see. You can't accomplish wonderful things with your life if you have no idea of what they are." – Brian Tracy

Dr. Vanda Amado

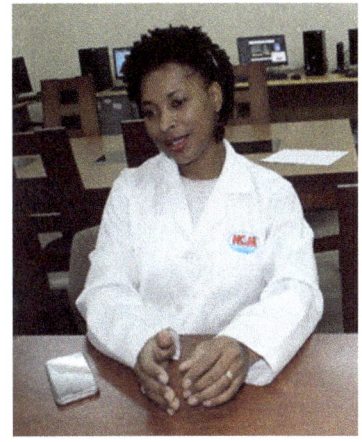

Dr. Vanda Amado is a pediatric surgeon at Maputo Central Hospital, Mozambique. She is also a professor of surgery at Eduardo Mondlane University in Maputo, Mozambique.

Born in 1978 in Mozambique, a few years after independence, Dr. Amado did not realize how poor her family was until she started school. In primary school, she wore slippers (flip-flops) to school and did not have a bag or any books. She remembers sitting on the floor and using boxes to write on. Life was better after her father found a nicer job, but they were far from wealthy. They were grateful to have a roof over their heads and were never hungry.

Dr. Amado's house was in front of a hospital. They sometimes housed family needing medical care at the hospital. She also had a paralyzed uncle who required many surgeries. As a young girl, she promised her uncle she would be a surgeon so she could help him. Dr. Amado's maternal aunt was a nurse and tried to influence her niece's interest in nursing, but Dr. Amado knew she wanted to be a doctor. As she progressed in her training, Dr. Amado saw the need for pediatric surgeons. There were no trauma experts and there was no pediatric surgery training in her country. Dr. Amado knew it would be challenging to find training outside her country, but this did not stop her.

There was only one medical school where she lived and there were 6,000 applicants for 100 spots. Dr. Amado was fortunate to be accepted into medical school. She found it difficult to adjust to the fact that she did not always have the top marks or was the best, but she learned to be content with herself. Dr. Amado worked extremely hard and always did her absolute best.

After graduating from medical school, Dr. Amado was assigned to the Namaacha District, which is close to the Swaziland border. It is a rural farming town where most homes do not have electricity. Here is where she learned to be a doctor! Dr. Amado was the only doctor, which meant she was on call every day. It was one of the most difficult experiences in her training, but it shaped her into the surgeon she is now. She learned many life lessons there and remembers receiving a call one Friday night from one of the sisters (nurses) telling her a pregnant woman came for care.

The sister told Dr. Amado the woman appeared to be around 37 weeks' gestation (pregnant) but did not seem ready to deliver. The patient was brought in by her husband so they could be transferred to the nearest town for care. Dr. Amado asked the necessary questions, but based on what the sister told her, it did not seem necessary to transfer the patient.

That night, Dr. Amado received a call saying the woman was in labor. She raced to the hospital in the middle of the night and discovered the baby was breech, meaning the baby was positioned to deliver bottom first instead of the proper head-first position. Dr. Amado was extremely nervous because she realized this would be an extremely difficult delivery. She was in a small hospital without the resources necessary to do a cesarean section (surgery to take the baby out through the abdomen).

To top things off, Dr. Amado discovered the patient's pacing husband was the mayor in the district, the most influential and powerful person in the community. They were 50 kilometers from the town, and it was too late to arrange transportation. During her examination, Dr. Amado realized the baby was a bit larger than she initially thought. She drew strength from deep within herself and delivered that 3.9kg (8.6 lbs.) baby. The mother and child did well. Dr. Amado learned an unbelievably valuable lesson. It is important to see and evaluate a patient when you receive a phone call like this. When Dr. Amado is on call and the sisters call about changes in a patient's condition, she makes it a practice to take the time to see and evaluate the patient rather than manage the problem over the phone.

After completing two years of rural service, Dr. Amado finished her general surgery training in Maputo. This was difficult because when she started residency training, she was five months pregnant. One male faculty member said, "Women should not do surgery. You should stay at home and take care of your husband and kids." One day, while walking into the hospital at the same time as this male faculty member, he pointed to her car and said, "Why are you killing yourself training to be a surgeon when other professions can give you a nice car like that?" She ignored him. Then he asked her how her night was because he knew she did emergency surgery in the middle of the night. He rudely said, "Now you know how it is to be a prostitute because you often have to do your best work at night." This man truly gave Dr. Amado a difficult time, but she persevered!

After finishing residency, Dr. Amado began thinking about how to find training in pediatric surgery. There were no training programs in Mozambique. She searched for places that would accept her and found a place in Barcelona, Spain. Her husband cared for their small children while she was abroad. She has been married for 14 years and they have a 13-year-old son and an 11-year-old daughter.

Dr. Amado traveled to Kenya for her pediatric surgery board exams in conjunction with COSECSA. She passed the first time she took the exams and became the first board-certified pediatric surgeon in Mozambique. Currently, there are four pediatric surgeons there. They are making strides.

When Dr. Amado returned home. She had difficultly establishing a pediatric surgery practice because she did not have support from her superiors and colleagues. It was challenging for her and she performed adult general surgery and accepted pediatric surgery on call opportunities for a while. It was exhausting. Eventually, things improved as she developed more confidence in practicing independently. Dr. Amado had to be strategic in developing herself and garnering support to build a pediatric surgical practice. Eventually, she was able to do strictly what she loves, pediatric surgery. Currently on a sabbatical in Solna, Sweden, Dr. Amado is working on her Ph.D. in global health studies at the Karolinska Institute.

Dr. Amado shares, "Be strong. Focus on what you want and permit yourself to shine. It will not be easy, but it will be worth it. Work hard and study hard and speak up for yourself in a strategic way. Find a support system. It is important for your success."

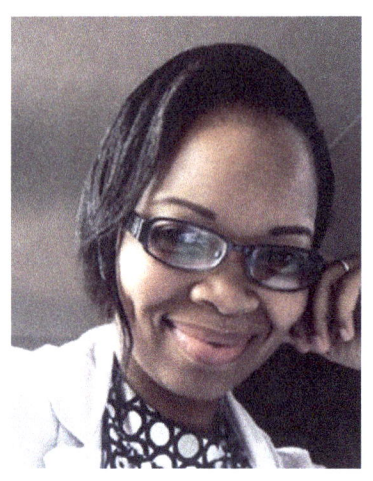

Dr. Patricia Shinondo

Dr. Patricia Shinondo is a pediatric surgeon in Zambia, Africa. She completed her undergraduate training in 2009 at the Kuban State Medical University, Krasnodar, Russia, and her pediatric surgery training at the University of Zambia, in conjunction with the College of Surgeons of East, Central, and Southern Africa (COSECSA). She became the first female Zambian-born pediatric surgeon in Zambia. She is part of the global pediatric surgery community seeking to improve access to children's surgical care and provide safe surgery for children in low- and middle-income countries.

Dr. Shinondo was born in Zambia and went to primary and secondary (high school) school there. As far back as she can remember, she always wanted to be a doctor. Looking back, she thinks her dad drilled it into her to be a doctor or one of the other major three professions preferred by African parents – banking, engineering, or law.

When she completed her high school A-levels, the government was offering scholarships abroad. The countries offered were Cuba, India, Russia, and China. Dr. Shinondo passed the exam required for scholarship eligibility and wanted to go to Cuba. However, when she arrived at the office to choose a country, Cuba was no longer an option. The only country with open positions was Russia. She spent her first year learning Russian and the remaining years in medical school in Russia. It took a total of seven years to complete her studies.

When Dr. Shinondo was home during her surgical rotations in her internship, one of the surgeons commented that she had good hands. He often told her she was skilled and good in the theater (operating room). This started her thinking about a career in surgery even though she did not necessarily enjoy the theater. She worked with obstetrics and gynecology (baby deliveries and women's reproductive health) but did not enjoy this, so she chose general surgery.

Dr. Shinondo knew, however, that she wanted to work with children and near the end of her second year of training, the pediatric surgery program was created. Four others and she joined the four-year program. Later, she entered the College of Surgeons of East, Central, and Southern Africa for a more established pediatric surgery fellowship. This was instruction parallel to the training Dr. Shinondo was receiving in her home institution at the same time. Two of the four trainees completed the training, a total of five years of pediatric surgery training. After her fellowship training, she passed her written and oral pediatric surgery board exams.

The language barrier in Russia was one of Dr. Shinondo's greatest challenges, as was adapting to the huge cultural differences. Racism added another layer of difficulty and several students quit and returned home. There were many students from African countries, so there was a community of people who looked like her and were experiencing similar challenges. She kept her head down and worked hard.

Dr. Shinondo honestly said, "It felt like a boy's club because I was the only girl in the class. I constantly had to prove myself. I do not think men have the same challenges as one does as a wife and a mother. It is not uncommon to hear odd remarks referring to how you should be at home and in the kitchen rather than in the operating room. At times, I felt older patients did not view me as a physician or surgeon because I am a female. I felt discriminated against."

She feels young women need to realize that this is a lifestyle and there will be challenges one will have as a female surgeon that male surgeons do not have. Everyone must optimize and prioritize time well. Women must prove themselves and not just be token members, because it is crucial to occupy space in the surgical world, have a seat at the table, and have a voice. Women must work hard and not want to be given positions just because they are female.

Confidence is crucial in medicine. Dr. Shinondo feels getting up when you fall is the greatest confidence booster. At times, you question your abilities and doubt yourself, but you must get through these moments because the falling and getting up is what makes you stronger. She did not get it right every time and remembers failing her first Masters of Medicine (MMed) exam; a required exam after completing residency and fellowship training. This was especially difficult because she was the only girl in her group and deeply felt the pressure of failing. She gave herself a short time to feel sorry for herself and then picked herself up and figured out what she needed to do to pass. After studying and working hard, she passed the exam. She cannot emphasize this enough; you must get back up and fight even harder! The exams only get harder, but it is so rewarding!

Since she was the first female pediatric surgeon in Zambia, Dr. Shinondo occasionally experienced impostor syndrome. It seemed when someone came looking for the voice of a pediatric surgeon, they almost always looked for a male pediatric surgeon to talk with to get an expert opinion, even if it was in regard to the hospital where she worked and her male colleague was at a different hospital. Dr. Shinondo still gave her opinion respectfully and made certain her opinion was recognized because, with time, current mind frames will change. She makes certain to be active and involved in meetings. She presents papers and is involved in her surgical society. Visibility is important.

Women must be seen to be heard.

The best advice Dr. Shinondo received along the way is, "Time is the best tool." For a long time, she could not find a way to use her time wisely. This was a problem until someone sat her down and helped her figure out how to use her time more efficiently throughout the day. They told her to leave work at work and be home when at home. They helped her figure out how to juggle time with family and career because there are more responsibilities as one advances in their career. Having a supportive spouse is critical if you are married and having a supportive family is also important. During her down-time, Dr. Shinondo is reading, Autism as Context Blindness by Peter Vermeulen.

Three people she would love to have dinner with and learn from are Oprah Winfrey, Barack Obama, and herself at the end of life to see how she did!

While so far Dr. Shinondo is the only pediatric surgeon in Zambia, there are three ladies are in training, and she is hoping there will be more. She is always encouraging young people to think about pediatric surgery.

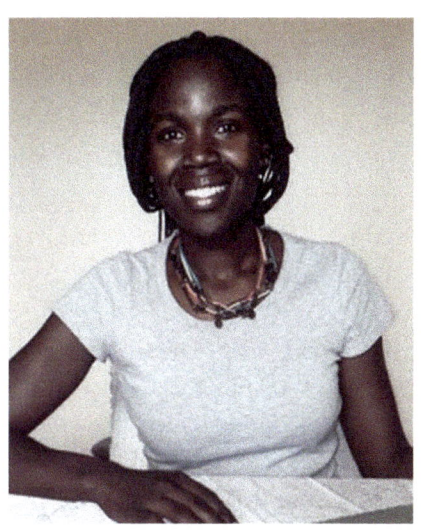

Dr. Phyllis Kisa

Dr. Phyllis Kisa completed her medical school training at Makerere University College of Health Sciences, Malungo National Referral and Teaching Hospital in Kampala, Uganda. She also remained there for her medical internship and general surgery training. She was accepted to the British Columbia Children's Hospital in Vancouver, Canada, for her pediatric surgery and pediatric urology fellowship. She is currently a pediatric and urological surgeon in the department of surgery and is a lecturer at Makerere University College of Health Sciences in Kampala, Uganda. She is the second pediatric surgeon in Uganda.

Dr. Kisa was born in Tororo, a town in Eastern Uganda. She grew up in many places in Uganda because of her father's job, but she predominantly lived in Kampala.

She did not always want to be a doctor. The education system in Uganda dictates the choices children have in future education. Dr. Kisa excelled in her O-level exams (in the British educational system, these are exams at the completion of four years of high school) and between her mother and teachers, they decided she would study physics, chemistry, biology, and subsidiary math.

Dr. Kisa wanted to study history and literature and be a tour guide, but she obviously did not win this argument and complied with her mother's choices, except she took art instead of math. These subjects dictated what she was able to apply for at the university. She excelled in her classes and was accepted to medical school at the Makerere University in Kampala, which was her first choice. Dr. Kisa breezed through medical school but only felt like she was in the right profession when she began her internship at a district hospital. Being responsible for patients, albeit under supervision, making the day to day decisions about their care, and seeing an impact, positive or negative, affirmed she was in the right place.

Dr. Kisa feels surgery chose her. As a medical student, an intern, and a general doctor, all she wanted to be was a pediatrician. It was her dream and she held on to it for the longest time. As a doctor working at Lacor Hospital in northern Uganda, Dr. Kisa worked in a surgical unit where she enjoyed the work, but still wanted to become a pediatrician. After working for Dr. Martin Ogwang for a short time, he mentioned she had surgeon's hands. He said it would be a disappointing waste if she did not pursue surgery in some way. He also said that many would like to have the gift she had but would never have it. Dr. Kisa protested.

He continued talking to her about surgery. He also had other surgeons visiting her hospital drum this idea into her, specifically recruiting Dr. John Craven of York, UK, and Professor Armin Pycha of Bolzano, Italy.

Eventually, he told Dr. Kisa he knew what she wanted, to treat children. He told her a career as a pediatric surgeon would allow her to be a surgeon but also to manage children. He emphasized that he would continue to support her in her training and, as promised, did continue to do so. This was her turning point. It took him two years to convince Dr. Kisa to pursue surgery and she applied for her general surgery training with the goal of becoming a pediatric surgeon.

Dr. Kisa ignored many of the challenges in becoming a pediatric surgeon because she expected a difficult path full of sacrifices. She believed that if she always did her best, her work would speak for itself and this has been her experience. Dr. Kisa's greatest annoyance (not challenge) were female trainees who did not pull their weight and always got away with a smile here and there but no actual output.

The best advice she received was, "Wherever you go, there will always be problems and people you cannot get along with. Always do your best and you will always get the best out of any situation and never regret a single moment of a given experience."

Dr. Kisa feels there is no one single greatest accomplishment in her life. But professionally, becoming the first fellowship-trained female pediatric surgeon in Uganda and the first, and currently the only, fellowship-trained pediatric urologist in Uganda, is on top of her list of greatest accomplishments. Her proudest personal moment has been becoming a mother to her two-year-old son.

A typical workday for Dr. Kisa usually begins with early rounds at 6:30 a.m. and grand rounds, where an invited speaker gives a lecture on a medical topic or a staff surgeon or registrar (resident) gives a lecture on a specific topic. They discuss difficult or puzzling surgical cases from 7 a.m. to 8 a.m. She then attends a weekly clinic from morning until lunchtime or early afternoon if it is a day she sees clinic patients. Her team sees and evaluates patients in the clinic who have appointments but at times they also see and evaluate patients who walk in without an appointment. On surgery days, Dr. Kisa is in the operating room from 8 a.m. to 4 p.m. The after-hours call responsibilities vary because the team divides the time between the partners. If time and money were not a factor, Dr. Kisa would still be a surgeon, but periodically she would work with a mobile clinic and a mobile operating room serving children in difficult-to-reach areas.

Finding balance is a challenge for Dr. Kisa like every other surgeon-to-be. When she first qualified as a pediatric and urological surgeon, there was no balance. It was work, work, and more work and poor eating habits to the point of malnutrition. But since having her son in 2017, she has learned to prioritize to create time for things. She finds that if one is deliberate about everything, then it is easy to find balance. She has a wonderful and supportive husband who helps her have a sense of balance. Dr. Kisa takes time to read novels and books like *Motorcycle Diaries* by Che Guevara. She loves traveling, meeting new people, listening to the music of the '70s, '80s and '90s, as well as classical music, watching musicals on stage, and playing Minesweeper/Hexaper.

Dr. Kisa added, "Many people believe that surgery is not for women and it is up to you to make them believe that you belong in surgery. There are personal sacrifices you will have to make to achieve your dream. Without wholehearted support of friends, siblings, parents, and partners, the training becomes a nightmare because it is rigorous. It is extremely important to always find a good social network of like-minded individuals. Nurture these relationships because these will get you through anything. Follow your heart, but also listen to people around you. Sometimes they know you better than you know yourself. Humility is a huge key to learning. Be eager to learn. If you are, people will want to teach you. Do take time to enjoy your hobbies."

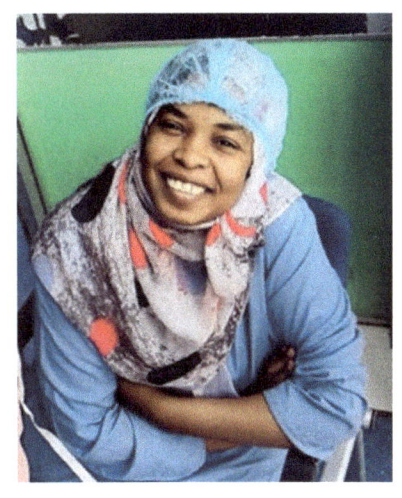

Dr. Wala Mohamed Ibrahim Rahma

Dr. Wala Mohamed Ibrahim Rahma is a specialist in pediatric surgery at Khartoum Teaching Hospital in Sudan.

She does not know why she chose medicine as a career but has been told that from as young as three years of age, she always said to her family and friends she was going to be a great doctor someday. She chose to be a surgeon because she wanted to relieve people's pain and have the immediate results that can be achieved with surgery. Dr. Mohamed Ibrahim Rahma's focus is surgery in children and her goal is to relieve their suffering. Pediatric surgeons are advocates for their patients who oftentimes do not know how to express themselves or speak.

On a personal note, Dr. Mohamed Ibrahim Rahma shared her personal challenges.

"Women do not belong in the operating room." "Women cannot work under stress." "A woman freezes when unexpected complications happen." These were the disappointing words she heard from a male registrar (resident) when, during her medical internship, she informed him she was ready to begin her surgical career. The greatest challenges she faced were destroying these false theories and concentrating on the fact that females are as talented as male surgeons.

Dr. Mohamed Ibrahim Rahma says her proudest moment is when one of her patients returns home healthy and happy. She is extremely pleased when her little angels (the children) play and grasp everything around them after being inactive for days because they were sick. She always thinks about these moments and talks about her patients when she meets with colleagues for coffee at the banks of the Great Nile River.

Five years ago, Dr. Mohamed Ibrahim Rahma attended a life coaching program. During this time, she began thinking about how she could contribute to her profession. She realized that to be great, you must help others to be great. She set a goal to help other pediatric surgeons. Now she is a pediatric surgery specialist who trains surgeons from other countries using evidence-based medicine (using evidence from well-designed and well-conducted research to optimize decision-making for patient care) and teaching surgical skills.

The best advice she received was when one of her teachers said, "Read the operation before you do it. I have been a practicing surgeon for 40 years and oftentimes I find something new in my reading. Learn from different sources and then develop your own style after graduation, based on all you have learned and from all your experiences operating with senior surgeons." This helped Dr. Mohamed Ibrahim Rahma choose the best techniques during her surgical training.

If Dr. Mohamed Ibrahim Rahma was not a surgeon, she would train teenagers on how to become public speakers because she loves to work with young people.

To find balance, Dr. Mohamed Ibrahim Rahma explains, if you love what you do and find a noble reason for doing it, you will find enough time to do other things. She works in different fields and enjoys every moment of her life, when operating in the OR (operating room), when holding the microphone on stage and speaking to a group of people, and when taking the pointer to give a lecture to her residents, students, and colleagues. She is happy. And she also finds balance by making time to do things she enjoys.

Some lessons Dr. Mohamed Ibrahim Rahma likes to leave with others. "Sometimes you need to be creative in how you manage negative talk from other people meant to discourage you from pursuing your dreams. I always tell young girls that you have to imagine that every bad or negative word that you hear is a balloon and you have a magic pin to prick the balloon and deflate it. You can then use the air from the balloon to fill up a bigger balloon that is taking you to your destiny. Work hard to improve yourself. Remember that the best investment is what you do to fulfill your goals and succeed. You must always set concrete or definite goals to work toward every day. Sometimes, you may have to divide the goals into smaller goals. It is important to have good and focused friends so you help each other achieve your goals. It is important to have friends that keep you accountable to working hard to achieve your goals. Whenever possible, take time to help others because we are all on the earth to serve each other.

"There is no royal road to anything. One thing at a time, all things in succession. That which grows fast, withers as rapidly. That which grows slowly, endures."
— Josiah Gilbert Holland

CHAPTER FIVE
Urological Surgery

Urology is the branch of medicine that focuses on surgical and medical diseases of the male and female urinary tract and the male reproductive organs. Organs under the domain of urology include the kidneys, adrenal glands, ureters, urinary bladder, urethra, and the male reproductive organs (testes, epididymis, vas deferens, seminal vesicles, prostrate, and penis).

Dr. Mumba Chalwe

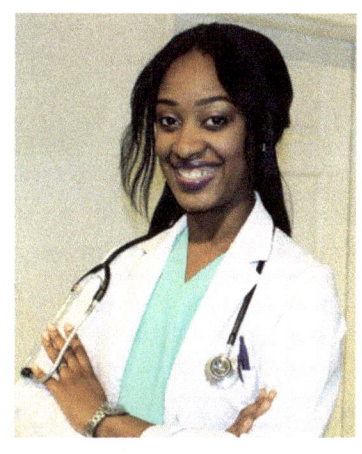

Dr. Mumba Chalwe is a consultant urological surgeon, a surgical sub-specialty that focuses on men's health as well as the urinary systems of both men and women. She practices in Zambia, Africa. She earned her medical degree at Ryazan Medical University in Ryazan, Russia. She completed a residency in urological surgery at the University of Zambia at the University Teaching Hospital in conjunction with the College of Surgeons of East, Central, and Southern Africa (COSESCA), Arusha, Tanzania. She was awarded the 2018 gold medalist status by the COSESCA for academic excellence.

This is Dr. Chalwe's story in her words.

Our African heritage is unequivocally a part of us, and I strongly believe we can thrive while embracing 'ubuntu' (Zulu) without it impeding our ability to soar high. 'Ubuntu' is best described as an African philosophy that emphasizes *being self through others*. It is a form of humanism that can be expressed in the phrase, "I am because of who we all are."

I dream of an Africa where girls are not rated based on

their levels of domestication but rather given a fair chance to achieve goals using our God-given abilities. This is an Africa where we no longer feel the need for validation through marital status, where we normalize feminine excellence to a point our gender is no longer an issue. There is strength in our curves, intelligence in our curls, and innovation in our delicate frames! My name is Mumba Chalwe and I was the first female urologist in Zambia.

I was always a nerd growing up and loved school. My mother watched the television show *ER* and I was drawn to it. She worked in the hospital as an administrator and cared for us when we were sick, tending to our minor, and not so minor, scrapes and bruises. I remember one pivotal moment in my life when I was at the hospital with my mom and saw a beautiful young Tswana female doctor in a sea of white doctors rounding. I was wowed. This moment had a huge impact on my future career choice. Seeing her made me realize it was possible to be a doctor. The choice to become a urologist was based on many factors. I love the challenges of surgery and wanted to defy stereotypes. At the time I trained to be a urologist, there were no female urologists in Zambia. This has changed. Currently, there are two female urologists in Zambia and six in training.

I completed my early schooling in Botswana and, after finishing secondary school, I attended medical school in Russia. Returning to the motherland, Zambia, I completed my two-year internship. These two years were divided into six-month sessions in internal medicine, general surgery, obstetrics and gynecology, and pediatrics. Afterward, I proceeded to complete my two years of community service in rural Zambia. Toward the end of my community service, I applied for specialty training in urology, a four-year residency. One of my fondest memories was when I started my urology residency and an elderly patient gave me a live goat as a thank you for my services!

Residency was more difficult for me because I had both my children by the time I completed my residency training. I met my husband, an orthopedic surgeon, in medical school. We had our first son one year before I started my urology residency and the second child one year before I finished my urology residency.

Being pregnant during my training was difficult. Sadly, I had a miscarriage late in the first trimester of my second pregnancy. My husband and I were devastated. For surgeons, the feeling of not being in control and being helpless is heart-wrenching. Despite this, we picked ourselves up and, somehow, we were able to try again. We were blessed with our second child.

Looking back at my residency, there were so many defining cases. I remember one in particular when I was on call on Christmas Eve. A patient presented with a gunshot wound to the abdomen. The general surgery resident started a laparotomy (opening the abdomen) but discovered that after repairing the injuries, the patient continued to bleed.

I visualized the retroperitoneal space (the space between the intestines and the back wall of the abdomen that contains the kidney, major blood vessels, and the pancreas) and found an expanding hematoma, an organized collection of blood. After discovering the hematoma, I called my immediate boss, who was not on call that night, but came into the hospital immediately to help. He was in a tux, no questions asked. I consider this true teamwork. It solidified my belief that I was in the right place. There were times I was riddled with self-doubt during my training, but I was surrounded by great mentors and support — men who believed in me and helped me succeed.

As a consultant, my week involves two operating days, two clinic days, one day a week for academia (teaching), and half a day for administration. I am on call every other week; these weeks tend to be hectic. I am often asked how I find balance as a wife, mother, and surgeon. There is no such thing as balance in my life. There is a great deal of teamwork. I am blessed with an amazing husband. We work together to make things work. We are both happy and satisfied with our home life and our careers. We live close to our hometown, so our extended family helps with childcare.

The advice I would give myself in primary school is, "If

you don't feel like you belong, or you feel like you are not pretty enough, continue believing in yourself and doing your best. You won't always be the ugly one." To my secondary school self, I would tell her that she is, "Good enough and does not need to prove anything to anyone." To my medical school self, I would say, "Relax, don't take everything so seriously." To myself during residency, I would say, "You don't need to kill yourself to prove that YOU can do it better, work longer, and are tough enough." Lastly, to myself during my first year as a consultant, I would say, "Just do your best. Always do the right thing and believe in yourself."

Finally, I think I have proven more to myself than anyone else that perseverance, dedication, a few tears, and above all, a good sense of humor will get you there. At the end of the day, humanity comes first. One must strive to never lose his or her humanity and never forget the basics. Treat everyone with dignity, respect, and kindness. Nothing should hinder your dreams and goals, not your age or gender or ethnicity. Nothing should stop you. Be your best and excel. Excellence will always reign supreme.

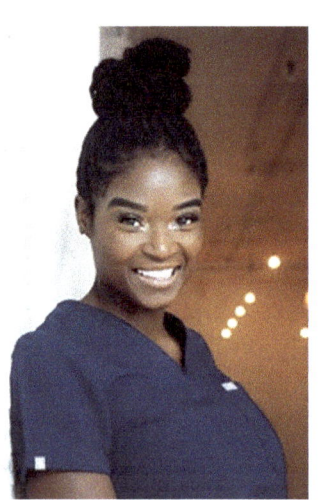

Dr. Fenwa Milhouse

Dr. Fenwa Milhouse is a fellowship-trained urologist specializing in female pelvic medicine and urogenital reconstruction. Also known as urogynecology, this focuses on the diagnosis and treatment of conditions affecting the muscles and tissues of the female pelvic organs.

She earned her bachelor's degree from the University of Texas at Austin and completed her medical training at the University of Texas at Houston. She was accepted for her urological surgery residency at the University of Chicago and afterwards, completed her fellowship in urogynecology at Metro Urology in the Twin Cities in Minnesota.

Dr. Milhouse has been one of those people who, being the good Nigerian that she is, grew up thinking she wanted to be a doctor. From the earliest time, when asked what she wanted to be when she grew up, she always said she wanted to be a doctor. Her mom was a nurse and this probably influenced her as well. In Nigerian culture, parents tend to push their children into certain industries, medicine is one of the main ones and Dr. Milhouse liked the idea of helping people. She has been a people-person all her life and helping people comes naturally. She never thought about doing anything else.

Dr. Milhouse did not know urology existed as a specialty until she was in medical school. She discovered urology on her first day and said to herself, "Oh, it is like the male gynecologist." At first, she was not interested in urology and considered other specialties as she rotated through the different areas of medicine and surgery while in medical school.

A crucial moment in Dr. Milhouse's choosing urology was during her second year in medical school. A urologist was scheduled to lecture and when the young black female urologist walked in, Dr. Milhouse was floored and asked herself, "This is the urologist?"

The urologist lectured and Dr. Milhouse was completely amazed by the idea of having someone who looked like her in a field she did not expect. Dr. Milhouse wanted to be like her and tells people it is because of this moment that representation matters. It matters because if you do not see yourself in that capacity, you do not know you can do something. She never knew about urology and this experience completely changed her career path. Now, she is a urologist. She loves what she does, and she would choose urology again if she had to choose again.

During her journey to becoming a surgeon, one challenge Dr. Milhouse experienced was internal self-doubt – internal impostor syndrome. This is a psychological pattern where one doubts one's accomplishments and has a persistent internalized fear of being exposed as a fraud. Despite external evidence of their competence, those experiencing this phenomenon remain convinced they are frauds and do not deserve all they have achieved.

Individuals with imposterism incorrectly attribute their success to luck or interpret it as a result of deceiving others into thinking they are more intelligent than they perceive themselves to be. While early research focused on the prevalence among high-achieving women, impostor syndrome has been recognized to affect both men and women equally.

At times, Dr. Milhouse still has difficult feelings such as, "What am I doing? I am not good enough like the rest of my colleagues. Why am I at the level I am?" She thinks this comes with being a woman. Women internalize things and second guess themselves because they are women of color, black women, surrounded by white men with tremendous confidence. She told herself, "You are here for a reason. You must fake it till you make it. You need to walk with your head held high and have the confidence that you belong. You are never assumed to be the doctor, let alone a surgeon."

To this day, she walks into the operating room and it is not assumed she is the surgeon. Once, Dr. Milhouse walked into a patient's room dressed in her white coat and the patient assumed she was there to retrieve his food tray. She had another patient who said, "Hi, Ms. Milhouse." She responded lightly with a laugh, "It's Dr. Milhouse." She is certain they would not call a male doctor, Mr., in the States. Dr. Milhouse is a humble person, but it is things like this that need normalized. She has noticed it is difficult being a female urologist dealing with men, but she has risen to this challenge and it has been great.

Dr. Milhouse is most proud of the woman she is now. She does not have it all but is content that she has a decent work-life balance as a wife, mom, and is able to do what she feels is meaningful work. She enjoys what she does and does not look for accolades as a gauge of her success. She is also proud of her family and knowing her patients feel she does the absolute best for them.

A typical work week includes Dr. Milhouse operating two days a week. These are full operating room (OR) days. Three days a week she sees clinic patients. On operating room days, she wakes between 5:00 a.m. and 5:30 a.m. is at the hospital for her first case at 7:30 a.m. She usually operates at two hospitals.

There are 14 urologists in her practice. They share on call duties by splitting the duties in half, so seven cover one area and the other seven cover another area. Dr. Milhouse is on call one day out of seven and has weekend call once every seven weekends. This is a nice schedule and she is at home for her on call responsibilities.

There are few true urology emergencies, however, there are some including testicular torsion, twisting of the testicle that results in cutting off blood supply to the testicle, and Fournier's gangrene, infection causing dead tissue in the genital area. These are both treated with surgery. Others, like penile fracture and an obstructing infected kidney stone may not be emergent, but they are urgent. Dr. Milhouse is in private practice, so they do not have residents. They do, however, have a great group of physician assistants who handle rounds, patient management, and consults during the day.

As far as balance goes, Dr. Milhouse considers herself a work in progress. At one time she was focused on her work and did not give proper attention to her marriage, her family, and her self-care. Her priorities were out of whack. Her spiritual, physical, and mental well-being needed to be prioritized. When she came home, she tried to be in the moment. She is doing better now and has a great husband who is understanding and because of his support, she can be her best self. She tries to work out three times a week and admits she could be better but is making progress. She tells herself to not be too hard on herself, just do her best!

She shared, "Seek out young mentors who are a few years ahead of you in training as quickly as you are able. Many of us do this alone and do not have people to lean on and glean experience and advice from. Especially now, in the age of social media, find someone who is doing what you want to do early in your training. Get mentorship early. You belong here. You are needed. We need physicians of color. You are a prized possession in this world of medicine. You may face self-doubt and self-consciousness, and this is ok. You are where you are supposed to be. Fake it till you make it. It does not mean be dangerous, it means to have the confidence that you belong and are on your path to become a doctor. Be confident and self-assured because when you are confident, others will have confidence in you, whether they are patients, peers, attending physicians, or others in the hospital."

And she sincerely adds, "As a new attending, do not be too picky about what cases you are doing. You are a surgeon and when building a practice, you need to go into the community and become acquainted with referring physicians. Do not be afraid to be busy. I extended my hours a couple of days a week to accommodate patients who are unable to come during regular hours. For some people it is easier to add weekend hours rather than late hours. Regardless, keep busy. Financially speaking, I wish I knew early in my residency about White Coat Investor (a great book and online tool to help managing finances as a physician in training and after training) so I could learn more about finances and take control of mine. Go to the website and learn about finances before completing your training."

Dr. Dumebi Iloba

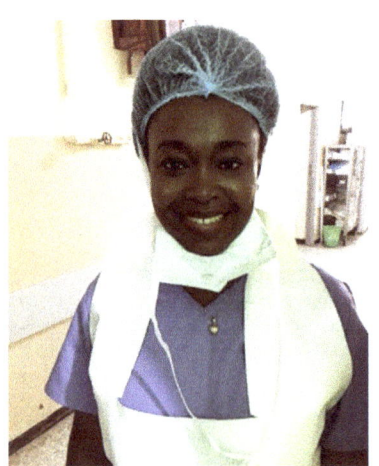

Dr. Dumebi Iloba earned her M.B.B.S degree (Bachelor of Medicine and Bachelor of Surgery), the equivalent of Medical Doctor in the USA, in 2008 from the University of Benin, Benin City, Nigeria. She completed her surgical residency training at the department of surgery, University of Benin

Teaching Hospital. Afterwards, she became a urology fellow at the West African College of Surgeons (WACS), Lagos, Nigeria.

She graduated as the best urology fellow in West Africa in 2018. She currently lectures at the University of Medical Sciences, Ondo State, and is an honorary consultant surgeon at the University of Medical Sciences Teaching Hospital Complex (UNIMEDTHC), Ondo State, Nigeria.

She is a goal-driven, conscientious, and diligent surgeon. She is passionate about teaching and research. She believes in teamwork, working sensibly, and loves mentoring people. She believes in equality and equity. Her special research interests are pediatric urology and andrology (male reproductive organ diseases). Her hobbies include spending time with family, cooking, watching movies, and traveling to new places.

Dr. Iloba chose medicine because she loves caring for people. She is a typical mother hen so she always knew she would be a doctor. Dr. Iloba chose surgery because she is better at what she can see and touch. Anatomy (the study of body parts) was her best pre-clinical course. Like she always says, "I cannot hold or touch hypertension. How can I treat it?" She chose urology because she loves men and feels they are the new endangered species. Everyone talks about female health and issues, but no one remembers the men. Even they do not have time for themselves.

In residency, time management was a huge challenge after Dr. Iloba married. Luckily, she has a supportive husband, children, and extended family. Her mom was willing to babysit for any reason. After all, they are her grandchildren. Her husband brought the children to the hospital for breastfeeding when she was away longer hours than expected and when the pumped milk ran out at home.

Dr. Iloba's husband never complained. She made things a little easier for him by buying groceries in bulk and cooking in bulk, so they did not have to shop or cook as often. Dr. Iloba feels God gives women, especially the ones who become surgeons, amazing multitasking skills. She read and studied everywhere — the kitchen, the recovery room, the operating room while waiting for surgery to start, the laboratory, and even the market. Anywhere! She found a way to merge all aspects of her life. For each different training phase, she carefully explained the nature of her responsibilities to her husband and family members, so they knew what to expect. Dr. Iloba frequently told her husband, "It won't be like this forever" and, at times, when she wanted to quit, he reminded her of these words.

On a typical day, Dr. Iloba wakes at about 5:00 a.m., says prayers, makes breakfast, has her bath, wakes and bathes the children, feeds them, and drops them off at school. She enjoys taking her children to school because it is one of the few bonding times she has with her children. She must judiciously utilize every second of her day. Her children tell her about their day at school and their friends and she tells them about her day at school (residency). Even today, her children call the hospital where she trained, mummy's school.

They understand their mother was a student just like them. Though they were young, this helped when she was away or spent time reading. She and her children often read together, which is another way they bond. After she takes them to school, she arrives at work, attends some academic programs and seminars, then Dr. Iloba begins to tackle the business of the day. This means she is either in theater session (the operating room), clinic, ward rounds, or lectures. When she is done for the day (because there are no closing hours for a surgeon), she heads home, makes dinner, bathes the children, feeds and puts them to bed, spends time with her husband, and then sleeps.

Dr. Iloba feels her very proudest moment and greatest accomplishment were in 2018 when she won the award for best graduating urology fellow in West Africa. She was presented the award at the West African College of Surgeons conference in Dakar, Senegal, January 2019. It was an awesome feeling because she did not set out to be the best. She truly and really loves urology and put her all into her training, exam preparations, and the examinations. It came as a shock and she received many calls from the college, colleagues, family, and friends. People kept asking, "Who is this individual who doesn't have a prostate and yet beat the guys who have one?" It was simply amazing.

Dr. Iloba finds balance by going all-out in every aspect of her life. She loves fiercely and works hard at everything she is interested in, always making certain to not neglect any one thing. This, however, can be difficult because urology can consume one's entire life. However, there are other parts of life that must not be neglected to be a functional adult. Dr. Iloba feels she must prioritize and multitask, giving due time to different aspects of life because this improves general functionality. As a woman, she works to maintain balance and prevent chaos. People are watching and waiting to say, "Aha! We said it! This is no job for a woman." She feels she cannot allow people like this to have the last laugh because it is not true.

Dr. Iloba helps her children with homework while making dinner. This way, they cook together, get homework done, and, above all, it is another way they bond. Things cannot always be done the way others do them. You find what works for you. Being a career mom has also helped her improve her focus and multitasking skills. And Dr. Iloba loves being a career mom.

As far as the recipe for success, Dr. Iloba feels support cannot be over-emphasized. She has a supportive husband and external family. Her younger sister, an accomplished, super-intelligent, and award-winning accountant, was her first nanny. Dr. Iloba had the opportunity to train in a bigger center, in a bigger city, but chose to stay close to home because her needed support came from her mother. Even when she completed her training, her support system again affected her choice of places for permanent employment. This is what worked for her.

Dr. Iloba's road was riddled with challenges. Her greatest challenge has been proving herself to colleagues and patients. As a woman, she feels she must work twice as hard to show she is capable of the almighty surgery training and even harder as a black woman. And even harder than hard as a black woman who looks meek and fragile, some words used to describe Dr. Iloba.

On top of everything else, as a black woman in a male-dominated specialty like urology, you can imagine how she had to work four times as hard as her male counterparts. She had to do this to prove she was capable and worthy.

Also, managing male patients, which are most of her patients, with genital and extremely sensitive issues such as erectile dysfunction, has been challenging for obvious reasons. To overcome this, Dr. Iloba is as professional as possible. She introduces herself and goes straight to the point. She provides as much information as she can while keeping things as simple as possible. This helps put patients at ease and helps them believe they are talking to a specialist and not a nursing student, as she was once called by a patient.

Another challenge Dr. Iloba faced was being hired as a consultant after finishing training. Most employers were not comfortable with a female urologist. They were unsure if their patients would accept a female urologist. Eventually, she was hired where the chief medical director was both willing and unbiased.

Dr. Iloba kept reminding herself she was good enough. She said to herself, "You don't need to be a man to operate." Also, she had to put in the time to become proficient by doing it over and over.

You become more proficient because you are exposed to patients, spend time with the other doctors, and are constantly learning and involved with the day-to-day tasks of being a doctor. When you become skillful and proficient in medical activities, you gain confidence. Dr. Iloba learned not to quit. She kept trying. She tried and kept on trying until she perfected each skill.

Also, Dr. Iloba had the best teachers one could ask for. They never lost their patience and were always willing to teach and teach again and again. They were always there to hold her hands (literally). They went so far as to join in extracurricular activities to increase the bond in the unit, which made the residents more comfortable with them as bosses and teachers. Dr. Iloba does not think there is anything worse than a boss who demeans his junior with words and actions. This results in a lack of confidence in learning doctors.

Dr. Iloba embraces failure by never giving up and always trying again. She remembers it taking her a while before she was proficient enough to begin and complete renal (kidney) surgeries independently, even when her contemporaries mastered them. The moment she failed and handed the knife to her senior surgeon, she plotted how she would do better for her next case. She is guided by the practice makes perfect mantra. She never thinks, "Well, this is not for me." She says to herself, "I haven't had enough practice."

To Dr. Iloba, mentorship means giving back. She had many mentors and they helped mold her into the woman, surgeon, mom, and wife she is today. She had the best teachers in urology. She calls them, "My fathers." They were loving and understanding and yet never failed to bring out the cane when she stepped out-of-line. She appreciates them deeply. Without them, she would not be writing this today.

And, while preparing for her membership exams, she discovered the first female urologist in her country who became another wonderful mentor for Dr. Iloba. Dr. Iloba did not realize there was only one female urologist at the time she began her training. Knowing this spurred her on. Her mentor gave Dr. Iloba valid advice on how to overcome the hurdles every female urologist faces.

This urologist still mentors Dr. Iloba today. Dr. Iloba is the third female urologist in her country and the first to be trained in her geopolitical region. So, mentoring others to join them is still a huge task. Dr. Iloba finds joy in giving back what she has received so freely and lovingly. She mentors young surgeons and ladies to become what they want to become. It is a privilege being involved in this beautiful method of giving back.

Dr. Iloba said, "Above all, I cannot overestimate the role of God in my life. I am proud of my Catholic faith and I try my best to please my Maker. He has given me everything I need. He guided me throughout my training and even now. At my lowest and highest times, I call on Him and He answers. I am forever thankful."

And advice she would like to share with up-and-coming black female surgeons as well as any other woman with a dream is, "Be strong emotionally and physically. Do not be too hard on yourself. You are good enough. Embrace challenges. Have good interpersonal relations and be humble. You do not want to make the already difficult journey even harder with rivalry, backbiting, and so forth. These are things that guided me through my training and even now, as a young consultant."

"I am grateful to those who did not take a chance on me. They, especially, sparked the fire that ignited my resilience. It is because of them that I learned how to adjust my sails and stay in the race. Each of us men and women will encounter challenges great and small in our careers. General Patton once said that he did not measure a man's success by how high he climbs but how high he bounces when he hits the bottom. Let's help future generations of surgeons male and female bounce higher."
Julie Freischlag, MD

CHAPTER SIX
Breast Oncology Surgery

A breast surgeon is a surgeon who takes care of patients with benign (noncancerous) and malignant (cancer) breast disease.

Dr. Jovita Oruwari

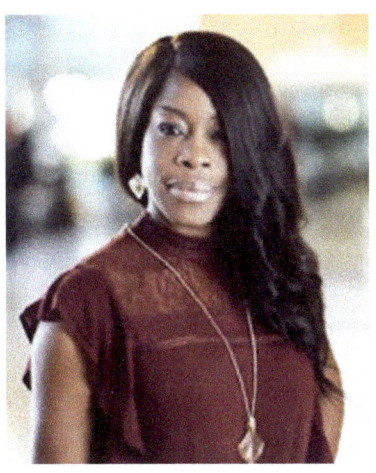

Dr. Jovita Oruwari is a board-certified general surgeon and breast oncology surgeon in St. Louis, Missouri. She earned her medical degree at the University of Medicine and Dentistry of New Jersey medical school (UMDNJ), Newark, New Jersey, and also completed her general surgery residency there. She finished a breast oncology fellowship at Brown University – Women and Infants Hospital in Providence, Rhode Island.

This is Dr. Oruwari's story in her own words.

In my second year of training, I was officially the surgeon in charge. My patient was on the operating table, and I was performing a particularly challenging axillary lymph node dissection – this is surgery to remove the lymph nodes in the armpit where breast cancer travels first.

Due to the extent of the cancer and scarring in this area, I remained calm and steady, taking one layer of dissection at a time to expose the lymph nodes. As I continued my dissection, I accidentally cut the axillary vein. This is a large and major vein in the axilla (armpit) we affectionately call big blue.

When this happened, the operating room staff panicked because there was a great deal of bleeding. I did not know it at the time, but the staff called a senior attending to help. I calmly asked for a 7-0 Prolene suture and a Castro needle holder. This is a type of small suture and a special instrument utilized by vascular surgeons (surgeons who repair blood vessels) to hold needles. I took the suture and finished repairing the vein as the senior attending entered the operating room and asked if I needed help. I calmly said, "No thanks." He left. All this happened in about three minutes. I completed the surgery and the patient went home without incident.

This was a particularly defining moment for me. I felt confident and in charge. I had great training and it came in handy when I needed it. This was the day I gained the respect of the staff and earned my surgeon's wings.

I am an oncologic breast surgeon. I perform surgery to remove cancer from the breast. I see women with all types of breast problems. About 30% of my practice is breast cancer and the remaining are benign breast diseases. I chose this specialty because it is a combination of women's health care and surgery. I enjoy the relationships I form with my patients long-term because I am with them the moment they receive the devastating diagnosis of cancer, and through their journey to survive with treatment.

Since I was three years old, I have wanted to be a doctor. My strength is in the STEM (science, technology, engineering, and math) field because I love the ability to think through problems and solve them. I attended medical school with the goal of becoming a gynecologist, a doctor for female reproductive health. But, once I completed my general surgery rotation, I was sold on surgery. I had the good fortune of having two great mentors in training who were breast surgeons that encouraged and inspired me to pursue a career in breast surgery.

I am also fortunate and lucky to have been raised by parents who did not see any limits where education was concerned. We were encouraged to study hard and aim high. Also, I married a man who believes in me 100% and is invested in my success.

I was a traditional student. After high school, I attended

college and majored in zoology and chemistry. I was accepted into medical school and chose a general surgery specialty, one of the most difficult specialties. Surgery training is usually an additional five years of instruction. I completed two additional years of training, mostly doing research. I spent one year in a fellowship for breast surgery. So, when I add it all up, I spent 14 years studying after high school to achieve where I am today.

Now, I practice full-time as part of a group of physicians and am married and have two grown children. Life is easier now that my children are both in college. When my children were younger, it was quite a balancing act being a mom, getting them fed, clothed, and educated, and being a doctor caring for my patients. My husband is also a physician and with both of us working full-time, we relied on family and nannies to help. We had full-time childcare from the time the children were born to when they started driving at age 16.

I enjoy my work, but I do not let it consume me. I do many things outside of work because balancing work and life is important to me. I am an avid reader and love writing, running (I have run in many half-marathons and 10Ks), cooking when I have time, traveling, fashion, shopping, and socializing. Lately, I have been regularly active on Instagram trying to educate, teach, and inspire on a larger platform.

I want to include what I would tell myself during my journey. In grade school, "Work hard, keep your eyes and ears open, and absorb all you can. Enjoy being a child." What I would tell myself in middle school is, "The habits you develop now will stay with you into adulthood. Make time for your studies and make time for play." What I would tell myself in high school is, "These are the years of education colleges are interested in. Work hard and maintain competitive grades, but do not forget that they also want well-rounded people. Make sure you have varied interests or extracurricular activities." What I would tell myself in undergrad is, "Keep your eyes on the prize. You are so close. Continue to work hard. There is no reason you cannot do this. Study hard and research the various medical specialties. If you have the opportunity to do research, do it. And if you know any doctors, shadow them during school holidays. Make sure they write letters of recommendation." What I would tell myself in medical school is "This is your chance to master the human body – to know its anatomy (parts of the body) and physiology (the normal function of those body parts) and to start to tie it into disease processes. This is a period that starts a lifetime of continued learning." What I would tell myself as an intern is, "Slow down. Take a deep breath. Remember to always respect the humanity of the people that entrust you to care for their health. They are not just numbers, but living, breathing people." What I would tell myself as a senior/chief resident is, "You have a responsibility to teach your junior residents." What I would tell myself my first year as an attending is, "Always be kind to the staff, patients, colleagues, and residents." What I would tell myself mid-career is, "Never stop learning. Keep an open mind to new ways of doing things, to new techniques and technology. You owe it to your patients to give them the most current treatment!"

And, the best advice I have for the next generation of girls in STEM is, "Just do it." It is an extremely diverse field of study with a wide range of options for careers and great options for leadership positions.

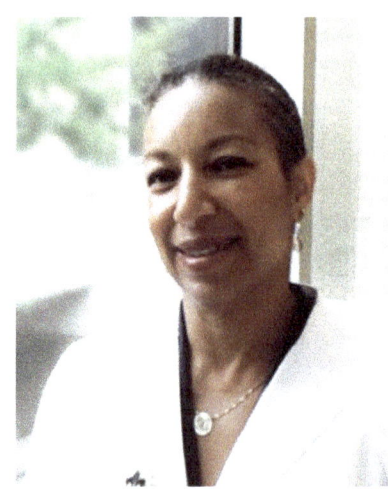

Dr. Shawn McKinney

Dr. Shawn McKinney is a professor of clinical surgery, director of breast services and a surgical breast oncologist at Louisiana State University Health Sciences Center in New Orleans, Louisiana.

A Southerner, Dr. McKinney grew up in New Orleans. She earned her bachelor's degree from Xavier

University, also in New Orleans. She did not realize how much culture and richness this city had until she left it. She took New Orleans for granted because it was her everyday life. She attended medical school at Morehouse School of Medicine in Atlanta, Georgia, and also finished her general surgical residency there. She completed her breast surgical oncology fellowship at Baylor University in Dallas, Texas.

Dr. McKinney thinks wanting to become a surgeon was something she considered later in life but wanting to become a doctor was something she dreamed of early in life. As early as she can remember, science interested her. She enjoyed learning about how things worked and did well in science classes. Her love for science was her avenue into medicine. She is an only child and there are no doctors in her family or physicians around her when she was young.

Her mother, however, worked in one of the general clinics as a secretary at the Veterans Administration Hospital in New Orleans. Sometimes after school, Dr. McKinney went to her mother's work, and there she met an older white male physician. This physician was nice, and he took her with him as he visited his patients. She was impressed by the way he talked to patients and how patients loved him because he was personable and friendly. He made people feel like there was an answer to whatever problem they had and that anything could be fixed.

At her young age, he showed her what a doctor is. This was her first exposure to hospitals and she admired him. His staff loved him, and patients loved him. He was a good doctor. Dr. McKinney was in elementary school but being around him sparked her interest in becoming a physician from that time on.

Dr. McKinney's parents exposed her to different programs and activities throughout her high school years that reinforced her interest in medicine. Her summers were divided between academic science-related programs and dance classes, her other love.

Most decide their path by the third year of medical school. Dr. McKinney rotated through all the departments that year and surgery was her last rotation. She figured she would find something to choose before she considered surgery.

There were several key things she knew about herself. Dr. McKinney likes working with her hands and she had little patience to pontificate long-term about certain situations. She likes the solution-driven aspects of medicine. She likes, "Here's a problem; what's the answer?" "What do we have to work through and how do we fix it?" Dr. McKinney knew these things about herself even as a student studying medicine. As she rotated through the different areas of medicine during her third year in medical school, she crossed off each specialty until the only one left was surgery.

Surgery was the one rotation where Dr. McKinney did not mind getting up early and going to the hospital. She remembers how she liked being at the hospital between 3-4 a.m. It was quiet and a good time to collect information about patients and study their issues to prepare for rounds. Some of her other classmates dragged in late and did not enjoy the early mornings and the work associated with surgical clerkship. Dr. McKinney could not wait to get behind the restricted double doors leading into the operating room. This was where she felt magic happened and wanted to be part of it!

Dr. McKinney knew being a black woman and doing surgery would be challenging. It was, and is, a male-dominated field, and there were no 80-hour work restrictions in the '90s. It was not uncommon to train for two or three years and then be told you were being let go. Nothing was guaranteed and there was little margin for error. This frightened her and there were times she did not think she could survive the training.

Since she liked procedures. Dr. McKinney considered other specialties such as becoming an emergency room doctor or anesthesiologist, but when she completed these rotations during her third and fourth years of medical school, she did not care for them.

She and her husband Gerald, who is originally from Chicago, met when he was an intern in the surgery program. She was a third-year medical student and experiencing turmoil about being a surgeon or not being a surgeon. When she finally rotated through surgery, he was one of the interns who was part of her team. While talking one day, he asked her what she thought she wanted to do with her life. She told him she liked surgery but was not confident about picking it as a specialty.

He said, "Well, you're just going to be a surgeon." She answered, "No, I do not want to be a surgeon. I have an anesthesia rotation lined up and ER (emergency room) also." She told him ER was looking like an option because it was a three-year residency and she would be finished.

He looked at her and said, "You'll be back." He saw how she performed in her surgery rotation and how much she loved being in the operating room. He knew she would be back to surgery and he was right. They married during her third year as a surgical resident.

It was important for her to not get pregnant during her residency because she did not want anything to interfere with her training. There was no way she would have been able to make it through residency had she chosen to become pregnant during this phase of her training. They had two beagle puppies and they were enough for Dr. and Dr. McKinney. Their schedules were unpredictable.

Gerald left the program before she did to complete a laparoscopic fellowship. Afterwards, she completed her fellowship. She chose surgery as her husband predicted because she did not want to have any regrets and knew she would have been heart-broken to look back and wish she had considered surgery if she had not. She tells students to follow their hearts and stay true to what they love, what makes use of their talents. The details work out if you follow your heart.

Training in the '90s was riddled with challenges. Dr. McKinney had doubts as to whether she would make it, if she would be supported, or if people would be able to give her what she needed to encourage her throughout the process. She chose a medical school that had professors and attendings that were predominantly black. She needed to see people who looked like her. Her future was plain to her and seeing them kept her going.

The 80-hour-work-week restriction became effective one month after Dr. McKinney finished residency in 2002. She trained in a busy urban setting at Grady Hospital in Atlanta, Georgia. The hours were long, days ran into each other, and she had to push through levels of exhaustion at times; but she was able to see and experience a great deal. When she needs to, she can push herself through bouts of exhaustion because of that training. It also prepared her to care for three children.

Dr. McKinney feels the greatest obstacle she encountered in training was being underestimated and stereotyped. Unfortunately, these have continued as ongoing challenges throughout her career. She thinks people expect her to be a certain way as a surgeon. In the past, the typical surgeon would have the reputation of being gruff, callous, and rude. During training, she was told, "You're not acting like a surgeon, you're too nice." There is a balance between staying true to your personality and who you are and having to prove and assert yourself as a trainee. People underestimate who she is and what she is capable of doing based on their own biases. She does not want to change who she is to fit into a mold of what people think she should be.

Even though Dr. McKinney is a phenomenally successful surgeon, she has struggled with impostor syndrome. She did not realize it was a thing until a few years ago. It is funny because she recently had a conversation about impostor syndrome with some girlfriends who are also successful black women. They discussed how they never feel like they are enough. They never feel comfortable just being fine with what they have already accomplished and being okay, even if they fail. Others are permitted to fail and are not labeled as a failure. So, they are always second-guessing themselves and fearful of failure. Sometimes it is exhausting to work so hard to be perfect and make sure nothing goes wrong when perfection is unattainable.

In fact, Dr. McKinney obsesses about perfection. To tell

the truth, she is constantly thinking, constantly ruminating. She is always wondering, "What if I had done things differently? Why didn't this go right?" She says to herself, "I've done this many times before and it's gone right. Why did this go wrong?"

Confidence is attainable, however. Dr. McKinney loved her fellowship training. She had a positive experience in Dallas during her fellowship and it solidified her specialty choice. She had mentors who believed in her and helped her have confidence during this training.

Her first job was in West Virginia. She was on her own and scared. She was hired to start a breast program from the ground up. They had a small building and offered mammograms, biopsies, and had a small breast clinic. There were plans to build a Cancer Center which would be completed by the next year.

They looked to Dr. McKinney as an expert to set up the breast clinic, and she rose to the challenge. This was a great experience for her. From viewing and revising blueprints for the breast center to picking the equipment, it was daunting for a first job.

She was young and just completed training, so she wanted to use the skills she gained, both clinical and administrative. She became more confident as time went on. This accredited, comprehensive breast center in Huntington, West Virginia, is still caring for patients today! Her 10-year experience in West Virginia gave her the confidence that laid the foundation for the remainder of her career.

Dr. McKinney and her husband lived apart for two years, but she managed to get pregnant during her fellowship year. Their first child was born two months after moving to West Virginia. Understandably, there was a great deal of stress – with a new job, in a new city, with no family, and a new baby. She would not advise combining major life events when planning things. They had two additional children, each two years apart.

In addition to the stress of a new job and new family, Dr. McKinney struggled with caring for herself. She feels children become your priority and she did not make herself a priority when her children were younger. And, when she started the breast program in West Virginia, she did not properly take care of herself because she worked too much. She worked in a fully booked clinic and on some days she was in the OR all day. Even though breast surgery is not an emergent surgery, things can still be busy.

Dr. McKinney's days at work were long and when she came home, she took care of her children and settled them and, after that, the day was over. Time for her? She did not think about it. Now that she is older and looking back, she could have limited how much she worked. But, as the only black female, she felt she had to prove herself. She felt she had to be available and create and continue a particular standard so she did not appear lazy. The pressure to succeed resulted in her neglecting herself, her health, and her marriage. This is one of the main reasons for the high divorce rate for married surgeons. Her husband and she were involved in the church and this helped keep them together and stable. Once they had their third child, she realized she needed more help, so they moved her parents in with them. This helped because she felt she had to be a superwoman but had to let that feeling go. She felt she had to be the best surgeon and the best mom.

Dr. McKinney remembers using a blender to make organic homemade vegetables for the baby. She did not need to do this and had to let go of the guilt of not living up to this picture of a perfect mom. She still struggles with self-care, but as she is getting older, it is becoming easier. She has decided to put her physical and mental health first and actively make herself do things that replenish her.

She feels her faith is her core for everything. Dr. McKinney does not have all the answers, but God does. She asks God to show up in surgery when she is struggling, and He always does. She prays a short prayer for her patients before every procedure asking for God's guidance; for Him to guide her hands, to make her aware, have her do no harm, and allow the patient to recover.

She knows, and has always known, that she is not truly in control. She is just an extension of His hands. Dr. McKinney asks that He allow her to use the knowledge He allowed her to gain to help each patient. Her faith is especially important to her. It is integral to how she views medicine as a whole and how she practices.

Not only does Dr. McKinney's field require a level of compassion, it also requires the ability to meet people where they are to guide them through a very scary process. A diagnosis of cancer can rattle the strongest patient. She thinks her faith, and being able to share her faith, and being able to open up and allow them to let go and let God during the process, is the way she shares her faith with patients. When patients say, "I'll pray for you," she says, "Thank you. Thank you so much. Absolutely, I will accept your prayer."

Dr. McKinney would love to have dinner with Michelle Obama. She read her book and was able to take her girls to Michelle Obama's speaking engagement at the Essence Festival in New Orleans in 2019. It was amazing just to hear her talk, hear her reflections, and how she navigated her eight years as the First Lady with a level of grace and restraint that is unimaginable. Dr. McKinney does not think she would have had the grace Michelle Obama did, amid the attacks she experienced. Everything was scrutinized; from her appearance to her character, and not to mention any policy the Former First Lady tried to promote.

Dr. McKinney does not know any other female, much less a black female, in Michelle Obamas's position who could have navigated through that experience as well as she did. Dr. McKinney is in awe of how Michelle Obama continues to show up as her authentic self in every situation and not lower her standard. She is comfortable in her own skin. Dr. McKinney thinks there are times we all struggle to show up as our authentic selves. Sometimes, she says to herself, "Be Michelle. Just be Michelle. For me this means that it is alright to be authentic and be true to who I am."

Dr. McKinney is currently reading historical books like,

The Half Has Never Been Told, by Edward Baptist. She must read in spurts because it is overwhelming. It documents how this country began, how the country was built on the backs of slavery, and how capitalism began.

She just finished reading, *The Checklist Manifesto,* by Atul Gawande, a book about how the timeout procedure protocol began.

Her husband and she usually read a Christian-based book for their couples' class.

She has also become interested in basic health, so she is reading the *Obesity Code* by Jason Fung, MD and recently finished *Deep Nutrition* by Catherine Shanahan, MD. Cell autophagy has recently fascinated Dr. McKinney, so she has been reading more about this subject. She hopes to use what she is learning to help patients on a practical level.

Dr. Miriam Mutebi

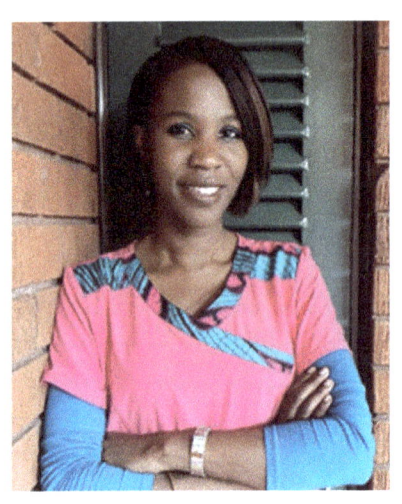

Dr. Miriam Mutebi is a consultant breast surgical oncologist at the Aga Khan University Hospital in Nairobi, Kenya. She received her medical degree from the University of Nairobi and completed her general surgery residency at the Aga Khan University Hospital followed by a two-year fellowship in breast surgical oncology. This included a year in the plastics and reconstruction unit at the University of Cape Town, Groote Schuur Hospital, South Africa.

She completed two years as a graduate surgical oncology fellow at the Memorial Sloan Kettering Cancer Center, New York. During this time, she trained as a clinical epidemiologist and health systems researcher at Weill Cornell University, New York.

Her research focus is on understanding the barriers to care for women with cancers in East Africa and in designing interventions to address these barriers. She is also the co-founder of the Pan African Women Association of Surgeons (PAWAS), whose aim is to provide mentorship and support to women in surgery and to advocate to improve women's health and surgical care on the African continent.

It was never an automatic decision for Dr. Mutebi to go into medicine and she finds it is her experiences that influenced her career choice. At the tender age of 18, she was torn between many different career choices, including medicine, journalism, law, and architecture. She spent time at hospitals, law firms, and publishing houses to find clarity before finally settling on medicine.

She completed her undergraduate training during the emergence of the HIV epidemic in Kenya. It was a period of great concern because, at that time, few patients had access to antiretroviral (ARV) medications (the medication used to treat HIV), making it heart-wrenching for patients and for the health workers who cared for them. Luckily, this has changed due to global initiatives like the President's Emergency Plan for AIDS Relief (PEPFAR).

Dr. Mutebi found herself gravitating towards surgery because it is a results-oriented profession and she felt she could make a direct and immediate impact on patients' lives.

During her surgical residency, Dr. Mutebi helped manage the breast clinic. She quickly realized her patients did not fit the mold she learned in school. The textbooks said breast cancer was a disease of much older women with several predisposing risk factors. She realized her patients were young ladies with many of the traditionally protective factors and were still getting breast cancer. She decided someone needed to help these women and needed to understand this disease better. This influenced her path to become a breast surgical oncologist and clinical epidemiologist and health systems researcher.

As a woman in surgery in Africa, it was difficult to carve

out a path where she could learn from other ladies. In many forums and many interactions, there is still a conscious or unconscious bias towards women in surgery. She is filled with gratitude to be able to disrupt these norms and break new ground for those coming behind, even though no one speaks about how this constant struggle is emotionally exhausting. Also, despite having wonderful and supportive colleagues of the opposite gender, Dr. Mutebi frequently feels isolated.

Dr. Mutebi built confidence by realizing that learning is a lifelong interest. So, to build confidence, she relies on the belief that her skills and knowledge are constantly improving through an iterative or repetitive process. She is always practicing and becoming more proficient. It also helps to stop periodically to reflect on and celebrate small wins and gains. She feels confidence is the culmination of these things over time that shows you just how far along your journey you have come and how much growth you have attained.

She also pushes herself to explore and try new things she would not ordinarily do or that take her outside her comfort zone. Dr. Mutebi is currently taking flying lessons that are difficult, but each progressive step helps her gain confidence. It does not need to be a plane; it could be a course one would never consider or as simple as speaking up during rounds. She finds that the more she challenges herself, the more she grows!

As an academic surgeon, it is always a challenge finding the balance between clinical work, training, and research, and life outside of work. Sometimes the best to-do lists go awry! Dr. Mutebi finds the first step is usually acknowledging that it is not possible to do everything, and tasks need to be prioritized. Sometimes, tasks do not need to be perfect, they just need to be done. Paradoxically, taking time to take breaks before returning to the task at hand helps her be more efficient at completing tasks and frequently gives her a fresh perspective on things.

Also, as an academic surgeon, Dr. Mutebi's day typically starts with residency teaching sessions, whether it is grand rounds (lectures on medical topics) or morbidity and mortality meetings

(meetings to discuss cases that have not ended well or are not responding well). After visiting patients on the wards, she either evaluates patients in surgical clinics or she operates. Afterwards, she frequently reviews patients on the ward again before heading to her office to work on administrative tasks.

It is difficult to limit Dr. Mutebi's greatest and proudest moments to just one. She feels there is usually a constellation of events to celebrate. Though the acquisition of academic accomplishments does give a sense of personal satisfaction, she finds some of her greatest moments are the ones spent at her breast clinic. She likes to say she is in the hope business, a much-needed factor when practicing as a breast cancer surgeon in Sub-Saharan Africa. This is because many consider cancer equals death.

For Dr. Mutebi, hope involves trying to demystify the process and let patients know there is treatment no matter what stage of cancer they are diagnosed with. The aims and goals of treatment may change depending on patient responses.

Most breast cancer is curative in early stages, and can be controlled in more advanced cancers, but something can be done to treat and control the disease and give comfort at any stage.

Dr. Mutebi's greatest moments are helping patients through the different stages of their cancer journey. This includes the privilege of removing their cancer and, together with a multidisciplinary team, seeing them through their successful treatment.

Also, many patients seen in her clinics do not have breast cancer but have concerns such as breast pain or nipple discharge they may attribute to cancer. The clinic is set up as a safe space and they use it as an opportunity to empower women about their breast health and awareness. They take time to address the concerns as to why this patient came to the clinic because their breast is frequently the least of their concerns. Often, they have other problems they want to discuss.

The team talks about many health and social concerns and it is amazing to see the transformation of a patient when they go from being a bundle of nerves to enlightenment, engagement, and understanding by the time they leave the clinic. These moments are priceless!

On the opposite end of the spectrum, Dr. Mutebi admits dealing with failure is never easy, but she tries to apply a few principles that help with her outlook during trying times. The first is, she realizes there is a huge potential for personal growth that occurs in times of adversity. Anyone can maintain a favorable outlook when everything is going well, but she finds that it is in difficult situations she learns the most about herself.

It provides Dr. Mutebi an opportunity to take stock of things and increases self-reflection. The first step towards dealing with failure is separating herself from the event. It is important to make the distinction between failing at something and saying you are a failure. Failing at something brings out the possibility that another attempt could be or could have been made with a potentially different outcome.

Next, she reviews what she learned from the incident and tries to explore different approaches that could achieve a better outcome. This encourages Dr. Mutebi to rethink the problems and motivates her to try again. To paraphrase Samuel Beckett, "Try again. Fail again. Fail better!!"

Dr. Mutebi shared her personal thoughts. "As surgeons, we do our best to minimize complications. However, one of my mentors once told me, 'The only surgeons who do not have complications are the ones who are not operating.' The reality most colleagues attest to is that even when one has done the best that one can, complications still occur due to a variety of factors including the heterogeneity of patients or comorbidities."

Dr. Mutebi counsels her patients on the potential for complications pre-operatively and lets them know that though complications are rare, they sometimes occur. She also tells them that the main thing to do when complications develop is to discover them quickly and manage them appropriately.

This upfront and candid discussion and regular communication throughout the management course of treatment helps the occurrence of complications seem less bewildering to the patient. Dr. Mutebi also discusses the complication and its management with her peers to see if there is or was anything additional she could have done, or if some other approach has worked for them. It is another opportunity for knowledge exchange and learning.

This is also why Dr. Mutebi feels mentorship is crucial and means supporting and empowering the next generation of surgeons. We have a collective responsibility to ensure that we transfer the skills we have learned. These skills go beyond the technical and include attributes like empathy and respect for the dignity of life.

It is ensuring that the model of a kind, competent, and ethical surgeon is carried forward and this can only be done through role-modeling. Not only do we need to pave the way for those coming after us, but we also need to ensure that we help them navigate and avoid the pitfalls we faced. This helps ensure the consistent development of a motivated, conscientious workforce engaged in addressing and optimizing the delivery of care to patients.

If Dr. Mutebi was giving advice to a young woman interested in following her dreams, she would say that there is no substitute for hard work. Invest early in a good and principled work ethic and it will be the foundation needed for a successful career. Never forget your humanity. As surgeons, we are given the privilege of managing people when they are most vulnerable. It is a responsibility that should never be taken lightly. Enjoy the journey. There is always something new to learn. The best surgeons are always questioning, reflecting, learning, and practicing his or her craft. Be yourself and do not be afraid to own your space. There is a tendency to want to be one of the guys and blend in but learn to find your authentic voice early. Speak your truth quietly and respectfully. You have as much right to be there as anybody else, so claim your light and shine!!

"I believe every human has a finite number of heartbeats. I don't intend to waste any of mine." – Neil Armstrong

Dr. Portia Siwawa

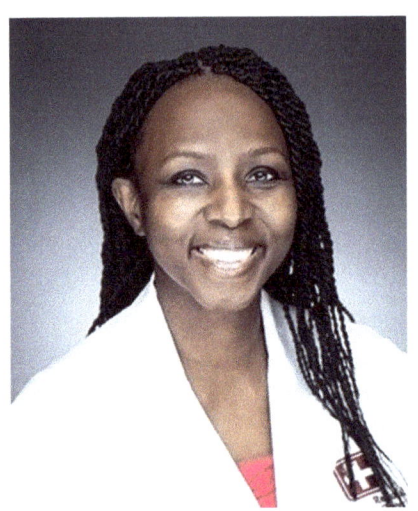

Dr. Portia Siwawa is currently a breast oncology surgeon in Georgia, USA.

She knew she wanted to be a doctor when she was six years old. Over the next 10 years of her life, the desire increased. When she finished high school in Botswana, she performed national service work and was assigned to a rural area to teach first and second graders. Some children came to class with health issues and there was no hospital nearby. There was a clinic, but it was staffed by people with no medical background.

Occasionally, a nurse arrived at the clinic and every other month or so, a doctor visited. It was at this time Dr. Siwawa decided she wanted to become a doctor. Originally, she wanted to be a pediatrician. It was not until her surgery rotation in medical school that the probability light bulb went off in her head. She loved everything about the operating room and taking care of surgical patients. Dr. Siwawa knew being a surgeon was what she was supposed to do.

Each year in Botswana, they picked a graduating high school student to receive a scholarship to study abroad. Dr. Siwawa was chosen and received a scholarship to study in the United States. In preparation for the American college, she attended a prep school in Connecticut for one year then earned her bachelor's degree from Mount Holyoke College in South Hadley, Massachusetts.

After graduating from college, she worked for one year and then received a scholarship to attend St. George's University School of Medicine, Grenada, West Indies. During her third year in medical school, everyone she spoke with said negative things about surgery, describing surgeons as mean and claiming surgery to be a difficult rotation. But when she rotated through surgery, she loved it. She loved working with her hands and enjoyed being in the operating room and appreciated the teamwork.

Dr. Siwawa was accepted and completed her general surgery residency training at the Brooklyn Hospital Center in Brooklyn, New York. Afterwards, she was matched with Texas Tech University in Lubbock, Texas, for her breast surgical oncology fellowship.

She was the victim of many negative remarks when she announced she intended to apply for a surgical residency. After starting her general surgery training, Dr. Siwawa realized she was a strong intern, but spent most of her internship taking care of patients on the wards instead of learning how to operate and spending time in the operating room. Often, when an intern excels in day-to-day patient care such as admitting patients to the hospital, making sure they have appropriate treatment for their diseases, and scheduling procedures as well as discharging patients, they may be denied training in the operating room.

While she loved and enjoyed the patients, Dr. Siwawa's heart was in surgery. She thinks patient care should be shared between all the interns and residents so that the training doctors receive equal exposure and time in the operating room. Unlike other areas of medicine, surgery requires doing surgery to learn surgery.

Dr. Siwawa had to stand up for herself because her training was being compromised. Even though she was efficient in providing patient care, her operative skills suffered because she was not practicing in the operating room. She was fortunate to have several black male attendings in her program who advocated for her. And they were not the only ones who advocated for her, attendings of other races did as well.

She is new at her current practice, but typically Dr. Siwawa has two operating days. She sees clinic patients two days a week and has a day she spends in meetings and works on administrative duties. Some weekends she has speaking engagements, health fairs, and outreach programs that provide breast cancer screening in communities that otherwise would not have access to these services.

The best advice she received from a mentor from Guyana was, "Whenever you are moving up the ladder in training, never forget to look down the ladder to pull up whoever is coming after you."

It is rewarding for Dr. Siwawa to be available for her patients through their journey. Knowing she has played a part in helping someone be well and get better makes her happy.

Advice she would give to others is, "Keep your head up. Do not take anything personally because then you will constantly be broken. Read, read, and read some more. Make sure you get excellent ABSITE scores. Find a mentor early."

Her final words are, "Dream big and you will do bigger. Will Smith said, 'If you stay ready, you don't have to get ready.' This means that opportunities can come from anywhere. This is an important thing to realize; that the chance to do something you really want to do can come when you least expect it."

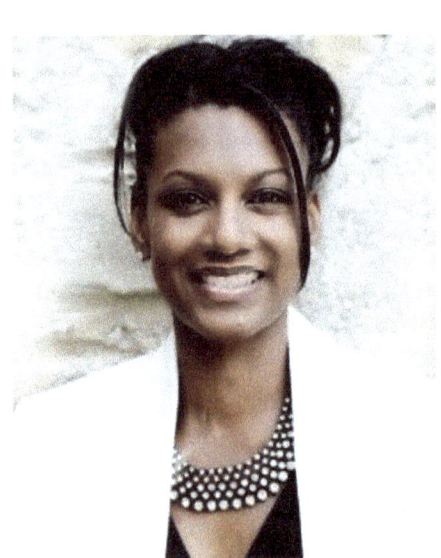

Miss Shireen McKenzie

Miss Shireen McKenzie is a consultant oncoplastic breast surgeon and head of year three at Leeds Medical School, University of Leeds, United Kingdom. Year three is the third year of the five-year program which focuses on increased clinical exposure.

Miss McKenzie cannot remember when she decided to be a medic; it was innate. When she was four years old, she told her aunt she would cut her up and make her feel better. She was either going to be a surgeon or a psycho.

Her mother was a nurse and when she was six years old, her babysitter bought her a nurse's bag. Miss McKenzie knew this was not for her. For the same birthday, her aunt bought her a belated gift, a doctor set. Now, she was hooked.

When she was 14 years old, an acquaintance of the family, a white male primary physician, gave her career advice. He did not discourage Miss McKenzie from medicine. He did do so for surgery, stating that as a black woman, she would be better off pursuing a career in gynecology, rather than surgery. Unknowingly, he probably strengthened her resolve to be a surgeon.

From the first week of medical school, she made everyone aware she was going to be a surgeon and never looked back.

Miss McKenzie completed her surgical training in Yorkshire, England. This training had a reputation for not appointing many females. There was a new consultant chairing the appointments committee for junior surgical training. He appointed four trainees, three were female. This was unusual.

Miss McKenzie continued to advance in her surgery training in the same region, again with very few females. They were a tight-knit group. During her time as a trainee, all her mentors were white males who gave her their utmost support. She heard about toxic environments where people were overlooked because of their race, religion, or gender. This was not the case for her. If Miss McKenzie worked hard and showed dedication, she was rewarded with support and superb training. Working in a large teaching hospital, she is still surrounded by some of these mentors who still offer great support when needed.

If she found herself in a tricky situation, Miss McKenzie did not automatically assume it was due to her race but reflected on why this occurred. She feels the real barrier she has had to face is related more to her gender and not from surgeons, but mainly from the nursing staff. She and her female colleagues notice the males experience an easier time in the theater (operating room) or on the wards, and this is not race-dependent.

In her current position, Miss McKenzie says every day is different! On certain days, she deals with research and university issues as head of year three. She has an all-day clinic another day followed by all-day theater (operating), and days she teaches medical students or trainees' surgical courses. She is also involved with the royal college of surgeons and various committees for her specialty. Theater is her best day, of course, and always has been.

Miss McKenzie started life as a budding transplant surgeon and completed her training in liver transplantation. At that time, being a breast surgeon was the last thing on her list of potential careers. Breast surgery was always seen as a career for those who could not operate, which she feels is a belittling way to think about females in general. However, in the United Kingdom, the specialty has evolved, and as oncoplastic breast surgeons, they all perform cancer surgery and various types of reconstructive surgery.

This is not only technically rewarding, but also emotionally rewarding for Miss McKenzie. Many women her age and younger are given the opportunity to spend more time with their families and potentially leaving them whole and healed is emotionally rewarding.

Miss McKenzie's proudest accomplishments are her three children. She took her consultant exams with two children under two years of age and was proud of this. And to think she never wanted children!

Her children keep her grounded and when things feel like they are spiraling out of control, they manage to manage her. This is a skill Miss McKenzie thinks her husband wishes he had! They bring laughter to the house and of course some tears, but they are an unexpected antidote to juggling life and work and the potential burnout and stress that sometimes comes with the life she has chosen.

The best advice Miss McKenzie has received is, "There is never a good time to do anything. Just do it."

The heart-felt lessons Miss McKenzie would like to share

with all readers and young women aspiring to greatness of all races, religions, and genders is, "Do not use your race, religion, or gender as a barrier. Do not make these an excuse for failing. If you are critiqued, do not automatically assume that person is against you, they may just want you to improve and reach your potential. Sometimes others looking from the outside can see what we cannot. Don't take yourself too seriously. Be kind, polite, and grounded. Good luck and never give up – unless it is your choice!"

"I have had to take a lot of chances to get there, and others have had to take chances on me. It has taken a good measure of fearlessness, some wonderful mentors, and an ability to adjust my sails to get here today."
– Julie Freischlag, MD

CHAPTER SEVEN
Colorectal Surgery

Colorectal surgery is a field in medicine dealing with disorders of the rectum, anus, and colon.

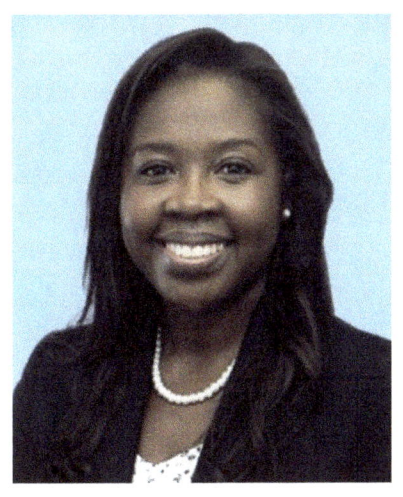

Dr. Gifty Kwakye

Dr. Gifty Kwakye graduated from Yale University in New Haven, Connecticut, with her Bachelor of Science degrees in both biology and psychology. She received her medical degree from Yale University in 2010 and earned a Master's in Public Health from Johns Hopkins in Baltimore, Maryland.

She completed her general surgery residency at the Brigham and Women's Hospital/Harvard Medical School, Boston, Massachusetts, in 2017 and her colorectal surgery fellowship at the University of Minnesota, Twin Cities, Minnesota, in 2018. Dr. Kwakye has been a clinical assistant professor of surgery in the Division of Colorectal Surgery at the University of Michigan, Ann Arbor, Michigan, since 2018.

As a resident, she received multiple awards including the Robert T. Osteen and the Partners Health System Medical Education awards for excellence in teaching. Also, her passion for global health was recognized with a Global Health Scholarship award from Johns Hopkins during her public health training.

Dr. Kwakye's clinical expertise is in the treatment of colon and rectal oncology, inflammatory bowel disease, anorectal disorders, and utilizing minimally invasive approaches to colorectal disease. Her interests are in the management of pelvic floor disorders including rectal prolapse and fecal incontinence.

Dr. Kwakye's mother was a nurse in a local polyclinic in Ghana, Africa, and was fondly known as Auntie Nurse in their community where she cared for people using their porch as a make-shift clinic. Some of Dr. Kwakye's favorite ways to spend the afternoon when she came home from school were assisting her mother debriding and bandaging wounds, comforting children and adults while they were given injections, and administering medications as part of national vaccination efforts for polio eradication.

She jokes that she did not choose medicine, it chose her, and it has been an awesome gift to be part of this profession. Surgery fits her personality better than other medical specialties. Dr. Kwakye needs to fix a problem presented and enjoy the gratification derived from positive immediate outcomes.

Many said she could not make it, or she did not belong and, without having black mentors to look up to or guide her, this made navigating through her journey more difficult. Dr. Kwakye has been fortunate to train in some amazing places, but with this comes the burden of being the minority among the physician staff and sometimes the patient population. This increases instances of micro and macro aggressions. Micro aggressions are comments or actions that subtly and often unconsciously or unintentionally express a prejudiced attitude toward a member of a marginalized group such as a racial minority. Macroaggressions are obvious negative comments or actions towards a marginalized group – a particular race, culture, or gender.

The best advice Dr. Kwakye received was "Take the Road Less Traveled." She credits all her successes to her faith in God, Who gives her the strength to accomplish all things and keeps her grounded.

Dr. Kwakye shared how she is not always confident. She is an introvert who, over time, has worked at being an extrovert. She started practicing being assertive with her inner circle of friends and family. Each day, she found one thing she could be more outspoken about. Now, she is working on saying, "No," and being proactive about crucial confrontations instead of avoiding them.

A typical day for Dr. Kwakye depends on the day. She is usually in the operating room or seeing clinic patients. One day a week is spent teaching, mentoring, and coaching since these are her roles in the medical school. Fridays are her academic days where she focuses on research and building skills to think about problems critically.

Three lessons she would like to impart for the up-and-coming young black female surgeon she wishes she knew going into this field are:

1. Use social media to your advantage. There are mentors available, maybe not in your immediate surroundings, but they are there. They are eager to talk with you, walk with you, and cheer you on.

2. Seek mentors, coaches, AND sponsors. Each person plays a different role and is critical for your success and advancing in the various stages in your career. Sometimes you are as qualified as the next person, but they have an advantage since they have someone in their corner who is advocating for them and making connections. Your mentor/coach/sponsor does not need to be a person of color, just someone who has your back and wishes you to succeed.

3. If you fail, try again, then try again! Cliché maybe, but it is absolutely true, "What doesn't kill you, WILL make you stronger."

Dr. Kwakye's greatest accomplishment is having had two beautiful daughters while she was a resident. It was probably the most challenging time in her life, but it was when she grew the most in strength, compassion, and resilience.

She is well-rounded and finds balance reading books such as *How to be an Antiracist* by Ibram Kendi.

There are three persons she would love to have dinner or talk with. First is her maternal grandmother who died when the doctor was young but lives on in the stories and fond memories many people share when they meet Dr. Kwakye. Her grandmother made a difference in many people's lives by being compassionate and generous. She had a gift for walking in other people's shoes. Second is Julie Freischlag. She is who Dr. Kwakye emulates regarding her leadership style, strength of character, excellence as a surgeon, and her ability to stay human and willingness to discuss her lows and lessons. Lastly, Michelle Obama. Dr. Kwakye feels she should run for President and has a unique way of bringing people together. People listen when she speaks!

Dr. Debra Holly Ford

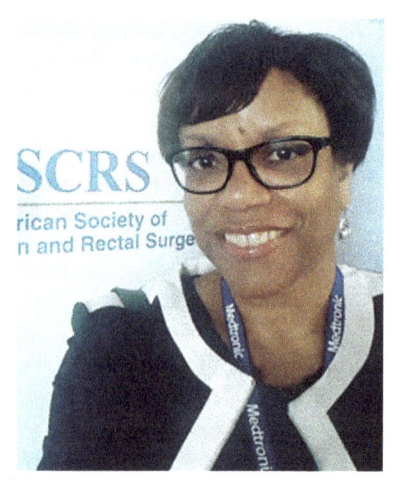

Dr. Debra Holly Ford is an amazing woman. Her chapter begins with a short introduction by editor, Dr. Praise Matemavi.

As I, Dr. Matemavi, interviewed the various contributing surgeons for this book, one question I asked, again and again, was who inspired them to the be best they could be. Amazingly, Dr. Ford was mentioned by every surgeon who met her! They all spoke fondly of Dr. Ford and how she inspired them to be great. They said Dr. Ford was one of the women who flawlessly balanced being a surgeon, a wife, and a mother. I was excited when she agreed to be featured in this book as an all-star black female surgeon, highlighting her career.

Some things the many doctors said inspired them were how intelligent Dr. Ford is and how thorough she is with patient care. Dr. Shuntaye Batson said just watching Dr. Ford inspired her to be compassionate and empathetic to her patients. It was wonderful to have such a positive example. Also, she was impressed to see women can be surgeons and they can do it well. Dr. Gina Jefferson mentioned that Dr. Ford was one of the surgeons who gave her a solid foundation that prepared her for her otolaryngology (ear, nose, and throat) training.

Dr. Ford inspired greatness in people around her, not only residents but also ancillary staff as well. When I talked with Dr. Nadege Fackche, she spoke about how amazing Dr. Ford is as a surgeon as well as a leader. She spoke highly of her dedication to education and said Dr. Ford is a surgeon's surgeon, meaning she is the surgeon that other surgeons want to be like and have as their surgeon.

Currently, Dr. Ford is an associate professor of surgery and vice-chair of the Department of Surgery at Howard University College of Medicine (HUCM) in Washington, D.C. She is head of the section of colon and rectal surgery and founding medical director of the Howard University Health Sciences Simulation and Clinical Skills Center. She is also the senior associate dean of Academic Affairs.

Dr. Ford is a native of Pine Bluff, Arkansas, and was educated through the public-school system. She received her Bachelor of Science degree in zoology in 1982 from Howard University and in 1986, earned her doctor of medicine degree at Howard University.

After graduating from the Howard University College of Medicine as the top-ranking medical student, she successfully completed a general surgery residency at Howard University Hospital (HUH) in 1991. In addition, she received further training in colon and rectal surgery at the University of Texas and Affiliated Hospitals in Houston, Texas.

Dr. Ford is board-certified by the American Board of Surgery and is the first African American female to earn board-certification in colon and rectal surgery in the United States. She is the first African American female to become a Fellow of the American College of Colon and Rectal Surgeons.

She has been a member of the faculty at the Howard University College of Medicine since September 1994. She has served on numerous national committees including the American College of Surgeons' Committee on Diversity Issues.

Dr. Ford has received many honors including the Kaiser Permanente Teaching Award and has been named to Black Enterprises 'America's Leading Doctors' and The Washingtonian Magazine 'Top Doctors in the Washington Metropolitan Area.'

Dr. Ford is actively involved in teaching every level of undergraduate and graduate medical education. She was a member of the HUH Graduate Medical Education Committee for 15 years and served as Associate Designated Institutional Officer (DIO). In addition, she is a member of the HUCM Curriculum Committee. She served a 14-year tenure as program director of the HUH general surgery residency where she guided the surgical training of more than 90 resident surgeons. She is an active member of the Association of Program Directors in Surgery and the Association for Surgical Education. Dr. Ford is a member of the Simulation Committee of the Association for Surgical Education and a member of the Society for Simulation in Healthcare.

The immediate past chair of the National Medical Association's Surgical Section, she is a member of the Society for Black Academic Surgery and the Washington Metropolitan Chapter of the American College of Surgeons (ACS). Dr. Ford is a past president of the local ACS chapter and has held every leadership position and committee chair in the local chapter. She has served as an American Board of Surgery associate examiner. In addition, she was a member of the National Board of Medical Examiners/USMLE Surgery Test Writing Committee for five years.

Dr. Ford has mentored many pre-medical and medical students. She frequently speaks to educate the public about colon and rectal cancer and screening. Dr. Ford has a surgical practice at Howard University Hospital. Her areas of interest are the prevention and management of colorectal cancer, diagnosis and management of inflammatory bowel disease, and the treatment of benign anorectal conditions.

CHAPTER EIGHT
Hepatobiliary and Pancreas Surgery

HPB (hepato-pancreatico-biliary) surgery is a subspecialty of surgery specific to benign and malignant diseases of the liver, pancreas, and biliary tree.

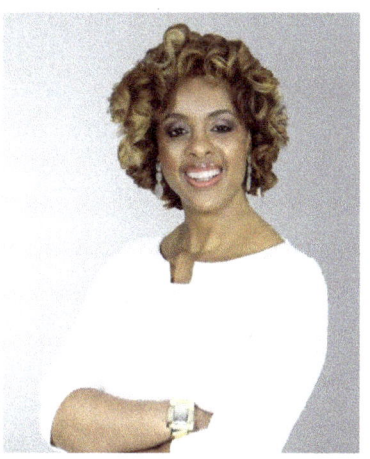

Dr. KMarie Reid

Dr. KMarie Reid is an accomplished hepatobiliary (liver and gall bladder) and pancreas surgeon, prolific researcher, patient advocate, and Operation Desert Shield Army veteran. Her award-winning research in the treatment of liver and pancreatic cancers has made her a respected authority in her field. She has more than 100 peer-reviewed publications and book chapters.

She earned her Bachelor of Science degree from St. Joseph's College in New York and her medical degree at Washington University in St. Louis, Missouri. She completed her residency in general surgery at the University of Pittsburgh, Pennsylvania, finished a fellowship in hepato-pancreato-biliary surgery, and a master's degree in biomedical sciences at the Mayo Clinic, Rochester, Minnesota, and finally, her Master's in Business Management at Brandeis University, Waltham, Massachusetts.

Currently, Dr. Reid is a professor of surgery at the Morehouse School of Medicine, Atlanta, Georgia. She also serves as the director of quality and chief for the section of liver, pancreas, and foregut surgery. She is the chief of surgery for Morehouse at Grady Memorial Hospital where she also serves as the medical director of quality. Before becoming a professor at Morehouse, she was a consulting surgeon and associate professor at the Mayo Clinic in Rochester, Minnesota.

Dr. Reid grew up in May Pen, Jamaica, and when she was a preteen, her family moved to the United States. Her grandmother came to the U.S. as a seamstress when in the '60s and '70s, there was an incentive allowing Caribbean individuals with certain skill sets to migrate to the United States, London, and Canada.

Once her grandmother settled in New York, she worked hard so she could afford for her children to join her. Dr. Reid's mother and three of her six siblings took her up on her offer. Here, Dr. Reid's mother worked and saved money.

When Dr. Reid's family came to the United States, they lived in the Flatbush area of Brooklyn, New York City, a neighborhood with many others from Jamaica. They were immersed in Jamaican culture. Dr. Reid did not leave her culture until she attended medical school at Washington University in St. Louis, Missouri. It was a huge culture shock.

Even though Dr. Reid grew up in the United States, the immigrant communities in New York are close knit. For instance, residents of Little Italy and Chinatown have strong cultural ties to their countries of origin. These are close communities that maintain their culture with different rates of assimilation.

So, even though she was not in Jamaica, Dr. Reid may as well have been because her church, her food, her community, her restaurants, and everything else was Jamaican. She is a Jamaican American woman and her family lives in Jamaica. Dr. Reid tries to go home once a year. This is the influence she grew up with.

Dr. Reid says she receives downloads from the universe and she listens to them. At eight-years-of-age, she wanted to become an astronomer. A voice told her, "No. You're going to be a doctor." Ever since then she walked the talk. She often said, "I'm going to be a doctor. I'm going to be a doctor." If you look through her graduation books, her classmates from elementary school through medical school signed, "Congratulations on being a doctor!" That is how much she spoke about it and lived it.

Her uncle, Dr. Sandford Prince, was 11 years older than she. He became an oral and maxillofacial surgeon. He attended dental school at Washington University. When Dr. Reid applied to medical school, she wanted to follow in his footsteps, so she applied to Washington University even though it was out of her community and region of the country. When Dr. Reid came to interview for medical school admission at Washington University, the dental school had recently closed. The dean of the dental school, however, was on staff and part of the medical school admission committee. He remembered her uncle was one of his best students. So, he was excited to say, "Yes! You're coming here," and Dr. Reid attended Washington University as a medical student.

There is one pivotal moment in Dr. Reid's career that impacted her greatly. A young plastic surgeon who still practices there, Dr. Susan Mackinnon, came to talk to Dr. Reid's second-year class about her surgical practice. She is a nerve reconstruction specialist who also performs facial surgeries. Dr. Reid remembers falling in love with the whole concept of being able to reconstruct a body part and improve someone's life. Instead of taking a vacation break between her second and third year of medical school as other classmates did, Dr. Reid shadowed Dr. Mackinnon and the other plastic surgeons. It was then that Dr. Reid chose to become a surgeon.

Dr. Reid chose surgery for her first rotation and had an incredible experience working with Dr. Timothy Buchman, who is now on faculty at the Emory University Hospital in Atlanta, Georgia. She also had the wonderful and life-changing experience of working with the famous hepatobiliary surgeon Dr. Steven Strasberg. Dr. Reid fell in love with how the liver looks and what it does. She was intrigued by the challenge of being a liver and pancreas surgeon and, as her career path continued, she chose this specialty.

Dr. Reid had much support along her career path, so much that if you asked how she was challenged during the different stages, she was not. She cruised through with support until she became an attending. During her early years as an attending, Dr. Reid experienced racism and sexism and, for her, the sexism was often worse than the racism.

Along the way, Dr. Reid heard things such as, "Women shouldn't be surgeons. Women should not be operating. Women shouldn't do this or that." In many surgical societies, there were closed doors to leadership for women and minorities, but this is changing.

Still, many times Dr. Reid is the only black woman in the room. There are not many black women surgeons, but they are working to change this. There are increasing numbers of women, but not the representation Dr. Reid would like to see for Black women.

After training, Dr. Reid was the only black person in her department for her first job. This was a rude awakening since she is from the Caribbean, where they do not culturally focus on race because everyone is a similar race. There are Indian and Chinese influences in the Caribbean because they came to live and work there after slavery, but no one focused on race. So, it has taken Dr. Reid 40 years living in the United States to see race the way black Americans see race. She still does not think she sees it as wholly as they do but she does experience it and understands the dilemma and the challenges.

Dr. Reid shared, "I came into residency with seven or eight manuscripts and finished my fellowship training with 20 to 30 publications in scientific journals. I was productive. When it came time to become an associate professor, the chair of the promotions committee of the institution asked, "What are you waiting on?" He thought I was more than prepared because of my 60 publications and it appeared I was waiting for someone else to tell me I was ready. As an academic surgeon, publications in peer-reviewed scientific journals show how productive you are and is a requirement for advancement in each stage of your career."

She adds, "One of the things I always say is, you have to be excellent. You cannot think you are playing the same game as everyone around you. No, it is not fair, but you must accept the reality of this and still strive to be excellent. You need to surround yourself with people who support you. If you are at a job and you are not being supported, you should leave and find another job. If you are in a supportive environment, you will flourish. One of the things I tell young women is to know what it takes to move from an assistant to an associate and from an associate to a full professor. Sometimes, the bar is low and sometimes, the bar is high. I cannot emphasize this enough. You must know the rules of the game (meaning, know exactly what you need to accomplish to advance to the next level in your career) and you have to play the game well and understand that no one takes you by the hand and leads you after your training is complete."

"Understanding that no one will lead you in your career requires shifting your mindset from being a student and being told what to do to taking your career firmly in-hand. You must understand what it takes to make career advancements. Once I understood you need a national reputation to be promoted to a professor because people with national reputations outside your institution write letters of recommendations for you, it led to my making sure I was on national committees for the surgical and medical societies I belonged to. I strove to do an excellent job on these committees. This is how others became acquainted with me and my work. Eventually, the chairman of the committee and some board members learned about me. So, when it came time to be promoted, they wrote letters of recommendation on my behalf. You need to create an infrastructure of support, which many black people do not do. They choose to be alone in the process with grandma praying for them at home."

We never want to underestimate the power or prayer by the ones that love us, but Dr. Reid feels, "This is not enough. This is not enough. This is not enough! Support from family is terrific when it is available, but you need to have support from peers and leaders in your field, and more than one."

In her own words, Dr. Reid shared her thoughts on how to be successful.

The first thing is you must be excellent. In Jamaica, we say, "Don't give nobody nothing to talk about you." Meaning, do not offer things that allow others to talk poorly about you. You cannot use the race card for your poor performance. If you are late for work and you are not doing your professional duties and you are doing a poor job taking care of patients, you are just a poor surgeon or doctor. No one can protect you. So, you must be excellent. This is what I am driving into our students, some of whom want to be spoon-fed and want people to do their tasks for them.

You must be excellent, there is no shortage of the need for excellence. This means you may be tired because you are writing papers after work and you cannot go on vacation with your buddies because you must study for your ABSITE exam. You may have to miss your friend's bachelorette party because you have a paper and an abstract due for a conference. It means you must sacrifice to get to your goal.

The second thing is you must create a vision board. This is because if you do not have a strong vision of where you are going, your actions and your decisions will not be in alignment with your visions. You will be all over the place.

I prepare a vision board annually and I have been doing this since I was a child. I knew what I wanted, and I spoke it into existence. So, speak what you want into existence and believe it is going to happen. I live a life of clear intention. Whatever I desire, I write it down. I visualize it. It is on a vision board. It is in my daily mantras and it is in my daily thoughts. So, my thoughts, my words, and my actions are all in alignment.

The third thing is to know the difference between a mentor and a sponsor. You need many. What does this mean? A mentor is someone who tells you what to do to get to the next step because they have been through these steps.

Sponsorship is different from mentorship. I have a story for illustration. I grew up in the era when hip-hop began in Brooklyn. I am hip-hop. When Jay Z was a young rapper on the scene, he worked with Jaz-O who introduced him to the famous rapper, Big Daddy Kane. Big Daddy Kane was huge to us during this time. He was not nationally known but locally, he was a powerhouse. So, this type of introduction is what a mentor may do. I am going to introduce you to this person of influence.

But what Big Daddy Kane did for Jay Z was a sponsor move. Big Daddy Kane took Jay Z on tour and not only allowed him to be the opening performance for his concerts, he also brought him on stage with him, performing with him and exposing him to his audience. This validated Jay Z because of his association with him. So, a sponsor is someone who endorses you and opens doors for you.

Early in my career as faculty, I had a sponsor, Dr. Michael Sarr, who talked about me and said, "She's the best. She is amazing. She is terrific. This is not because she is a black woman, it is because she is KMarie Reid. She is amazing and she should have this." He put his credibility on the line and used his power and influence to open doors for me. This is a sponsor.

I have always been confident. It is because of the love from my family and extended family I had growing up. I had five uncles and an aunt and my grandmother and my mom that loved on me so hard, it helped me develop into a confident person.

When I was born, my grandmother said to my mom, "She's going to be a jewel in your crown." So, hearing this story and having this blessing on my life from such an early age made me a confident person. Later, I discovered the secret identity of my biological father when I was 30 years old. I am glad I had the opportunity to meet, know, and adore him as I do now.

My favorite operation is the Whipple procedure, also known as a pancreatico-duodenectomy mostly used to remove cancers from the head of the pancreas. I also love liver resections. I love it all. I love gastrostomies, removing part of the stomach for cancer or ulcers. They are simple and quick. But I still consider a Whipple my favorite if I had to choose just one!

I feel becoming a doctor is my greatest accomplishment. There was no other path for me. There was only the dream I could do it and I did it. Despite many obstacles, I figured out a way to do it.

Another of my proudest moments and my greatest

achievements was receiving my MBA and delivering the commencement speech. Prior to earning my Master's in Business Administration (MBA), I took a sabbatical. It was a year or two to invest in myself emotionally, physically, spiritually, and to complete my MBA.

In what little free time I have, I tend to read self-development books that deal with personal improvement and leadership. I am reading *Success Principles* by Jack Canfield and *Daring Greatly: How the Courage to be Vulnerable Transforms the Way We Live, Love, Parent, and Lead* by Brene Brown. I am also reading, *In Search of Sisterhood: Delta Sigma Theta* and *The Challenge of the Black Sorority Movement* by Paula Giddings. I go between these simultaneously. I am constantly reading something.

"Nothing replaces excellence and you must be committed to working hard. There are many sacrifices you will make but, if it is your passion, these choices come easily. If it is not your passion and you find yourself combating and fighting to do it, then it is probably not in alignment with your true self and desires. You need to be in alignment with your true self, so it is imperative that you take the time to know who you are."

"I alone cannot change the world, but I can cast a stone across the water to create many ripples." – Mother Teresa

CHAPTER NINE
Endocrine Surgery

Endocrine surgery is a surgical sub-specialty focusing on surgery of the endocrine glands, including the thyroid gland, the parathyroid glands, the adrenal glands, glands of the endocrine pancreas, and some neuroendocrine glands.

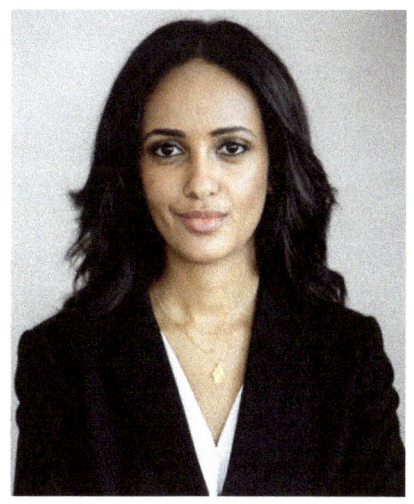

Dr. Aida Taye

Dr. Aida Taye was accepted into the BA/MD Early Selection Scholar program at George Washington University in Washington, D.C., where she graduated *magna cum laude* and was elected to Phi Beta Kappa at George Washington University. Early selection is a program that allows students to earn a combined bachelor's degree and medical degree at the same time after high school, taking six years instead of the usual eight.

Dr. Taye completed her residency in general surgery at the Albert Einstein College of Medicine Montefiore Medical Center in Bronx, New York, where she was appointed academic surgical chief resident. During her time at the Albert Einstein College of Medicine, she also held the position of general surgery resident representative of the Graduate Medical Education Committee.

Following her residency, Dr. Taye completed a one-year fellowship in endocrine and metabolic surgery at the Icahn School of Medicine at Mount Sinai, in Manhattan, New York City, under the direction of William B. Inabnet III, MD.

Her current research interests include efficient and cost-effective localization of parathyroid adenomas, molecular characterizations of intermediate thyroid nodules, and secondary hyperparathyroidism after gastric bypass surgery. She has been published in peer-reviewed journals for her work in endocrine disorders and she has also presented her work at conferences across the country.

Dr. Taye's clinical interests include the treatment of benign and malignant diseases of the thyroid, parathyroid, and adrenal glands. She is also interested in general surgery, minimally invasive surgery, and bariatric surgery.

She is passionate about sustainable global surgery programs. This means rather than short-term mission trips to developing countries to provide much-needed surgical care, Dr. Taye wants to help local programs develop surgical services and train doctors to provide the care on a long-term basis. She has worked in Ecuador, Sudan, Ethiopia, and India.

Dr. Taye grew up in Addis Ababa, Ethiopia, and moved to the United States when she was 14 years old. Medicine was her top career choice because she excelled in sciences and was affected by the lack of standard medical care in her city. A family member, in need of a kidney transplant, traveled overseas because dialysis and transplantation were not available 20 years ago. Now, there are renal transplant options in Ethiopia.

When she attended medical school at George Washington University, she was accepted to the BA/MD program as a sophomore. This allowed her the opportunity to spend summer breaks working with overseas medical missions before entering medical school. Surgery seemed to be a critically needed specialty along with additional skills to treat medical and surgical emergencies. By the time she was in her first year of medical school, she decided she wanted to be a surgeon. On her first day of medical school, she met a female surgeon at a meet-and-greet. Dr. Taye told her she was interested in surgery and this surgeon invited Dr. Taye to shadow her in the operating room. This early exposure, especially with a female surgeon, was an important encouragement for her.

Initially, Dr. Taye wanted to be a transplant surgeon. After exposure at a transplant center in New York City, she ruled transplantation out. However, the experience confirmed her excitement to consider a different surgical training in New York City. Here, there was diversity in patients, pathologies, traumas, and exposure to different specialties. She contemplated vascular surgery during residency. Eventually, she discovered she enjoyed endocrine surgery. Dr. Taye feels graduating from her general surgery residency was her proudest moment.

Dr. Taye is excited by the complex work-up of patients leading to surgery and an opportunity to operate on various parts of the human body. She also had endocrine surgery mentors who inspired her; one was the president of the American Association of Endocrine Surgeons at the time.

Looking back, Dr. Taye feels her greatest challenges were her financial challenges. Finding funding for her schooling was a challenge.

If she had to choose only one surgery to do, she would choose a laparoscopic adrenalectomy, the removal of an adrenal gland through a small incision with the use of a small scope.

Dr. Taye admits she still experiences impostor syndrome occasionally when she finds herself at the lectern or on a panel at surgical meetings, sitting next to highly accomplished people. It lessens with time as her confidence and knowledge grows. As a surgeon, any complication, even the ones no one can control, can bring about this temporary feeling. Dr. Taye knows impostor syndrome is universal. Even men and older surgeons experience it. It comes when physicians find themselves growing to the next level, having a novel experience, or experiencing failure.

The most important lesson Dr. Taye feels she has learned is knowing how to fail well. There will be many failures in life, and it is important to remember there is always a plan B for everything.

Dr. Taye works at finding balance. Both she and her husband are passionate about physical, mental, and spiritual health. They do not drink alcohol and they cook mostly plant-based meals at home at least five days a week. They make time to exercise and spend time with friends. Dr. Taye also spends time reading. Two books she is currently reading about personal finance and investing are *Your Money, Your Life* by Vicki Robin and *Playing with FIRE* by Scott Rieckens. She also enjoys reading popular memoirs such as *Educated* by Tara Westover.

Dr. Taye's words of encouragement are, "Work hard. Nothing replaces hard work. Find a mentor. They do not have to look like you. Don't be afraid to fail."

"Everyone can rise above their circumstances and achieve success if they are dedicated to and passionate about what they do."
— Nelson Mandela

CHAPTER TEN
Neurosurgery

Neurosurgery/neurological surgery focuses on the prevention, diagnosis, surgical treatment, and rehabilitation of disorders affecting portions of the nervous system including the brain, spinal cord, peripheral nerves, and cerebrovascular system.

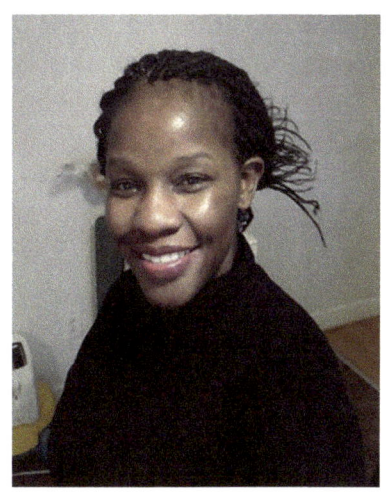

Dr. Juliet Sekabunga Nalwanga

Dr. Juliet Sekabunga Nalwanga is a neurosurgeon at the Mulago National Referral Hospital in Kampala, Uganda, Africa. After finishing medical school, she completed her internship at Lira Regional Referral Hospital Lira, Uganda, and Mulago National Referral Hospital before completing her additional training in general surgery at the Mbarara University of Science and Technology, Mbarara, Uganda. She completed a neurosurgery residency at Mulago National Referral Hospital and wrote an essay detailing her journey to becoming the first female neurosurgeon in Uganda.

This is Dr. Juliet Sekabunga Nalwanga's story.

God designed us to carry out His purpose on earth and many different people come into our lives along our journey to help us fulfill this purpose. My name is Dr. Juliet Sekabunga Nalwanga. I believe in Jesus as my personal Lord and Savior. I am a mother of one and I am Uganda's first female neurosurgeon.

I was born and raised in Uganda. My father was a pediatric surgeon and my mother was a clerk at Mulago Hospital. Despite having parents in the medical field, I spent most of my childhood with my mother's family. My father did not live with us. We were poor and my mother struggled to pay my school fees. Often, she did not have money for my schooling until one month after school started. This made me late for school. Amazingly, I still managed to be top of my class at the end of the school term.

At times, the head of the school allowed me to attend without my mother paying the fees, hoping she would pay later. At home, my mother, my two brothers, my two cousins, and I lived in a one-room house. Sometimes, we did not have food to eat. Thankfully, we had a small house in a low-income section of the town where we lived, though the house was not habitable.

As a young girl, I dreamed of working at the Bank of Uganda because we were told bankers are rich people. We had extraordinarily little, but I have fond memories of our family. We loved each other and shared what little we had.

During my last year of primary school in 1995, one of my aunts, Dr. Jane Bosa Ssewanyanna, who was the director of the Makerere University Hospital, decided to take me into her home and pay for my schooling. I completed my primary schooling and was recognized as the best student that year. My secondary school years were filled with turmoil. I succumbed to peer pressure and my grades dropped. It was a time of self-discovery as my body was changing and I was under the influence of my ever-changing hormones. Secondary school can be a defining point in life, and I learned it can make or break future career aspirations.

I lost my mother in 1999 and, shortly after, my father died. It was during this difficult time I made a decision that would shape my life. During my earlier years of secondary school, I loved history and thought I would become a lawyer. The notion of becoming a lawyer faded as I watched City of Angels starring Nicholas Cage and Meg Ryan. This movie changed my life. I saw her passion as a surgeon, and I knew then I wanted to become a surgeon.

I told my aunt, Dr. Bosa, about my passion to pursue a medical career. God is amazing. As soon as I made my decision to study medicine, our Uganda Certificate of Education results were released, and I was the best female student at Ndejje Senior Secondary School in December of 1999. I had the great grades required to obtain a position to take the classes I needed to attend medical school, such classes as physics, chemistry, and biology. It was not easy, and I struggled at times but had enough points to be accepted into medical school.

As a first-year medical student, I still had no idea what I wanted to be. At first, the anatomy lectures were frightening. We cut dead bodies. But, as time went by, this became my favorite subject. During our third year, we went to patient wards and I loved pediatrics and general surgery. However, we lacked mentors in those two disciplines. Internal medicine, on the other hand, had so many mentors I thought to myself, "Maybe cardiology would be my next option." I continued pushing myself to be the best I could be and by the time I completed my fifth year of medical school, I was certain I wanted to pursue internal medicine.

After undergraduate training, my first internship rotation was general surgery. I met a wonderful surgeon in the Lira Regional Referral Hospital named Dr. William Ocen. He loved to teach. My passion for surgery was slowly being reignited, but my heart was still in internal medicine. When I rotated through internal medicine at Mulago National Hospital, my views changed. There were so many deaths and at times, we did not know the cause of death. I found this disturbing.

During rounds one morning, I met Professor Kijjambu. He was a lecturer (teacher) at Makerere University. He had known my father, who was his teacher. He invited me to the surgeons' meeting where I was warmly welcomed to the department. I felt like a returning prodigal child because I had been running away from my calling of going into surgery.

As they say, the rest is history. I trained in surgical rotations at the Kampala International Hospital in Bushenyi and the Mbarara Regional Referral Hospital. Then, I joined Mbarara Hospital as a general surgery resident and lecturer at the university. As residents, we taught medical students. During my training, I met people who inspired me and believed in me.

My general surgery training was not a smooth ride. My son was one year old when I began my training. There were times I was on call for 36 to 48 hours and because my pay as a resident was insufficient, I worked part-time to afford living expenses and care for my child. Sometimes we were apart for 72 hours.

Later that first year, I decided to concentrate on my studies and my son, so I quit my part-time work. This came at a cost because it was difficult to make ends meet, but I was able to spend more time with my son, especially when I was not on call.

I am grateful for my general surgery lecturers (teachers), Professor Alcides Lopez (Cuba), Professor David Kitya, Professor D. Bitariho, Dr. Sr. Justine Najjuka, Dr. Gerald Tumusiime, and Dr. Deus Twesigye for teaching me the craft of surgery and encouraging me throughout my training.

After completing my general surgery training, I rotated through neurosurgery. It was then I discovered my passion for neurosurgery. I spoke to Professor Kayanja about the neurosurgery scholarship position available in Mulago under the College of Surgeons of Eastern, Central and Southern Africa (COSECSA). He was supportive and instrumental in helping me secure a position.

I met the team in Mulago led by Dr. Michael Edgar Muhumuza and the Duke Neurosurgery team led by Professor Michael Haglund. In my heart, this was another example of God's faithfulness. He always makes a way where there seems to be no way.

The new team was phenomenal and to this day, I see them as my neurosurgery fathers. I will never forget Dr. Joel Kiryabwire, Dr. John B Mukasa, and Dr. Hussein Ssenyonjo.

The neurosurgery fellowship I began in September 2013 and finished in December 2017 was more challenging than my general surgery residency. I was one of two fellows. This meant we were on call every other day and in the operating room (OR) when we were not on call. The schedule was hectic. I lost contact with most of my family. I had no time off. I had to believe God and trust He would see me to completion of the program because there were so many times I wanted to give up. Despite being the only female in training, I never felt mistreated. My colleagues and I were treated the same.

I took my written examination in September 2017 and my oral examination in December 2017, followed by graduating as Uganda's first female neurosurgeon.

Near the end of this fellowship, I received another scholarship to Wisconsin (USA) for two months and this opened more doors for a position to train in pediatric neurosurgery at the Hospital for Sick Children in Toronto, Canada, where I am currently completing a one-year fellowship in pediatric neurosurgery.

During my undergraduate years, becoming a surgeon seemed so difficult and, amazingly, I fainted during one of the surgical procedures. During my internship, I met several surgeons who made me believe surgery was a possible option. Being the only female during my training and the first left me with a great sense of accomplishment. It is difficult when no one who looks like you has gone before you to ask questions about how they made it.

Being a pioneer taught me to encourage myself daily and know that going through the different challenges was preparing me to uphold those who would follow in my footsteps. This inspires you to excel in integrity, diligence, honor, strength, and accountability and to be disciplined. God has always been my greatest Encourager; the faith within to believe the unbelievable and dream the unthinkable. I had to believe in myself and know I could make it. I always tell myself, "God has not brought me this far to leave me. He is faithful and He will complete that which He started in me."

"If you can't fly, then run. If you can't run, then walk. If you can't walk, then crawl. but whatever you do, you have to keep moving forward."

Martin Luther King Jr

Dr. Claire Karekezi

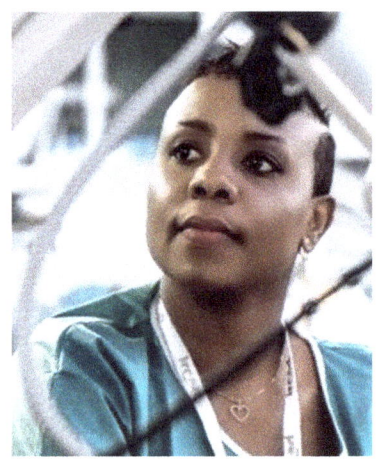

Dr. Claire Karekezi is a consultant neurosurgeon at the Rwanda Military Hospital, Africa. She obtained her Doctor of Medicine degree from the University of Rwanda, College of Medicine and Health Sciences in 2009. She graduated as a neurosurgeon in 2016 from the Mohamed V University, World Federation of Neurosurgical Societies (WFNS)-Rabat Training Center for African Neurosurgeons in Morocco, Africa.

She completed a clinical fellowship in neuro-oncology and skull base surgery at the University of Toronto, Toronto Western Hospital, Canada. Upon her return home to Rwanda in July 2018, she became Rwanda's first female neurosurgeon. She has been featured in multiple newspaper articles and television and radio programs. She was a TedExEuston presenter and her topic was *Joining the Ranks of Neurosurgery: Her Impossible Dream*!

When Dr. Karekezi came home, she was offered a position at the Rwanda Military Hospital where she was challenged to create and oversee the neurosurgical department. It was difficult to organize things without an existing neurosurgery department. There were the challenges of hiring a team, purchasing equipment, and beginning to see patients and performing operations without these things in place. It was especially difficult because Dr. Karekezi was used to the equipment and the resources being fully available the way they were in Toronto during her fellowship.

Dr. Karekezi was alone for almost one year until another neurosurgeon newly trained was hired. Now there are six neurosurgeons for the whole country of about 12 million people. All are in the capital city of Kigali based at the Rwanda Military Hospital, one of the largest referral hospitals in the country.

The journey to becoming the first female neurosurgeon in Rwanda began for Dr. Karekezi as she grew up in Butare until she was six years old. It was then that her family moved to Kigali. In high school, she was an excellent student. Students with high exam scores majored in mathematics or physics. She was a mathematics major which meant she studied physics, biology, and chemistry. This major fit well with her because, initially, she wanted to be a pilot or work for NASA. Dr. Karekezi also grew up thinking she would become a doctor someday. She did well on her exams and most people who scored high pursued a career in medicine.

Dr. Karekezi returned to Butare and, after finishing six years of medical school, she completed her general practitioner assignment in Kigali. This is a mandatory two-year program, but she was able to complete it in one and a half years.

During her fourth year in medical school, Dr. Karekezi applied for an externship in Sweden. She intended to study radiology but was only offered neurosurgery because it was summertime and most departments did not receive foreign students. She met the head of the neurosurgery department, Dr. Jan Hillman. Most of his residents were away for holiday and he had also recently returned from holiday. The department consisted of him, his scrub nurse, and one operating room nurse. Dr. Karekezi worked with him and his team.

Dr. Hillman changed her life in just one month. He took time to teach her and helped her understand more about her own country by asking her questions for which she did not know the answers. It made her research and report back to him. He was the first person to see a light in Dr. Karekezi and tell her she could be a neurosurgeon. His belief in her made her believe in herself.

When she returned home, Dr. Karekezi focused on becoming a neurosurgeon and searched for neurosurgery training programs. She doubted she could become a neurosurgeon because there were no programs in her country. At that time, Rwanda had one neurosurgeon for 11 million people, and it seemed impossible to train abroad. Dr. Hillman stayed in touch with her and wrote a letter of recommendation when an opportunity presented to apply for training in Morocco.

One year before graduating from medical school, she applied to Oxford, England, to complete a neurosurgery elective. Dr. Karekezi received an email from the coordinator that even though she was almost a year late applying for this position, she granted Dr. Karekezi a position to rotate at Oxford on the neurosurgery service. This was a miracle.

The rotation was educational in many ways. There were seven or eight trainees following the professor. Dr. Karekezi remembers how everyone else seemed so established and advanced. It was a one-month elective and she worked hard. During this time, she realized her knowledge of the anatomy of the brain, spinal cord, and peripheral nervous system was not strong, so she spent a great deal of time in the library studying and preparing for surgical cases.

One day, while learning about subarachnoid hemorrhages, one of the fellows mentioned the World Federation of Neurosurgical Societies (WFNS). He advised Dr. Karekezi to read about the classification system of subarachnoid hemorrhages (bleeding in the brain). When she read the assigned material, she was taken to the website of the World Federation of Neurosurgical Societies which opened the world of neurosurgery training for her. It was there she discovered the different training programs available and immediately emailed the program director at the Rabat Reference Center for Training Young African Neurosurgeons in Morocco telling him she was interested in his program.

After finishing her rotation in the United Kingdom, she returned home. Dr. Karekezi did not receive a response from the program director in Morocco. She continued emailing him and he finally responded!

Dr. Karekezi was working as a general practitioner when her letter of acceptance arrived. They wanted her to start training right away. She was accepted to train at the World Federation of Neurosurgical Societies (WFNS)-Rabat Training Center for

African Neurosurgeons in Morocco. This neurosurgery training program was part of the Mohamed V University, so she was required to be a student of the University separately, which turned out to be an unexpected challenge. When she received her acceptance letter, she wrote the Minister in Rwanda requesting sponsorship to train in Morocco. This was granted.

During her training, the director of the neurosurgery training program often told her he liked her perseverance and persistence and how he remembered her long emails. Dr. Karekezi almost lost faith because it took so long to be accepted. She did not realize how acclaimed the director was in the world of neurosurgery until she was in training. In Morocco, education is free. She only needed money for living expenses. Dr. Karekezi was the first Rwandan to be in Morocco for specialized medical education.

Training was difficult, but she persevered. The challenge of acclimating to a completely new system and culture was greater because Dr. Karekezi was away from her family. She made friends and adapted to her new environment. One thing she learned was the importance of attending conferences and courses specific to her craft because this was where she met people that became her mentors. She applied for a Women in Neurosurgery award to assist with expenses to attend an international neurosurgery conference and flew to San Francisco, USA, for this conference.

While in San Francisco, she met a surgeon who became one of her mentors when she eventually went to Toronto, Canada, for specialty training. Soon after her residency, Dr. Karekezi was the recipient of the AANS International Visiting Surgeon Award and this took her to Brigham and Women's Hospital in Boston, Massachusetts, for three months. Here she met incredible neurosurgeons and learned from them. She went on to Mount Sinai Hospital in New York after leaving Boston and it became another great networking and educational opportunity.

Dr. Karekezi was accepted for a fellowship in skull base

and neurooncology at the University of Toronto in Canada. This was a one-year fellowship from July 2017-June 2018. She returned to Rwanda after this fellowship to start a neurosurgery program at her institution.

She trained in Morocco for five years, but Dr. Karekezi never noticed a difference in the way she was treated compared to her male counterparts. It was during her fellowship training she felt she was treated unfairly. Dr. Karekezi had a crisis of confidence because there was one time she looked at herself and thought, "I am from Africa. I am black and a woman in a male-dominated field. I do not belong here."

This was short-lived because, soon after, she met two professors who became the best mentors a girl could ask for, Dr. Fred Gentili and Dr. Mark Bernstein, who sponsored the scholarship she received to travel to San Francisco as a resident.

Though Dr. Gentili is a world-renowned neurosurgeon, he is a humble person who made a huge impact on her growth as a neurosurgeon. His trust in her empowered her. It is a challenge for people to trust someone especially when they are new. He boosted Dr. Karekezi's confidence and was one of the greatest mentors she has ever had.

Dr. Karekezi faced challenges coming home. It has always been a challenge to prove herself. She shares, "When you come home, everyone looks at you and wonders what you are capable of, especially when you are a woman surgeon. I remember many people coming to my theater (operating room) when I performed my first surgery. Being the first woman neurosurgeon in the country and having a great deal of media coverage made me feel tremendous pressure to succeed."

Dr. Karekezi remains in contact with her former mentors. So, whenever she has a complex case, she has people to discuss the case with. She knows what she can do and what she is not capable of doing with the equipment and resources she has. Dr. Karekezi began with simple cases and is gradually accepting more complicated ones.

As everyone knows, neurosurgery is a complex specialty

that requires a dedicated team to care for patients. At first, Dr. Karekezi did not have residents or medical students, so she did everything herself. She pulled drains, wrote notes, changed post-operative dressings, and completed patient discharge paperwork. Everything. Her first year was challenging in terms of coming home to Rwanda after training for nine years abroad and proving herself as a surgeon. Now that the foundation is laid, she is at a point she can grow as a surgeon.

A typical work week for Dr. Karekezi is she operates on Mondays. She has one or two surgical cases depending on how long they run. On Tuesdays and Thursdays, she sees patients in the clinic and operates as needed if an emergency presents. On Wednesdays, she has teaching rounds and discharges post-operative patients when they are ready to go home. On Fridays, she sees her private practice patients and operates on them. She usually has five-six cases per week.

Dr. Karekezi feels her greatest accomplishments are having completed 95 surgeries in the first 12 months practicing alone and building the neurosurgery program from the ground up.

The best advice she received is to be patient and keep persevering. Dr. Karekezi's mentors told her to not allow people to bully her and to fight for what she believes in. She was advised to start slow with easy cases to develop confidence in herself and her team, and to work toward more complex cases.

Dr. Karekezi is extremely busy, but she takes time to read a good book. Presently, she is reading Becoming by Michelle Obama.

"We have to mentor and fight for the younger girls that look up to us and help them achieve their wildest dreams. As Winston Churchill said, 'Success is not final; failure is not fatal: it is the courage to continue that counts.'"

"Success is walking from failure to failure with no loss of enthusiasm." -- Winston Churchill

Dr. J. Nozipo Maraire

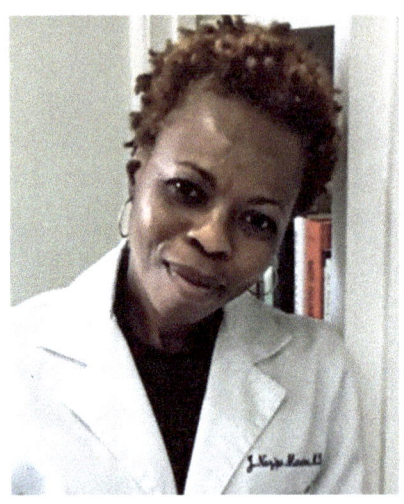

Have you ever read about someone and somehow knew that even though they are famous and accomplished, you would meet them one day? It has been 12 years since I, Dr. Praise Matemavi, discovered Dr. J. Nozipo Maraire's book, *Zenzele: A Letter for My Daughter.* I was a second-year medical student at Michigan State University College of Osteopathic Medicine in East Lansing, Michigan. It was a rare phenomenon to see a Zimbabwean woman thriving and finding a place in this complicated world of black female surgeons, in this land we now called home.

Even though I did not have anyone who resembled me that I knew was a surgeon, I had Dr. Maraire. I read every article written about her I could find. She unknowingly became a mentor to me. I often read and re-read one of the articles written about her in the *Yale Medicine Magazine* titled, *The Many Worlds of Nozipo Maraire.* This provided a glimpse into her world as she balanced training as a neurosurgeon, obtained a master's degree in public health, and wrote a best-selling novel. To me, she is the epitome of what living one's best life and seizing the day means: the meaning of going after one's dreams and passions, working hard, and striving for greatness, whatever greatness means to you.

Throughout my general surgery residency, I found myself referring to Dr. Maraire's article for inspiration. This encouraged me to work hard and showed me that anything you set your mind to is possible. I am humbled and blessed to know Dr. Maraire and was excited when she agreed to be featured in this collection.

Dr. J. Nozipo Maraire's novel, *Zenzele: A Letter for My Daughter,* was published in 1996 and was a *New York Times* "Notable Book of the Year" and a *Boston Globe* best-seller. It has been published and translated into more than 14 languages. This is how she is described by Penelope Lively in a 1996 *New York Times* review, "A Zimbabwean mother writes to her daughter, Zenzele, a Harvard student, telling the story of her life and thus reflecting the upheavals of her country and indeed her continent over the last 30 years. Maraire herself said at the time: 'Since I've written the book, I've met a lot of young Africans who've told me it's the first time they've read a book in which they recognize themselves, the generation of children who made the transition from pre-independence to the struggle for independence and the post-independence era, and the ensuing cynicism that inevitably followed. We remember apartheid when we were not allowed to shop in certain stores. We are lost between the traditional African culture and modern culture. We do not know how to incorporate them, and there are no role models. The world is so Western, and we want to retain our core identity.' "

Rose Spaziani also wrote a tremendous article about Maraire in the *Columbia Medicine Alumni News and Notes* publication titled, *Returning Home to Zimbabwe*, that captures the essence of her journey to becoming a neurosurgeon and what makes her such an incredible woman.

In the article by Rose Spaziani she wrote. Dr. Maraire was born in what was known as Southern Rhodesia, a British colony. Educational opportunities were limited for blacks in Zimbabwe, and her father went abroad to college. At age 8, Dr. Maraire joined him and over the years lived in Seattle, Toronto, and Jamaica.

After Zimbabwe became independent, Dr. Maraire went home for a brief time before continuing her education in Wales, where she earned the equivalent of a high school diploma before entering Harvard to study biology. Her fascination with how the brain is wired led her to medical school.

Graduating from Columbia University College of Physicians and Surgeons in New York, she completed her neurosurgery residency at Yale University. Here she was one of several hundred graduates vying for the single residency spot and only the second woman to complete training there. Women represent only 5% of practicing neurosurgeons certified by the American Board of Neurological Surgery. The numbers were even lower when Dr. Maraire was a medical student. "I was at Columbia at a time when being a female neurosurgeon raised eyebrows," says Dr. Maraire. "I am grateful to people like Dean of Students Linda Lewis and my student adviser, Dr. Donald O. Quest, who encouraged me to pursue my dream."

After her residency, she completed a fellowship in pediatric neurosurgery at Beth Israel Hospital in New York, then worked as an attending neurosurgeon in Delaware, Ohio, and Oregon before returning to Zimbabwe in 2012 with her husband Allen Chiura, a urologist, and their four children.

Nothing could have prepared her for the vast discrepancy she found between the United States' health care system and the resource-starved system in Zimbabwe. "The Zimbabwe hospital system is in tatters," says Dr. Maraire. The country's economy relies mainly on agriculture and mining, and the unemployment rate has been reported as high as 95 percent; nearly three-fourths of the population lives below the poverty line. "There are more than 14 million people in the country and only six neurosurgeons. People are dying of basic conditions."

Dr. Maraire gave an example of a child with hydrocephalus, which put the child at risk of losing her eyesight, going into a coma, and even death. "The treatment for hydrocephalus is such a straightforward procedure in America that a junior resident usually does it," says Dr. Maraire. "You put a shunt in the tummy to drain the water that is accumulating in the brain. I never thought of the cost of shunts before, but then I realized that the families here can't afford them." A shunt costs the equivalent of a combined monthly household income of parents in Zimbabwe. Dr. Maraire contacted Econet, an international telecommunications company serving Africa, and pitched the idea of partnering on a shunt program at Harare Hospital. If Econet agreed to buy and donate shunts to the hospital, she would insert them for free.

"Seeing this girl walk after she had the shunt procedure was amazing," says Dr. Maraire about the program started in 2014. "One of the most important things I learned from my time working in the United States was to ask: 'Who can I partner with to make a difference?' This boldness is part of the mindset in America and has made me think outside the box." Her boldest plan yet led her and her husband to build a 10-bed hospital in Harare, the country's capital city. It will have additional specialists in orthopedics, gynecology, and general surgery. "We're doing it ourselves, brick by brick with the little we are able to scrape together month after month. We'll bring together the best of Western medicine and holistic African medicine in one place." In addition to performing surgery two days a week, Dr. Maraire runs a wellness clinic two blocks from where the hospital is being built. Then, there is the smartphone app she is creating.

"We need neurosurgeon innovators," she says. "If we are just technicians, we'll be pushed out by robots. We need to be at the forefront of innovations for patients." Conceiving the need for an app took shape over many years. Dr. Maraire found information about the latest medical treatments and resources easy to find in big U.S. cities, but when she worked in southern Oregon, she found herself in a place that medical device companies rarely visited. She felt isolated and began to think about ways to keep neurosurgeons informed. The goal of the app, called Cutting Edge Neurosurgeon, is to create a place where neurosurgeons can find the information they need: clinical research breakthroughs, basic science articles, and recommendations for new surgical devices. The app also will have a resident education component and a way for neurosurgeons to track their certification renewals.

The app has been tested at Weill Cornell, the European Association of Neurological Societies, and the Latin American Federation of Neurological Societies.

Dr. Maraire is a dynamite woman and thrives on her "wonderful, crazy life," as she calls it, even though striking the right balance often feels elusive. She shared, "There are days when I'm at work for 18 hours and save someone's life and feel like a goddess of neurosurgery, but then I realize I haven't seen my kids all day. Then there are days when I go to soccer games and cook dinner and I miss being in the operating room."

Dr. Coceka Mfundisi

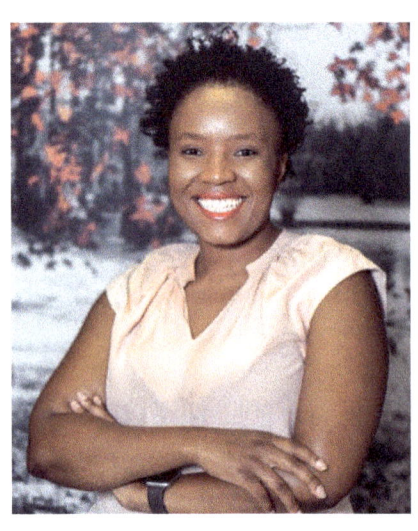

Dr. Coceka Mfundisi is a specialist neurosurgeon at the Busamed in Modderfontein Oncology and Orthopedic Private Hospital in South Africa. She graduated from the University of Cape Town (UCT), South Africa, with a Bachelor of Medicine and Bachelor of Surgery. She completed her training as a specialist neurosurgeon at the Colleges of Medicine of South Africa and became an Admitted Fellow of the College of Neurosurgeons of South Africa. She also earned a Master of Medicine in Neurosurgery from the University of Pretoria, South Africa.

Dr. Mfundisi became the first woman to qualify as a neurosurgeon from the University of Pretoria in its more than 100-year history. She is the second black woman admitted as a Fellow of the College of Neurosurgeons of South Africa.

She previously served as a member of the Road Accident Fund (RAF) Appeal Tribunal at the Health Professions Council of South Africa (HPCSA) and was also a member of the Golden Lions Rugby Club Medical Committee.

Dr. Mfundisi's other notable achievements include being a recipient of the Goldman Sachs Global Leadership Award, and she is an author of a scientific paper published in the *South African Medical Journal*.

She is a member of the World Federation of Neurological

Surgeons (WFNS) subcommittee on Global Neurosurgery and is director of her practice. She also serves as a non-executive member of the South African Neurosurgical Society representing young neurosurgeons. She has ventured outside medicine and is a director of her company, Elimu, dealing in property and student accommodation.

Dr. Mfundisi's job entails surgical treatment of neurological conditions affecting the head, brain, and spine, including the spinal cord and its nerve roots. Achieving success at the level of a practicing neurosurgeon was not smooth sailing, but determination kept her going.

She decided to become a doctor when she was seven or eight years old. What inspired her is she was able to count to 100 and a supportive and encouraging aunt told her she could be a doctor because she was able to count to 100. Her aunt said this as they stamped mielies (the process of turning corn into cornmeal) in the rural areas of Engcobo. Engcobo is a town in the Eastern Cape province of South Africa.

Looking back, she thinks her aunt planted the idea about becoming a doctor because there were no doctors where she grew up. Her only exposure to doctors was when they drove to town for care for Dr. Mfundisi's asthma with their local general practitioner, a black woman.

After high school, Dr. Mfundisi was confused about what she wanted to do. During her first year at the University of Cape Town (UCT), she majored in engineering. During this first year, she did not enjoy engineering and switched to medical school, which she liked.

Dr. Mfundisi's interest in neurosurgery began when she was in her third or fourth year in medical school. She loved neuroanatomy and neurosciences and also loved complex topics. She struggled with neurophysiology in her second year during the physiology program, but she worked hard and passed her exam.

She liked anything to do with the brain, whether it was psychiatry, neurology, or neurosurgery. What makes it exciting is that it is like working a puzzle as you try to figure out what is wrong with the patient without looking at imaging taken via a CT scan.

Dr. Mfundisi felt she had an excellent understanding of the brain and spinal cord. She liked to fix things and work with her hands, so she decided psychiatry and neurology were not for her. She thinks what solidified her decision to pursue training in neurosurgery was when she met Dr. Sichizya who took on a mentorship role for the black medical students at UCT. One day, Dr. Mfundisi evaluated a patient with a meningioma (tumor of the brain) and Dr. Sichizya invited her to the theater (operating room) with him to observe as he operated on this patient. The improvement was so quick, this is when she said, "This is the thing I want to do."

The challenges Dr. Mfundisi faced, and is still facing, are not vastly different from challenges any other South African who looks like her faces. It is difficult and unpleasant to be ruled out, not because of your abilities, but because of who you are. This hurts and is discouraging but, with the right support, you can accomplish whatever you set your mind to. This is not only support in your training or job, but also in your social network and from family and friends. Growing in a demanding career can be physically exhausting. Dr. Mfundisi is tired much of the time because of the long hours she works. But she loves what she does and cannot imagine herself doing anything else.

Even though there was only one black female neurosurgeon in South Africa at that time, she enjoyed the challenge of walking in uncharted territories. Dr. Mfundisi was often told she would not last six months before succumbing to the pressure and rigors of training and quit. The training can be intense, but the challenges of misogyny and racism had to be overcome. Because there were not many women in the specialty of neurosurgery, it felt like a lonely journey.

There was an elderly neurosurgeon who once advised that this specialty was not suitable for a woman like her. However, Dr. Mfundisi was not going to be deterred, so she continued despite such discouraging remarks. She is glad she pushed harder because this is a fascinating specialty that can provide excellent outcomes. It can also lead to heartbreak for the surgeon when things do not go well.

Seeing the differences she makes in the day-to-day life of her patients is Dr. Mfundisi's motivating force to continue as a neurosurgeon. Seeing that she inspires others to pursue something greater for themselves is exciting and motivates her as well.

Dr. Mfundisi would like to share with all the young women reading and dreaming big dreams, "Persevere and never give up. Always work hard. Know that some things are going to be difficult, but also know that there is much support around you. Learn to silence the negativity and negative voices because, unfortunately, there are always people who want to discourage you. Hang on to the positive voices and those who are there to encourage you to be your best self. When things get tough, push harder. Oftentimes, you realize you are doing ok. Social media has made us all closer. Reach out. The first mentee I successfully mentored is now a neurosurgeon and contacted me on social media. Do your research. Read about careers you are interested in and what you need to do to achieve that goal. Believe in yourself. Your current situations and current placement say nothing about your talent and your possibilities. Look at me, a girl who grew up in the rural areas who learned to count by picking corn while my aunt stamped mielies. Here I am now in a nice and very enjoyable career.

CHAPTER ELEVEN
Trauma and Critical Care Surgery

Surgical critical care is a specialty of surgery and a primary component of general surgery related to the care of patients with acute, life-threatening, or potentially life-threatening surgical conditions. Surgical critical care not only incorporates knowledge and skills of non-operative techniques for supportive care for critically ill patients but also a broad understanding of the relationship between critical surgical illness and surgical procedures.

Dr. Violet Onkoba

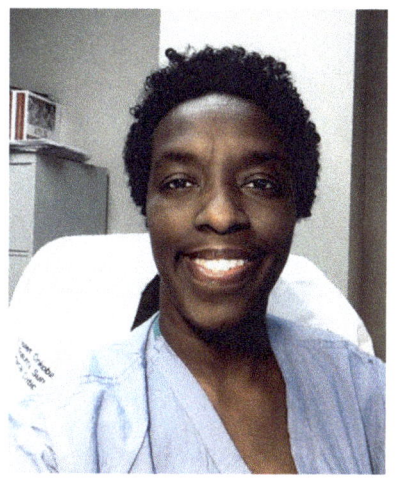

Dr. Violet Onkoba is a trauma and critical care surgeon at the Detroit Medical Center (DMC) in Detroit, Michigan. She earned her bachelor's degree in Studio Art from Union College in Lincoln, Nebraska, and a Bachelor of Science degree in Medical Technology from the University of Nebraska Medical Center in Omaha, Nebraska. She received her medical degree from AT Still University School of Health Sciences, Kirksville College of Osteopathic Medicine in Kirksville, Missouri. She completed a general surgery residency at Sinai Grace Hospital-DMC and a critical care surgical fellowship at Henry Ford Hospital in Detroit, Michigan.

Dr. Onkoba grew up in Kenya, Africa. She realized she wanted to be a doctor when she was in the seventh grade. Her mother cared for sick children and this was her first exposure to the healthcare field. When she was growing up, she originally thought she wanted to be a neurologist and then she thought she wanted to be a cardiologist. When she was older, she wanted to be a heart surgeon and build a hospital for the children she heard about that went to other countries for cardiac surgery. At that time many people in her country took their children to India, the United States, or the United Kingdom for medical care that was not available in Kenya. This motivated her to want to make a difference and change things in her country. As she grew, she wanted to be a heart surgeon and build a hospital for the children she heard about that went to other countries for cardiac surgery. She finally decided on trauma and critical care surgery.

Dr. Onkoba's first serious case as an attending was caring for a gentleman who sustained a gunshot wound to the neck. She was proud that he recovered well after surgery. Dr. Onkoba will never forget that day. Her first resident assisting her passed out. The second resident who relieved him also passed out. Then, the third resident must have been hungry because he also passed out! Three residents passed out! She called one of her partners to assist her. They did a great job!

As a black woman in surgery, there are some challenges she feels are unique. First, how others respond to you and how you are viewed are hugely different for a black woman than for a male surgeon. If she is assertive, it is often viewed as being aggressive or mean. Dr. Onkoba remembers male residents behaving the same as she and their behavior was considered appropriate and as getting the job done.

As an attending, she has not personally experienced any difference in the way she is treated as a female surgeon and this is probably because she has learned to do the very best she can and not care about how people perceive her or treat her.

Dr. Onkoba feels it will always be a challenge to be a black woman in surgery until there are more black women in the field. There have been times when she entered a patient's room, introduced herself as the surgeon, evaluated the patient, and was later told the patient said they had not been seen by a doctor. Some patients and family ask her how long she has been a doctor, and if she is sure she knows what she is doing. Dr. Onkoba doubts they would ask a white male surgeon this.

She feels the reason for this is because patients have not seen many black women surgeons and are not comfortable with the notion that black women can be whatever they dream of becoming. Always doing an excellent job is paramount because you will always be remembered as the black doctor if something goes wrong. Now, if patients do not receive her well as their physician, she offers to have one of her colleagues care for them because this is no longer a battle she is willing to fight. Dr. Onkoba has so many other things on her plate and patients to take care of.

A typical day for Dr. Onkoba includes of caring for patients in the different areas of the hospital, in the surgical intensive care (SICU) and on the trauma unit. During her SICU week, she rounds between 8 to 9 a.m. She and her team complete procedures such as placing central lines, arterial lines, doing tracheostomies, bronchoscopies, and sometimes they have patients that need to return to the operating room for various procedures. Then, she sees clinic patients if there are any scheduled and she touches base with the residents throughout the day to supervise and help them do whatever is needed. Dr. Onkoba rounds again in the evening with the residents before going home. They examine and treat patients as necessary.

During her trauma week, she is busier. The team rounds around 7 a.m. and responds to trauma codes in the emergency department (ED). These include, but are not limited to, gunshot wounds to any part of the body, car accidents, falls from a height, and pedestrians struck by cars. Dr. Onkoba's team sees patients in the ED and hospital units as consults, which means other doctors ask their opinion for various surgical concerns such as patients bleeding in their gastrointestinal tract, wounds not healing well, or other serious conditions like perforated intestines. They are asked to evaluate anything that may need a surgeon to decide if surgery is indicated or not.

Dr. Onkoba also performs surgeries and teaches residents to do operations throughout the day. These are surgeries they are consulted on in the trauma area or other consults they evaluated. She usually finishes work by 6 p.m. The days she is on call, she stays in the hospital until the following day.

She considers her beautiful and wonderful 18-month-old son her greatest personal accomplishment. Professionally, her greatest accomplishment is achieving her dream of becoming a surgeon despite not having a clear path.

Dr. Onkoba was in the unfortunate position of having to figure things out on her own because no one in her family is a physician. Now, she is passionate about mentoring high school students interested in medicine. When she came to the United States, she attended college and worked full-time, but did not understand the system. Dr. Onkoba persevered despite the challenges she faced.

It was difficult to start in a new system as a college student without the financial resources needed to focus her efforts on school. Dr. Onkoba had to balance her full school load with a full-time job so she could pay for her schooling. Adjusting to a new environment was also challenging, but she worked hard and kept her dream of becoming a doctor alive.

The lessons Dr. Onkoba would like to impart on the up-and-coming black female surgeons are, "Network with other black female residents. I had a strong support system at church, and this helped while I completed my residency training. Mentorship is extremely important. Find a mentor. You must excel in everything you do! Find someone who has done what you want to do and learn from them. I cannot emphasize this enough. You will be successful. As a new attending, do not be afraid to ask for help. Find a great mentor and someone to discuss cases with, someone who can be a back-up and provide insight when you face a difficult case or patient. The first five years are when you learn the most and you want to set yourself up for success."

Dr. Onkoba finds balance in life amid all the responsibilities she has. She has a supportive husband. Before they married, they talked realistically about her career path. He needed to be comfortable with her unpredictable work schedule when she is on call. She let him know she would not be able to be a traditional wife and needed a partner to help with child-rearing and home responsibilities. He often brings the baby to the hospital when she is on call so they can spend time together.

Dr. Onkoba designed eight most essential areas of her life and put these on her calendar. It is something she does daily to keep these eight areas balanced. Her eight areas are: Body (health and fitness) – What does she need to do today to keep her body healthy and fit? Mind and Emotions (psychology and beliefs) – She is intentional about her thoughts. It is important to have positive thoughts. Relationships (intimate) – How does she want to show up in the lives of her husband and son? Family – What can she do to cultivate her relationships with her family (parents and siblings)? Social/friends/fun –What does she need to do to feel connected to her friends? What can her family do that is fun; maybe dinner with family friends? Business/Career – What does she need to do to become more proficient at her job? What does she need to read and what additional skills does she want to acquire? Money/Finances – She worked hard to pay off her student loans and she is constantly learning about finances and investing. Spirituality (religion, meditation practice) – Her faith is especially important to her. She is intentional about time spent with God. The truth is that Dr. Onkoba does not believe balance exists in her life, but she is happy and fulfilled.

Dr. Qaali Hussein

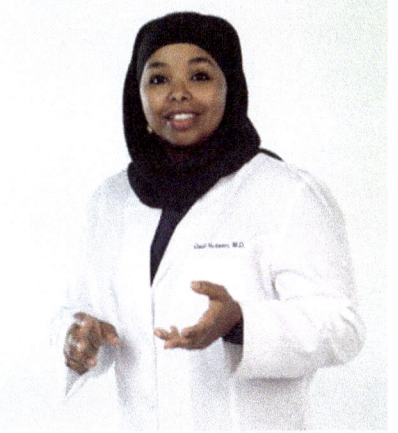

Dr. Qaali Hussein is board-certified as both a trauma and an acute-care surgeon, as well as a surgical intensivist. She graduated with her bachelor's degree from the University of Texas at Austin with honors in human biology before attending medical school at the University of Texas Medical Branch in Galveston, Texas. Dr. Hussein continued to Baylor College of Medicine in Houston, Texas, where she completed her residency in general surgery and her fellowship in surgical critical care.

After completing her training, she relocated to Florida in 2015 to practice at the Blake Medical Center in Bradenton, Florida, a level-two trauma center. While there, she was the managing director of the intensive care unit and chair of the hospital's Critical Care Committee. She also provides as needed coverage for trauma and acute care surgery for understaffed hospitals throughout the country.

In addition to her busy professional schedule, Dr. Qaali is a wife and the mother of six children she birthed during her intense training years in general surgery. She strongly believes that maternity-leave policies and the accommodations for pregnant women in the workplace are inadequate and changes are in order. She writes and speaks about the lessons she learned to empower women to make these needed changes from within their organizations. Her outside interests include spending time with her family, cooking, reading, and working on crafts with her children.

Dr. Hussein grew up in Somalia until she was seven years old and then war broke out. As her family was leaving Somalia with her grandmother, their truck was shot at and her grandmother sustained gunshot wounds to both legs. They were forced to return through the war zone to take her to the hospital because she was bleeding to death. Her grandmother was cared for at this hospital and she lived.

This was Dr. Hussein's first experience with trauma. Her family moved to Kenya and eventually to Houston, Texas, USA, to be with family. Dr. Hussein's grandmother always encouraged her in her quest to become a trauma surgeon because she seemed to have a knack for it. Her initial experience with her grandmother's injuries drew her to trauma. Dr. Hussein liked the fact that if someone is bleeding to death, you can do something to help them.

One of the challenges Dr. Hussein faced early in her journey was that there was a contradiction between her performance and the counseling and guidance she received. Academically, she performed well and worked hard but, the advice she received was, "Regardless of her grades, motivation, and hard work, the hijab would hold her back from succeeding." This meant people would discriminate against her based on her religious beliefs rather than give her a fair chance based on her performance.

Dr. Hussein had to choose between continuing with her dream wearing a hijab or not wearing a hijab. In her pre-medical studies, she was not in the click with resources and material they shared. She is certain this was because she was a hijab-wearing Muslim. Dr. Hussein felt left out of the secret society and that she did not belong. No matter how hard she worked it seemed she would never be good enough.

As a society, we teach people to conform to an accepted standard. Dr. Hussein wants young girls to know that it is alright to be themselves and not listen to negative people; being true to themselves. If someone does not accept you for who you are, then you do not belong there. Dr. Hussein wants to empower young women to set their own standards; bring their whole selves to the table and not compromise who they are. She feels if others do not accept you for who you are then they do not deserve you.

Two of her greatest challenges as a Black Muslim woman in training were that she was underestimated, and she was made to feel like she was a token. Some people insinuated that she was there only to fill a diversity quota. Always fighting against this stigma compelled her to work harder than everyone else and to read more than anyone else and to be better than everyone else just to be at the same level as everyone else. Unfortunately, there were instances where she was treated unfairly because of how she looks, but this did not stop her from excelling. What it did was force her to work harder so she could prove the people wrong who did not believe she belonged.

Dr. Hussein strongly feels mentorship is important. When

she was in medical school, her dean was a black woman who saw something in her and pushed her to be her best self. Having a tribe of women like her during medical school was such a blessing. One of her friends was from the Ivory Coast and the other from Cameron. They are still her best friends to this day. Through everything, Dr. Hussein had great family support. Having support outside medical school is key.

The best advice she received while in medical school was from one of her chief residents who took her under his wing when he saw how excited she was about surgery. He was a husband and father and his wife often brought their children to visit him at the hospital. When she was contemplating her career choices, she told him she wanted to be a mother and was concerned about surgery as a career since it did not seem conducive to motherhood.

He said, "Residency is a finite amount of time and it will end. Your lifestyle is what you make it. Do not choose a residency based on how long or how tough the training is going to be. Choose something that you are passionate about and that you will be happy doing for the rest of your life." This was great advice and she has passed it on to countless young women regardless of what specialty they are interested in. She advises others to be open and express their interests and find mentorship along their journey.

Dr. Hussein married after finishing medical school. She met her husband while working for an outreach program during her third year of medical school where they raised funds to help clinics in Somalia. Her husband was the IT specialist for that program.

A few months after starting her internship, she learned she was pregnant. It was challenging because it was stressful. Dr. Hussein was often told she would never be able to finish a surgical residency because she chose to become pregnant. No women had become pregnant and returned to her program, so there was no maternity leave policy. They looked to the OB/GYN department for guidance because they had more female residents and did have a policy. Dr. Hussein was away from her residency training for four weeks after having her first baby. Returning was a challenge because she felt she was being punished for having been gone for four weeks. There was little support during training, but she remained grounded because she knew she worked hard and did well.

Dr. Hussein was pregnant with her second child during her second year of residency. She was told at that time, "At this rate, you will never finish residency." At one point she was asked if she wanted to switch to internal medicine or family medicine because her priorities had changed since she chose to become pregnant again. She was disappointed by the remarks but continued to put her head down and work hard. She did not allow the negativity to affect her work.

When she was a third-year resident, she took her education in her hands. As third-year residents, there was control over the operating room schedule. Dr. Hussein had a chief resident who was training in vascular surgery, so he was interested in vascular cases. This allowed her to operate a great deal that year. The third year was the only year she did not have a baby because it was the most difficult year. That year she operated like crazy! Dr. Hussein had to take ownership for her learning because she was easily dismissed. No one was willing to go out of their way to invest in her education, so she had to create an environment for herself to thrive.

She did not become confident during her training until she started seeing the impact of her decisions. She isolated herself from social media so she could focus on her studies in whatever spare time she had. She downloaded book chapters on her phone as PDF files so she could read anywhere and was well-read.

Dr. Hussein remembers as a third-year resident, one patient on the medical service had a massive upper gastrointestinal bleed, which is bleeding in the stomach and the first part of the intestines. He was vomiting and defecating blood. He was unstable, hypotensive (low blood pressure) and tachycardic (fast heart rate).

The medical service was managing the patient. After finishing her rounds (seeing her hospital patients) with her team, she returned to check on the patient and found him unchanged and hypotensive and tachycardic. The only blood transfusion he received was the one she ordered when she initially evaluated him. She assumed the care of the patient and placed a central line, a large intravenous line that ends in a large blood vessel feeding into the heart and started resuscitating him. He was severely acidotic (this refers to the pH balance in the blood) which occurs in patients who are ill and patients who have lost a great deal of blood.

The patient was originally admitted with necrotizing pneumonia but was bleeding to death from this upper GI bleed. Dr. Hussein took care of this patient all day and all night. They eventually took the patient to the operating room at 2 a.m. and the gastroenterologist performed an endoscopy (looking into his stomach and the first part of the intestines with a small scope and camera) and found the source of his bleeding, a duodenal ulcer. The duodenum is the very first section of small intestines.

They opened the patient's abdomen, easily ligated the gastroduodenal artery (GDA), and stopped the bleeding. He was taken to the intensive care unit. His acidosis improved, and he was extubated (removal of the tube in his windpipe (throat) assisting his breathing). That morning, after the patient was awake and his condition improved, he fired Dr. Hussein because she was wearing a hijab! Despite this, she became more confident in her abilities as a surgeon.

A typical work schedule for Dr. Hussein is block scheduling. This means she works seven days and she is off for seven days. She has a nice schedule. Her children are old enough to get themselves ready for school in the morning. Her husband and she are a great team and they tag team.

When the children were younger it was a hardship to get them all ready, but it is much easier now. Dr. Hussein has learned to manage her time well because of being a mother.

Her faith is a vital part of her life and she is currently reading the book, The Productive Muslim: Where Faith Meets Productivity by Mohammed Faris. Another book she recently read was Deep Work by Cal Newport.

Praying and meditating is an essential part of her life and it makes her more productive and gives her purpose. When she was struggling throughout her journey, her faith is what kept her grounded. Dr. Hussein puts all her faith in Allah (God) and this has always propelled her forward.

There are three key persons Dr. Hussein would love to have dinner with and learn from. First is her grandmother because she was full of wisdom. She was a child bride and was married when she was 13 years old to her husband who was 40 years old. Grandmother had five children. When her grandfather died, grandmother remarried and had five more children. She had six girls and four boys. She made sure her children were well-educated and independent. She sent them abroad to study. Grandmother was ahead of her time. She was an incredible woman! Dr. Hussein admired her strength and courage. Also, Dr. Hussein would love to have dinner with Malcolm X because of his transition and his ability to change his mind and to be open-minded. Lastly, Martin Luther King Jr. is on her list because he chose peace in the face of hatred to arrive at the bigger goal.

Dr. Hussein would like to share, "Do not compromise your values. You are the author of your destiny. Society has their idea of who you should be, but only you can decide who you want to be and how you want your life to be. If I left it to others, I would have either been a stay-at-home mom with six children or a single, unmarried surgeon with no children. But, as I said, you are the author of your life and can decide what you want. I knew what I wanted, and I worked hard to make it all happen at the same time."

"You walk one step at a time, and so you must achieve milestones one at a time, whatever your role in life turns out to be." Kathryn Anderson, MD

Dr. Shuntaye Batson

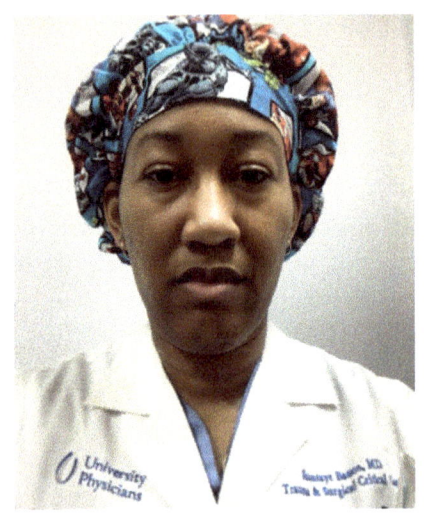

Dr. Shuntaye Batson is an associate professor of surgery in the Division of Trauma, Critical Care, and Acute Care Surgery at the University of Mississippi Medical Center (UMMC) in Jackson, Mississippi. She earned her Bachelor of Science degree in ecology and evolutionary biology from the University of Tennessee, Knoxville, and continued to Howard University in Washington, D. C., for medical school.

She remained at Howard University for her general surgery residency and after completing this, she was accepted to the Georgia Health Science University in Augusta, Georgia, for a trauma and critical care surgery fellowship. She is a recipient of multiple scholarships including the American Medical Association Foundation (AAMC) Minority Faculty Career Development Scholarship. She is involved in community service and community development.

Dr. Batson is a preceptor for the health careers development program at the UMMC and is active in her local Association of Women Surgeons (AWS) chapter. She is a member of the American College of Surgeons, Society of Black Academic Surgeons, and Eastern Association for the Surgery of Trauma.

Dr. Batson grew up in Gulfport, Mississippi, about two-and-a-half hours south of Jackson on the coast, east of New Orleans. It is a fishing community and there is a military base there, so it was a robust community. She is the oldest of three children. She grew up in a single-parent household but had a great support system because she was also raised by her grandparents (so she actually had three parents). Her grandparents were not college-educated. Her grandmother finished high school but always regretted not going to college, and her grandfather had a third-grade education. Her mother was an accountant so Dr. Batson grew up knowing she would have a career.

The first time Dr. Batson recalls saying, "I am going to be a doctor," was in high school. It was a random statement. A teacher asked what she wanted to be and the first thought she had was doctor. She is certain she was influenced by *The Cosby Show*. Her sister said she wanted to be a lawyer, so Dr. Batson was left with being a doctor as a profession. She enjoyed and loved her science courses and thought becoming a doctor was a good way to apply this love.

Dr. Batson knew she wanted to be a surgeon when she attended a lecture given by Dr. Debra Ford at Howard University, Washington, D.C., as a second-year medical student. She was so impressed.

Dr. Ford demonstrated that not only can women do it, but they can also do it well. Dr. Batson's first third-year clerkship was general surgery and she loved it. The first procedure she scrubbed in for was a pneumonectomy (removing one lung). As she held a clamp on the lung and ripped a piece of tissue off, she thought to herself, "Oh my gosh, I just killed someone." The scrub tech whispered to her, "It's ok," and took the lung tissue from her trembling hand. Dr. Batson did not realize you can remove someone's lung and they will live. She enjoyed the teamwork and atmosphere in surgery. From then on, she was committed to surgery.

As a black woman in surgery, her greatest challenges have been internal, feeling like an impostor. Dr. Batson wondered if she was good enough to be a surgeon. Once she knew impostor syndrome is not real, but an idea based on past experiences, she developed strategies to not believe the negative voices and kept encouraging herself. She is a good surgeon and will continue to strive to be an even better surgeon each day.

Dr. Batson feels there is no perfect balance in life. Her priorities often shift on a daily or weekly basis. She has learned to accept this constant change. She is learning to separate her personal life from her work. For her, once she crosses the Pearl River on her way home, she tries to leave work behind and focus on herself, the person that she is with or without her career. Sometimes it does not work well, but she tries.

Dr. Batson has also learned to take time off for rejuvenation; just taking a vacation which is something she never used to do. She always has a goal to accomplish and this drives her. In this past year, her biggest goal was learning to swim! She has thoroughly enjoyed it. She is currently reading the book, *Tough Love: her Story of the Things Worth Fighting For* by Susan Rice and is working her way through the entire Bible.

Three lessons Dr. Batson wishes she had known to go into surgery are, "Trust your instincts and know that your path is your path and it will be different from everyone else's and this is ok. Learn about impostor syndrome so you learn how to manage it early on. Never downsize your dreams!" and finally, "Your complexion, your story, everything about you is not a curse, it is a blessing!"

"Disciplining yourself to do what you know is right and important, although difficult, is the highroad to pride, self-esteem, and personal satisfaction." – Margret Thatcher

CHAPTER TWELVE
Obstetrics and Gynecological Surgery

Obstetrician-gynecologists (OB/GYN) are physicians for the medical and surgical care of the female reproductive system and associated disorders. They serve as consultants to other physicians and as primary physicians for women.

There are also subspecialties in obstetrics and gynecology, requiring additional training: maternal-fetal medicine specialists are obstetricians/gynecologists who are prepared to care for, and to consult on, patients with high-risk pregnancies; and reproductive endocrinologists are capable of managing complex problems related to reproductive endocrinology and infertility, including aspects of assisted reproduction, such as in vitro fertilization (IVF).

Dr. Keisha Bell Catchings

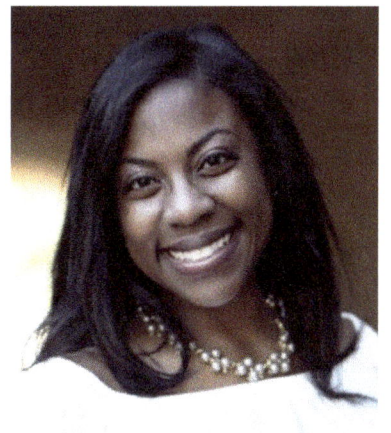

Dr. Keisha Bell Catchings is an assistant professor of obstetrics and gynecology at the University of Mississippi Medical Center, Jackson, Mississippi. She received her Bachelor of Science degree in biology cum laude from Tougaloo College, Tougaloo, Mississippi, in 2005; her Master of Science degree in biomedical science in 2007; and a Master of Science degree in biomedical science in 2007. She earned her medical degree from the University of Mississippi Medical Center (UMMC) in Jackson, Mississippi.

She completed her internship and residency in obstetrics and gynecology at UMMC where she was chief resident her final year. After graduating from residency, she joined MomDoc, Inc. in

Arizona where she practiced for a year.

As an active member of the American Congress of Obstetricians and Gynecologists, Dr. Bell Catchings has received numerous awards including the UMMC Department of Obstetrics and Gynecology Chief Resident Award, the Best Teaching Resident Award, and the Society for Maternal-Fetal Medicine Award for Excellence in Obstetrics. She has also received the Council on Resident Education in Obstetrics and Gynecology National Faculty Award for promoting high standards of residency education. Her research interests include the prevention of recurrent preterm birth in Mississippi.

This is Dr. Bell Catchings' story in her words.

I was born to Harvey Gales and Leesha Bell in February 1983. I lived with my Granny, Katherine Gales, for about five years when I was four or five years of age while my mom worked hard to make a better life for us. My granny is my heart.

I decided I wanted to be a physician when I was six years old. I was blessed to have parents, grandparents, aunts, and uncles who believed in my dream, even at that young age. They told me I could be whatever I wanted to be. My dream was nurtured from that time forward.

Through the years I participated in majorette dance as a Jackson Steperette, ballet, and piano. I returned to live with my mom at age nine. I was an honor student and was in the APAC (Academic and Performing Arts Complex) program from fourth grade through high school.

I decided I wanted to be an OB/GYN in the ninth grade after watching Dr. Catherine Hamlin, an OB/GYN, on the *Oprah Show*. She discussed the Hamlin Fistula Clinic she opened in Ethiopia to help women who developed vesicovaginal fistulas after childbirth. My friends were aware I wanted to become an OB/GYN physician and they, along with my family, encouraged and supported me. They even made future appointments with me.

I graduated from Murrah High School in May 2001 and began my undergraduate studies at Tougaloo College in August

2001, thankful for a full Presidential Scholarship. I never learned to study in high school because learning came easily to me. I scored well on the ACT having only read the small handout they provide when you sign up for the test.

College, however, was different. I struggled initially because I thought I could treat it the same as high school. I was wrong. By the end of my freshman year, my GPA was lower than what was required for the scholarship. I petitioned the Provost to allow me to attend summer school to attempt to improve my GPA. Though I did well in summer school, it was not enough to keep my scholarship. I was forced to take out loans to pay for the remainder of my education and I continued to struggle with learning to study. I earned a poor score on the MCAT when I took it during my junior year and applied to medical school my senior year.

I needed a letter written by a chairperson in the biological sciences department to apply to medical school. The chairperson did not know me but met with me to discuss my plans and goals. During this meeting, he told me he planned to write a letter stating he did not think I was ready for the rigors of medical school. I was devastated.

My granny was having problems with her lungs and was in the hospital preparing to undergo a lung biopsy when I discovered his intentions. I vividly remember going to the hospital to tell her what he said and how because of this, my dream would likely not come to fruition. She was livid and said a few choice words.

She underwent surgery later that day, aspirated and coded, but was revived with CPR. However, this was the beginning of a two-month hospital stay, including being in the intensive care unit. She was unaware of who we were while she was in the hospital, and we never had an opportunity to discuss it again.

Around Christmastime that year I prayed for God to give her at least a moment of clarity so I could talk to her and know that she knew who I was. Shortly after, I received a phone call early one morning to hurry to the hospital because she was awake.

I jumped out of bed, threw on the first clothes I could find, and high-tailed it to the hospital. I walked in and she was watching television.

I said, "Hey, Granny!"

She said, "Hey," and continued to watch the television. I asked if she knew who I was and she said, "Yeah, Keisha. I don't know why y'all keep asking me these stupid questions."

I laughed out loud and cried. I still cherish that moment and thank God for allowing it to happen. The moment was fleeting because later that day she reverted to not knowing us. Things went downhill from then and on January 13, 2005, a family decision was made to make her a comfort care patient. She died that day surrounded by her children and me. I was her baby too. She loved me so much and I knew it. I was devastated that she left this earth knowing I would not be accepted into medical school and without seeing me graduate from college. It breaks my heart to this day!

I was not accepted into medical school but was offered a position in a post-baccalaureate program (post-bac) at UMMC, which I accepted. A post-bac program is reserved for students working toward a second bachelor's or master's degree or for students who want to strengthen their application to apply to a graduate or professional school like medical school or pharmacy school.

I completed the post-bac program, took the MCAT again, and obtained a worse score than the first time. I graduated with my master's degree in May 2007, but I was not accepted into medical school. I was crushed. I remember telling my mom that maybe being a doctor was not in-the-cards for me and maybe I should dream a new dream. She encouraged me to not give up and that it would happen in God's time. I did not believe it.

On June 21, 2007, baby Jai was born to a close friend. She was struggling and I wanted to help, so baby Jai came to live with me when she was three days old. I had a new, beautiful baby. I never had a baby shower or any of the usual things when people have a baby. I figured it out as I went along.

Around August that year, I began working as a Regions bank teller. I applied to medical school for the third time and told myself it would be my last time. In December 2007 I received an email that I was accepted at UMMC. God blessed me just as I was about to give up. I realize now that the reason He did not allow me to be accepted before was because His plan was for me to raise Jai. If I was in the throes of medical school, I may not have felt that I could raise her. He waited so He could bless me with the best gift I have ever received, my baby girl.

I began medical school in August 2008. I struggled the first two years because even though I studied all day and all night, I had difficulty retaining the information. I struggled so much I missed earning a 75% score in physiology by 3/10ths of a point and was required to go to Georgetown in Washington, D.C., for six weeks between my first and second years to retake it.

I finished the course with a B. At the end of my second year, I saw a specialist, took a two-hour test, and was diagnosed with ADD (attention deficit disorder), the impulsive type.

I was provided with tools to help create a study plan to fit my needs. I performed averagely on my USMLE Step 1 board exam, but with the tools provided to help me study, I was able to increase my USMLE Step 2 board exam by more than 20 points. Throughout medical school, I balanced being a mom and being a medical student. People always ask how I did it, but this is difficult to answer because when you must do something, you just do it.

I learned to work hard and sacrifice from my mom. She did it because it was her only option. There were many times I brought my daughter to the hospital with me to study and she watched movies on her I-pad, ate snacks, and slept on her sleep mat on the floor in the classroom wing. I applied and interviewed for my OB/GYN residency during my fourth year of medical school and was matched with my first choice, the University of Mississippi Medical Center (UMMC).

I graduated from medical school in May 2012. My entire family was there wearing shirts with my name on them that read,

"I'm with the doctor." They rang cowbells (since I was becoming Dr. Bell) as I walked across the stage. The love was palpable, and I knew they were so proud of me. We even made the cover of the university magazine because of it.

My residency training was difficult. There were many challenges and many struggles. There were times I thought I was not going to make it, yet I made it through. Residency graduation was such an amazing experience, the realization of a lifelong dream. I was blessed to receive my certificate of completion and the Chief Resident Award, the Best Resident Teacher Award (voted on by my fellow residents), and the Society for Maternal-Fetal Medicine Award for Excellence in Obstetrics.

I was so surprised because I still do not see myself as one of those people considered for awards. I do not know why this is, but I feel tremendously blessed that I was not only considered but I was chosen. I was overwhelmed with emotion because I felt that after all these years of hard work God was saying, "Well done."

I also had the opportunity to present the award I created in my daughter's name: The Jai Williams Board Award that pays for one rising senior resident's written boards each year. This is a resident starting their last year of training. I know what it is like to struggle financially in residency and wanted to give back. Since I did not have an opportunity to prepare a speech that night, I gave generalized thank yous. Here is the speech I want to share. The speech I wish I had said at graduation.

Thank you so much to everyone who is here in support of me tonight. There is no way that I could have made it through this if it were not for the people at my table tonight, as well as those who could not be here because of ticket constraints. To my mama, from whom I learned a fierce work ethic and the art of sacrifice, thank you for your love, support, your constant prayers; for always being there for me and Jai even when you are 2,000 miles away. Thank you for reminding me that I am still your baby girl when I say that it makes no sense that you are still having to help me at the age of 33. If I become half the woman you are, I will be blessed.

Thank you to my daddy who always told us, "Whatever you are in life, be the best at it. If you are a garbage man, be the best one." I have carried that with me throughout my life. To my grandma, thank you for ensuring I did not starve. To my aunt Yolanda and Uncle Aaron, thank you for your unwavering support, encouraging words and financial blessings throughout my journey. Thank you to my Aunt Jerry for your unwavering support, encouragement and for German chocolate cakes. To my brothers and sisters, I hope that I have set a great example for you; and that you know from watching my journey that anything is possible. To my cousins, thank you for supporting me and always letting me know how much I inspire you. To the man in my life, thank you for coming into my life at a time when I had determined that I would be alone for the rest of my life and for showing me that that was not the plan. Thank you for loving me through this and always letting me know how proud you are of me.

To my friends who could not be here, thank you for the calls, texts and Facebook posts of encouragement and for always believing in my dream. Thank you, also for continuing to invite me to events, even when you knew I would not be able to make it. That meant more to me than you know. To all the aforementioned, thank you for keeping me in your prayers. To my Thirsty Thursday crew, thank you for being such an important part of my life. I would not have made it through without those vent sessions.

To the little love of my life, my baby girl, thank you for being on this journey with me. When I have wanted to give up, I have looked at your sweet face and remembered that I am not just doing this for me. I pray that seeing me work so hard will inspire you to do the same in the future. I always worry about the damage residency has done to you with having to get up at 4 a.m. some mornings so that I could round and me missing important events at school because of work. I pray that instead of being scarred, you will be able to look back and say, "My mama set a great example for me." When you came into my life, I thought that I was being a blessing to you. Instead, you were a blessing to me. I love you more than words can say. Right now, you do not know what life is like outside of medical school and residency, as you were only one when we started. I am looking forward to showing you what real life is like. We are about to have some awesome experiences because of mama's hard work and the sacrifices we've both made.

Thank you to the attendings who have participated in my training; for teaching me the art of medicine and surgery. Thank you to Dr. Owens for being in my corner; for being a listening ear and a shoulder to cry on. Thank you for believing in me when I did not believe in myself and for that fantastic introduction that you did for me tonight.

To my co-residents, I am so glad to have been on this journey with you. Thank you for allowing me to be your chief resident and be our voice. It has been such an honor and a privilege. Rising third years, remember what it was like to be an intern and be kind to the incoming interns even when you are frustrated. Remember that it is possible to be tough on a person and show love at the same time. To the rising senior residents, remember that patience is a virtue and that those below you will be looking to you as an example. Be a good one. To all of you who will be here next year, be kind to one another and remember to talk to one another when you have a problem. To the #1 night team, you two are fantastic physicians and it has been such a pleasure to have been a part of your training. I know you will continue to make me proud. I love you and I will miss you all.

To the fantastic nurses and ancillary staff that I have had the opportunity to work with and get to know over the last four years: Thank you for being a part of my journey. Thank you for being on my team and working with me to provide the best patient care we can. Thank you for the encouragement, love, and support you have given me over the years. We have laughed, cried, and saved lives together. I love you all so much. You all mean more to me than you will ever know.

To my classmates, the class of 2016, it has been a privilege to share this journey with you. You all are fantastic physicians. The cities to which you are taking your talents will be all the better because you are providing care in them. I wish you the best.

To the patients that I have had the honor and privilege to care for, thank you for allowing me to be a part of some of the most wonderful and most heart-breaking parts of your life. Thank you for the many lessons that you have taught me, not only medical lessons but also life lessons.

Lastly, to My Lord and Savior: Thank you for every dark time, every valley, every "NO," every heartache and every ounce of sorrow because it makes me appreciate the tremendous blessings you have bestowed upon me even more. Looking back on my journey, I realize that ALL of it was necessary for me to become the woman and physician that I am today. You are so awesome, and You just continue to show this in my life daily. I thank you for my tests that have given me in my testimony. I thank you for every storm that has given me rainbows.

I have NO DOUBT that God is real. If He is not, I would not be who I am today. There are not many people who can say that a dream they have had since age six has come true. I pray that my granny and my granddaddy (who passed in November 2014) are sitting at the Lord's side and were able to see me graduate on Friday and know I finally made it. I hope I make them, as well as the rest of my family, friends, and supporters proud.

I want to leave you with this: I love butterflies. They are so beautiful and symbolize a new creation or new beginning. There is a story called the *Lesson of the Butterfly* about a man who saw a butterfly wriggling and writhing, struggling to get out of the cocoon. He decided to help by cutting the cocoon open and freeing her. However, the butterfly's wings were all wrinkled, dragging the ground, and she was never able to fly. It is the struggle that allows the butterfly to get her colors and fly. So, the struggle was necessary for her to be the beautiful, colorful, airborne butterfly God designed her to be.

Today, as I stand here looking at my beautiful wings (my accomplishments) and preparing to take off into the world as an attending physician, I am thankful to God for my struggle. I am thankful for those who stood on the side encouraging me and cheering me on as I fought my way out of the darkness and flew toward the light of my dream. The struggle was, indeed, necessary.

You are enough!
Keep your eye on the prize!
Enjoy the journey!
This too shall pass!
This is where you are supposed to be.

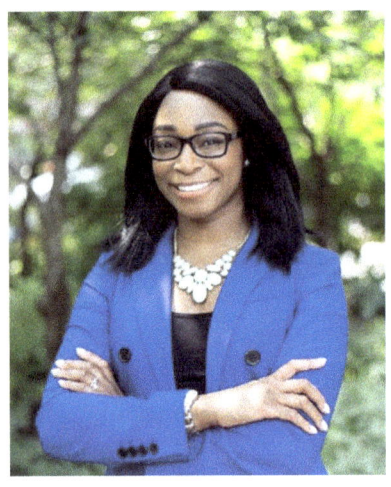

Dr. Tosin Odunsi

Dr. Tosin Odunsi is an obstetrics and gynecologist (OB/GYN) who has had a non-traditional path. After graduating in 2008 from Cornell University, Ithaca, New York, she started her master's education in Public Health at Thomas Jefferson University, Philadelphia, Pennsylvania. She continued to medical school at Meharry Medical College, Nashville, Tennessee, and completed her MPH between her second and third year of medical school. She graduated from Meharry in 2014.

Sadly, Dr. Tosin became a young widow during her intern year of her OB/GYN residency in June 2015. This significant life experience has given her the courage to be transparent with her struggles and serve as a life motivator. She has since found love again and remarried. She has found beauty in her new normal. She is a coach to many and encourages people to live a full and intentional life.

Dr. Tosin is originally from Nigeria. Her family moved to England when she was a child and to the United States when she was eight years old. From what she is told, she has wanted to be a doctor since she was three years old.

Her parents supported her but never forced her into medicine. Dr. Tosin's father is a gynecologic oncologist and guided and encouraged her along her journey. Seeing how much he loves his job encourages and inspires her. He still wakes up at 5 a.m. even though he does not necessarily have to and the passion he has for his job is always apparent.

Dr. Tosin's first memorable exposure to medicine was when she was in the seventh grade. She fractured her wrist and the orthopedic surgeon who cared for her inspired her to become a surgeon. How he fixed her problem with skill and gentleness was incredible and she wanted to be able to do the same for others.

She also volunteered at Roswell Park Cancer Center in Buffalo, New York, where her dad works. She had the opportunity to work with cancer patients, talking with them and passing out books. Later, Dr. Tosin also developed an interest in global health and wanted to incorporate this into her career.

When she began medical school, Dr. Tosin thought she wanted to be an orthopedic surgeon and she was the president of the orthopedic surgery club for two years. Then, during her third year in medical school, she rotated in obstetrics and gynecology. It was then she realized she wanted to do this instead of orthopedics. She felt she could have more impact and incorporate her MPH in this field because there are still problems with disproportionately higher maternal and fetal mortality rates among black patients in this country.

She likes this field because she can provide care for her patients throughout their entire lifecycle. She can take care of a lady during puberty, during her pregnancies, during menopause, and beyond. It is great to have the opportunity to care for multiple generations in the same family.

Dr. Tosin enjoys operating and this is probably the direction she is pursuing, moving away from obstetrics. She would like to focus her career on minimally invasive gynecology surgery. She loves fixing a problem and having instant gratification. She feels most comfortable when she is in the operating room and views surgery as an art. She is always learning from other surgeons and working on fine-tuning her style and technique to be more efficient.

Dr. Tosin would love to create a niche in fibroid and endometriosis management and treatment, both medical and surgical. This is because fibroid masses disproportionately affect African Americans and because of her personal struggle with endometriosis. It can take up to seven years to reach a diagnosis. She wants to advocate for women who look like her and are often overlooked.

Dr. Tosin has faced many challenges along her journey. She separated these challenges into academic and personal challenges. As for academic encounters, she has been a repeat test taker most of her medical journey. She took the MCAT (Medical College Admission Test) three times. She took both USMLE Steps 1 and Step 2 twice and had to take USMLE Step 3 four times!! Looking back, she says it took a lot of grit and tenacity to continue trying again despite the disappointment associated with failure.

Failing the USMLE Step 1 was the most devastating event for Dr. Tosin because there was so much hype about it being the exam that was going to determine her future career. When she received the results, she went through a deep depression she had never experienced before. She felt hopeless, useless, and worthless. To top it off, she only failed by two points.

She has a supportive family that encouraged her and reminded her of who she is and that an exam would not destroy her life. Dr. Tosin had to physically remove herself from Meharry where she was attending medical school. She needed time away. Her late husband and she were in a long-distance marriage at the time, and they had a home in Delaware. Her parents gave her the idea to take a year off to go home, retake the exam, and finish her MPH degree. This time away helped rebuild her confidence.

These are the times that test your faith. It is blind faith because it may not work out and you put in so much time and energy into your schooling. But this is what faith is. You must believe that even if your path ends up with your not becoming a physician, God will open another door.

For personal challenges, she lost her late husband Don the last week of her intern year. Her whole world came crashing down. Much of Dr. Tosin's identity was in becoming a physician and being Don's wife. When Don died, the bulk of her identity was gone. She faced the challenge of figuring out who she was during the remainder of her residency training.

Dr. Tosin walked away from God for almost a year because she was hurting so much. She could not even go to church. She was only 28 years old and devastated. It took time for her to find her way back to God. He was always there and waiting with open arms. She believes losing a spouse is one of the worst things that can happen to anyone, especially at an early age. If you can bounce back from that experience, a deep resilience is set for that person's life.

Another challenge Dr. Tosin faced was with impostor syndrome. Until she started her new job as an attending, she never felt she was smart enough or deserved to be a physician. She thinks the idea came about when she struggled with calculus in high school. She did not understand calculus, even with tutoring. This is when she began having feelings that she was not good enough or smart enough. These thoughts lingered until the end of her residency training. She was competent but not confident in herself. She needed time after residency to process everything and undo the years of negative thoughts.

Dr. Tosin has learned to speak life into her soul and spirit. She reminds herself she has been trained well and has everything within herself to succeed. She feels that for most new attending physicians the greatest fear is making a mistake that will result in the loss of a patient.

The reality is that physicians are human. No one is perfect but she knows that she will always do her best to care for patients the greatest way possible and call for help from more experienced surgeons when she needs help. She is at a hospital where she feels supported and respected. If she does not know something, she reads about it and finds answers. Plus, she seeks answers from those who have been practicing medicine longer than she.

One of Dr. Tosin's passions is mentorship. During her entire residency, she wore a mask and never presented her true self. She did not want to falsely come off as an angry black woman. She also did not talk about race. She had one black resident friend in another department who she felt comfortable discussing race-related issues with as they pertained to her training experience. It was nice to have someone who understood and helped her analyze frequent micro aggressions because she was experiencing the same issues.

Dr. Tosin regrets not advocating for herself but says this with caution because the truth is that people in power can retaliate if you call them out. It can be difficult when you see others who do not look like you have an easier time. So, for black girls, you must always be on your 'A' game. You must work three times as hard as everyone else to get half the recognition. You must not be on time, but early. You must be better than everyone else. She wishes she had someone who would have told her this when she started.

Dr. Tosin has been unofficially mentoring since college. She has mentored many women, but in March 2018 she started feeling alone and isolated because there were no physicians or residents who looked like her in her department.

She created The Mentorship Squad (TMS) which is a community of U.S.-based Black and Latinx women seeking mentorship along their journey to becoming U.S. physicians. The mission of TMS is to increase the percentage of Black and Latinx U.S. women physicians because these groups are markedly underrepresented. Dr. Tosin matches mentees with practicing physicians of the same demographic who are also passionate about mentorship.

Dr. Tosin feels sponsorship is the next level of mentoring, someone going to bat for you. If someone does not match into a residency, their sponsor can advocate and make phone calls on their behalf. A sponsor must trust you and is more invested because sometimes they put their reputation on the line.

Now that Dr. Tosin has full control and autonomy of her life, she has more choices for how she spends her time. She is adamant about prioritizing her mental, emotional, physical, and spiritual wellness. Occasionally, she finds time to read for fun, and started reading *Grit* by Angela Duckworth. It is a great book about perseverance and determination. This is one way she finds balance.

Dr. Tosin read a disturbing statistic in the American Association of Medical Colleges in October 2019 stating 40% of women physicians switch to working part-time or leave medicine completely within six years of completing their residency training. Physician burnout is real, and by taking care of herself, she can hope to enjoy her career for a long time.

Two people Dr. Tosin would love to have dinner and talk with are her grandmother and her late husband Don. The last of her grandparents to die, her grandmother was a kind person and cared for everyone. Her house was always filled with people and was always giving. She was a praying woman and Dr. Tosin felt comforted by her faith. Her grandmother reminds her to be prayerful, grateful, and generous. Dr. Tosin's late husband, Don, died suddenly. She would want him to see where she is now. When they were courting, he promised her dad he would support her through her journey to becoming a physician and would make sure she achieved her goal. She wants him to see she made it to the finish line!!

If Dr. Tosin had to pick only one operation to do, she would pick a laparoscopic hysterectomy for simple postmenopausal bleeding. This is an operation to remove a uterus through a small incision using a long flexible scope. And, if she could choose the music in the operating room, she would pick Sade, but she would love to blast Afro beats. She is not brave enough to do so at this time. Who knows, maybe she will start.

Dr. Tosin's final words to all the young women dreaming dreams are, "You have everything within yourself to succeed. God has gifted you with the knowledge and skills and/or the ability to acquire the skills you need to become the best surgeon you can be. As with life, surgery is not about competing or comparing yourself to others. It is about learning, improving, and becoming the best version of yourself!"

Dr. Fatu Forna

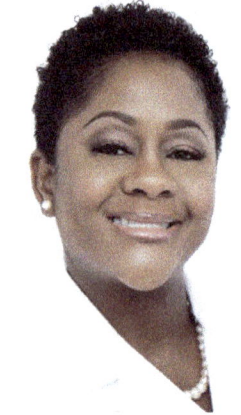

Dr. Fatu Forna earned her undergraduate degree from Florida A&M University, Tallahassee, Florida, and her public health degree from the University of North Carolina at Chapel Hill School of Public Health, Chapel Hill, North Carolina. She received her medical degree from Duke University School of Medicine, Durham, North Carolina, and completed her obstetrics and gynecology residency at Emory University School of Medicine, Atlanta, Georgia.

Dr. Forna served four years as a Medical Officer in the U.S. Public Health Service at the Centers for Disease Control and Prevention (CDC), Atlanta, Georgia, after completing her residency training. While at the CDC, she worked with HIV prevention programs in the United States and countries around the world.

She has also served as the Chief of the Department of Women's Services for Kaiser Permanente in Georgia, and as the Lead for Reproductive and Maternal Health at the World Health Organization in Sierra Leone.

Dr. Forna has authored numerous articles on sexually-transmitted-diseases (STDs), maternal and child health, and HIV prevention and care.

She is currently an obstetrician and gynecologist in practice in Atlanta, Georgia. Dr. Forna is married to a pediatrician and has four children.

She was born and grew up in Sierra Leone, Africa. Sierra

Leone has always had one of the highest maternal and fetal mortality rates in the world. As a child, she grew up hearing stories about women and babies dying during childbirth. She heard things such as, "It was the first baby, she'll have another one." Even though she was young, this narrative influenced her to want to do something to change this. Dr. Forna wanted to be a doctor since she was six years old.

Her family always referred to Dr. Forna as a doctor and so this must have also imprinted in her mind that it was what she was supposed to do with her life. Her father had a library with many books, but she was mainly fascinated by medical books.

Dr. Forna clearly remembers the night before her 11th birthday. Her mother began to labor. She remembers the anguish she felt and how she was afraid for her mother to leave because so many women died in childbirth. Dr. Forna slipped into the car that took her mother to the hospital because she believed she could prevent her mother from dying if she was with her. Dr. Forna wanted to be the type of doctor that would keep mothers and babies safe, so obstetrics and gynecology was the only thing that made sense to her.

When she was 15 years old, the war in Sierra Leone was just beginning. Dr. Forna finished high school early because she skipped two grades. There were no medical schools in her country at that time. Since her mother knew she wanted to be a doctor and nothing else, her mother arranged for her to move to Tallahassee, Florida, to live with her sister, Dr. Forna's aunt. This way she would have an opportunity to study medicine. Dr. Forna discovered later that a medical school opened in her country the year before she left.

Dr. Forna arrived in Florida with one suitcase that contained all her belongings and two other suitcases with shoes, bags, and African clothes to sell. She received $1,500 from these sales. In her mind, $1,500 was not enough to live on and go to college, so she was determined to earn a scholarship. At 16 years old, she finished high school in Florida and her aunt used the $1,500 to pay for Dr. Forna's first semester college fees. Dr. Forna earned a scholarship because her GPA was 5.0 during her one year in high school.

By Sierra Leone standards, she was from an affluent family. Her parents had good-paying jobs. Her mother was a lawyer and her father was a politician. Regardless of their affluence, it was not enough to pay for her schooling in the States, so she needed to maintain good grades to earn and keep scholarships to help pay tuition.

Dr. Forna faced many understandable challenges adjusting to life in America as a teenager moving to a new country. Her uncle's job took them to Iowa where he was a professor at the University of Northern Iowa in Cedar Falls, Iowa. They also lived in Cedar Falls, which is not remarkably diverse.

It was difficult to come from Africa, where race is not an issue since most people are black, to a place where hardly anyone looks like you. Dr. Forna was not well-prepared for this adjustment. What she knew of America was what she saw on television, which is not realistic. She was able to make some friends, however, including a few foreign exchange students from other countries.

Dr. Forna's aunt and uncle did not like living in Iowa, so they moved back to Tallahassee. She had two choices for schooling close to home with reasonable tuition, so Dr. Forna chose Florida A&M University. This is one of the best decisions she made.

At Florida A&M University, she found a great community; faculty members that cared about her growth and success and supported her. For her, having a community of support was critical because she was young. Dr. Forna joined the sorority Alpha Kappa Alpha Sorority Incorporated. She had a great experience during her undergraduate studies.

Though she was offered a full academic scholarship to the University of Florida in Gainesville, Florida, for medical school, she chose Duke University in North Carolina. This was because when interviewing for medical school, she met an amazing woman at Duke who was the dean of admissions, Dr. Brenda Armstrong.

Dr. Armstrong's mission was to diversify the school, so she invited Dr. Forna and other underrepresented minority students to Duke after their interviews for a second look over a weekend. Dr. Armstrong talked about her vision and showed Dr. Forna and the others how they would be supported throughout their studies. Another positive thing was they had a joint program with the University of North Carolina where Dr. Forna could earn a Master of Public Health concurrently and still graduate in four years with a combined MD/MPH degree.

Dr. Forna's Master's in Public Health is in maternal-child health and her research was in reduction of maternal mortality in Sub-Saharan Africa. She completed an internship at the World Health Organization (WHO) in Geneva, Switzerland. It was perfect for her. This experience opened doors for her to do exactly what she wanted to do, travel to African countries combating maternal and fetal mortality and working with the CDC.

When she completed her residency at Emory University Hospital in Atlanta, Georgia, it was a happy and positive experience. Most of her family was in Atlanta so she decided she wanted to be closer to them. The CDC is there and at the time, her interest was in doing a research fellowship.

When Dr. Forna interviewed for residency, she met a faculty member named Dr. Dennis Jamison who is now the chair of obstetrics and gynecology at Emory. During her residency, she worked at the CDC doing health research. During her interview, she told Dr. Jamison she wanted to do exactly what she was doing, working as an OB/GYN and doing research at the CDC. This was one of the reasons Dr. Forna wanted to train at that location. They had a multicultural patient base with many African patients. Whenever one came into the clinic, Dr. Forna's colleagues teased her that one of her African sisters was there to see her.

Dr. Forna's dream came true and after residency, she

completed a two-year research fellowship at the CDC which allowed her to go to Malawi as part of her studies. She loved it so much at the CDC, she ended up staying for another two years. This allowed her to travel to other African nations including Kenya and Uganda. Like she said, it was a dream come true.

Being extremely fortunate, Dr. Forna and her husband recently worked in Sierra Leone for a couple of years. They moved their family home so they could spend time with her father because his health was failing. She was excited to be home and work on decreasing maternal and fetal mortality rates and is glad they made the move because her father died. She was able to spend his last years with him.

Her husband is a pediatrician and he also worked in Sierra Leone for one year, but it became difficult financially, so he moved back to the States. When she moved back, she accepted a position at Kaiser Permanente, where she is happy.

Dr. Forna's role is to help redesign their department to improve the quality of perinatal (all the care for a pregnant woman) care and decrease maternal morbidity and mortality. She is doing something similar as before, just in a different setting. She spends half her time doing clinical work and half her time concentrating on administrative duties. She has four children, one girl and three boys. The oldest is 14 years old and the youngest is seven years old.

Dr. Forna is a busy lady, but she is creative and talented and does some unique things. She is a writer and has puberty parties. Sometimes she feels like she is just existing because of the exhaustion from wearing so many hats. One thing that helps is realizing you can do it all, just not all at the same time. She gave herself permission to not be a superwoman. For example, she loved working at the CDC and loved traveling to different countries in Africa, but if you are breastfeeding and you have a baby, it is difficult and not practical. So, she had to give up the CDC because she wanted to be with her babies and breastfeed.

She knows that when they are older and if she still wants to do the job she did before, she can. Also, Dr. Forna has always had help raising her children. She had a village to support her. She may have moved out of Africa, but she never left the lifestyle where you have your family help raise your children.

At first, her grandmother lived with them to help care for the children, and at various times they had help from different relatives. Dr. Forna found ways that worked for her and her family. If she did not have time to clean the house, she hired a housekeeper. When she wanted African food for her husband, she catered it. Initially, she thought she could do everything, but it was not working. Figure out what works for you and your family, not what everyone else says is what you should be doing.

In terms of her writing, she authored a book for teenage girls called, *From Your Doctor to You: What Every Teenage Girl Should Know About Her Body, Sex, STDs, and Contraception.* This book gives teens the tools they need to protect their sexual and reproductive health.

Dr. Forna also adapted the book into a curriculum for pre-teens and teens and started hosting puberty parties. Growing up in Sierra Leone, no one talked to her or her peers about the changes one experiences as we get older, whether it is menstrual periods or sex. Her parents never discussed these things, so she had to figure things out on her own. Dr. Forna wanted to write a guide for girls. In fact, her daughter helped her with the book. As she wrote, she gave her daughter pages to proof-read.

For her puberty writing, Dr. Forna created PowerPoint slides and talked to her daughter about the changes she was experiencing. She is certain she helped her daughter understand her body and growing up more than most African parents do with their teenage girls. Dr. Forna decided to invite her daughter's friends and their moms. It became a party with food and cake, and everyone talked and Dr. Forna answered questions.

Initially, her daughter was horrified when Dr. Forna told her she wanted to have a puberty party for her and her friends, but Dr. Forna did it anyway and they all enjoyed it. Dr. Forna uploaded a short Facebook video clip and people started messaging her to host a puberty party for their children. The video has almost a million views. It has been incredible. Dr. Forna is terribly busy and realized she could not host the parties in person, so she created an immensely popular online course so parents all over the world can access the material.

Dr. Forna is also the author of a bestselling children's book series called *Puppy Princess Sheba*. She was motivated to write this series when she realized there are a limited number of books with black children in them. Since she and her family love to travel, she wanted to travel in the books. She wanted her children to see themselves in books and show them how beautiful Africa is. In these books, she chose several African countries and picked something special from each country. She was intentional in her choices.

For instance, for Nigeria, she chose a picture of Lagos with the skyscrapers to show children around the world that Lagos is as cosmopolitan as New York. For other countries, she chose unique animals to that country or the beautiful beaches there so the children could learn and enjoy reading. Dr. Forna also learned a great deal during her research; she was not aware that the largest church in the world is in Africa. She had so much fun creating the series. Dr. Forna feels writing was her calling, but as the oldest child, she felt a sense of responsibility to become a doctor, so she figured out how to combine writing with her medical career.

Dr. Forna feels her greatest accomplishment is realizing that life and your career are a journey and there are many milestones to achieve. At the end of the day, it is not about the milestones. It is not about the destination but enjoying the journey. It has taken her a while to figure this out. For example, when she moved back to Sierra Leone, she thought that was it, they were moving back home for good. It did not work out well for her family and she had to readjust that goal.

In addition to all she has accomplished, Dr. Forna has created a special foundation, a non-profit called the Mama Pikin Foundation. She and her husband are both from Sierra Leone and when they went home to help with health care, they noticed many women delivered their babies at home because they were ashamed to go to the clinic because they did not have anything to wrap their baby in.

This led to an even higher rate of maternal and fetal deaths because some of these women were birthing without experienced help. The beds in the rural clinics and hospitals were old with torn bed sheets. Dr. Forna and her Mama Pikin Foundation developed a delivery bucket.

Each bucket contains a sheet of plastic to provide a clean surface area for delivery, a Lappa (cloth) to wrap the baby, and soap. Each kit costs $7 and at the time this book was created, they have distributed more than 10,000 buckets. The buckets have been phenomenally successful in decreasing maternal and neonatal infections and provide an incentive for women to come to the clinics to deliver.

Dangerous home deliveries have been decreased substantially in the areas served by the six Mama-Pikin Foundation-supported clinics. The women who once delivered at home now come in to deliver with a midwife because they know they will receive a delivery bucket and also because the foundation pays for a motorcycle taxi to bring them to the clinic when they are in labor. It is not practical for a woman to walk a long distance when they are in labor, so transportation has been helpful.

Dr. Forna has three key persons that she would love to have dinner with and learn from. First is Barack Obama because she thinks he showed the world what is possible. When you have a goal and you aspire to something bigger than you could ever imagine, and you plan and you work towards it, it is possible. Michelle Obama is second on the list because she is a phenomenal woman, probably more amazing than her husband. She took a back seat while he ran the country and now, she is doing her own amazing things. Also, the president of Rwanda. She just loves him. Dr. Forna is not from Rwanda so there may be intricacies she may not understand that may make him unpopular among his constituents but for her, from the outside looking in, he is someone who was able to take a country that was poor post-war and bring the people together, allow them to heal, and transform the country into a stable society and economy. Rwanda is at a point where they are doing well. When she went to Rwanda, Dr. Forna was amazed at the way the country has transformed. She would love to sit and talk with him and find out how he led his country to this level of reformation.

Dr. Forna added another person, her grandmother who helped raise her children. Her grandmother was not educated; her family was poor from a young age. Grandmother sold produce at the market to help support her family. When she was young, she married a Nigerian man who was a trader and had another family in Nigeria. He left for extended periods of time, so she created a business and put all six of her children through school. She valued education and knew that for her children to have a better life than she had, they needed to be educated. Grandmother's children did well. Dr. Forna's mother was a lawyer and her siblings also had great careers. For someone with little resources who could not read or write, Dr. Forna's grandmother worked hard and was determined to provide a better future for her children. Dr. Forna is grateful.

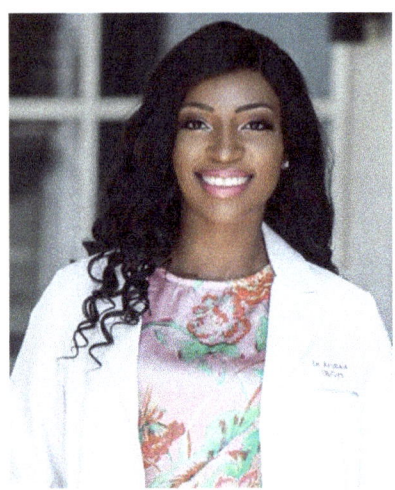

Dr. Ruth O. Arumala

Dr. Ruth O. Arumala is an obstetrician/gynecologist and women's health advocate with a solo practice in Mansfield, Texas. She obtained her Bachelor of Science in cellular and molecular biology/genetics at the University of Maryland, College Park, Maryland, as a Gemstones Scholar on a Banneker-Key full academic scholarship.

She also earned a Bachelor of Science in psychology from

the University of Maryland, College Park, Maryland, and continued on to the Mercer University School of Medicine, Macon, Georgia, where she earned a Master of Public Health. She has a Health Administration Leadership Certificate from the University of North Carolina, Chapel Hill, North Carolina, and a Doctor of Osteopathic Medicine from Rowan University School of Osteopathic Medicine, Stratford, New Jersey.

Dr. Arumala completed her obstetrics and gynecology residency at Georgetown University, Washington, D.C., Medstar Washington Hospital Center in Washington, D.C. She received the following awards recently, her second year as an attending obstetrician and gynecologist: 2020 National Minority Quality Forum's 40 Under 40 Leaders in Minority Health; 2020 *Fort Worth Magazine* "Top Docs" Tarrant County; Ob-Gyn, 2020 Texas Super Doctors Rising Stars; and 2020 Women in Medicine's "Top OB/Gyn" Forth Worth. She is a member of the American College of Obstetrics & Gynecology (ACOG), American Association of Gynecologic Laparoscopists (AAGL), North American Menopause Society, and American Academy of Cosmetic Surgery (AACS).

Dr. Arumala offers comprehensive women's health services focusing on the medical and surgical management of pregnancy, fibroid masses, poly-cystic ovarian syndrome, infertility, sexual dysfunction, and menopause. She is passionate about empowering women to live a healthier, more fulfilling life through improving health literacy. She is a proud Nigerian-American raised in Salisbury, Maryland. She incorporates her myriad of experiences to offer the best and evidence-based care compassionately to her patients. In addition to patient care, Dr. Arumala is the hostess of the *Pretty in Pink Podcast: A Modern Guide to Women's Health and Wellness*. She embodies the *Pretty in Pink* woman as she exudes confidence through her voice, elegance through fashion, and strength through fitness.

One of her favorite things to do as a child was being dropped off at her mother's office after a long, stressful day at school. In her checkered school uniform and with her over-sized backpack, Dr. Arumala pranced down the hallway past all the other doctors' offices then made a swift right turn into her mother's office. Although her heart swelled with pride every time she saw her mother as a physician, one experience remains imprinted in her memory far more than the others.

Dr. Arumala's mother had a busy practice as a family physician in Port Harcourt, Nigeria. The number of people traveling in and out of her mother' office always impressed her. One specific day, a young man came searching for her mother. He spoke to the receptionist, or the unit clerk as she was called, asking to see her mother, Dr. Arumala. He did not have an appointment.

At the same time the polite woman explained that her mother had a full clinic schedule, her mother walked out of her office into the hallway with a patient. The man saw her and beamed with a wide smile. He rushed past the receptionist and started lavishly thanking her mother. She was too far away to hear each word but from what she could decipher, he was thanking her mother for caring for him when he was ill a couple of weeks prior.

He proceeded to describe a scenario that challenged the trajectory of Dr. Arumala's life. He thanked her mother for not only caring for him, but for also paying his clinic and hospital bill. Her mother had given him money for public transportation, to buy food, and fill his prescription. Her mother is unaware that this act of kindness formulated the foundation of how her daughter practices medicine today.

Dr. Arumala's road to medicine began in high school, where she excelled academically with minimal effort, particularly in science classes. Simultaneously, she was attracted to things that involved creating while using her hands. One of her side jobs in college was styling hair. She taught herself to braid, cornrow, twist locks, roller-set, and more. Dr. Arumala could look at an image and easily recreate it.

When she began medical school, she considered dermatology. In addition to the fact that the only physician she routinely saw was a dermatologist due to her persistently horrific acne, she also loved the cosmetic aspects of dermatology. As she continued in medical school, Dr. Arumala realized she would spend more time learning medicine than surgery if she chose dermatology as a career. She knew she was gifted surgically because she could recreate almost anything using her hands.

In the middle of her second year in medical school, six months before taking the USMLE Step 1 exam, her favorite person in the world, her brother, Samuel Arumala, died at 24 years of age. This devastating and life-changing event shook her to her core. It compelled her to truly investigate the path she would choose because she felt she needed to live out his legacy while living her life.

Still confused about her path, she took a year off from medical school to do research in dermatology and telemedicine. In addition to providing the necessary time for her to grieve without the additional stress of medical school, she secretly had time to reevaluate her path. During this year, she chose to pursue a career as an obstetrician/gynecologist.

OB/GYN, particularly gynecologic surgery, has created the avenue for her to impact the world. Her love for her patients transformed into women's health advocacy and a passion to prepare the next generation of OB/GYNs.

Dr. Arumala feels the challenges faced by black female gynecologists mirror that of black females in any field that is not traditionally ascribed to her. Her field is increasingly female, so her blackness seems more offensive than her being female. There is an expectation that all her conjectures, assertions, and instructions are shrouded in the image of the angry black female. In addition, her youth (or youthful melanated skin) does not always portend a peaceful transition in and out of the OR.

She was warned and adequately prepared by her mentors how to navigate her first year as a black female surgeon. One mentor advised Dr. Arumala to choose simple cases in the operating room to enable her to build rapport with the operating room (OR) staff in each new operating environment she encountered. Their trust in her skills came with time and she feels she had to prove herself more as a black female. Her mentor also encouraged her to practice professionally and consistently outside of the OR. This allowed Dr. Arumala to navigate the inevitable complications every surgeon encounters with more complex cases.

Most of her difficult days in training were due to false accusations, inaccurate blame, or plain hazing. (Yes! This is prevalent in medical training today.) Dr. Arumala shared her difficulties with her physician mother who also faced racism and sexism in her workplace. They shared these experiences. In addition, she worked out her stress and frustration at the gym.

Dr. Arumala has confidence. She feels confidence is deeply rooted in skill. The more you master your craft, the more comfortable you are taking over cases and pushing boundaries. But over-confidence is detrimental in most fields, and particularly so in surgery. Nevertheless, she still deals with impostor syndrome almost daily. As a woman of faith, she prays about her feelings of inadequacy and asks for the strength to be resilient and persevere. She also finds time to read her Bible to help her with life's challenges and keep close to God.

A typical day in the life of Dr. Arumala is anything but typical. She claims if you are a solo OB/GYN like she is, you know there are no typical days. On days she operates, she wakes between 3:30-4 a.m. She reviews pertinent information about patients including laboratory results and imaging for her cases. She also reviews the procedures and relevant anatomy. Then, she heads to the OR. After her cases, she sees patients in her office and/or rounds on her patients on labor and delivery, post-partum, the floor where the mothers who have delivered their babies are, or post-operative units.

On non-operating days, she wakes around 5 a.m. and does her morning ritual which includes prayer, reading her Bible, and working out. She heads to the office around 8:30 a.m. because her clinic appointments begin at 9 a.m. She usually sees patients in her office but may be called for a baby delivery or patient in the emergency department (ED), particularly when she is on call twice a week.

Dr. Arumala's schedule seems hectic but it is how she likes to live: a disruptive plan.

If she had to choose only one operation to do forever, it would be a total laparoscopic hysterectomy (removal of the ovaries and cervix through three to four small incisions using a scope to remove the organs) for issues ranging from abnormal bleeding to chronic pelvic pain. This major surgery can provide definitive treatment to many women while maintaining sexual function, urine and fecal continence, and ovarian function.

The procedural steps are almost always predictable because internal anatomy does not change. But as with any surgery, there may be things particular to the case that make the case complicated or interesting.

The best advice Dr. Arumala has ever received is to ALWAYS remain humble and hungry. Humility keeps her grounded. Hunger makes her grow.

The best advice Dr. Arumala can give is, "Take every opportunity to practice your craft. Do not take an easier route during training. Stay for the late, difficult cases. Anatomy is key. Study it often. Analyze your cases. Critically review your surgeries. What did you do well? What can you improve? Are there more efficient techniques? Better tools?"

And Dr. Arumala's final words to all young women are, "Dear black girl, we need you! The world needs you! Your community needs you! Through those almond-shaped brown eyes, you see the world with a unique perspective. Your strength and resilience are unmatched. Ignore the naysayers even if they look like you or share your gene pool because you are worthy of living your dream."

CHAPTER THIRTEEN
Gynecologic Oncology Surgery

A gynecology oncologist is an OB/GYN who has specialized training in cancers of the uterus, ovary, cervix, and vulva.

Dr. Kemi Doll

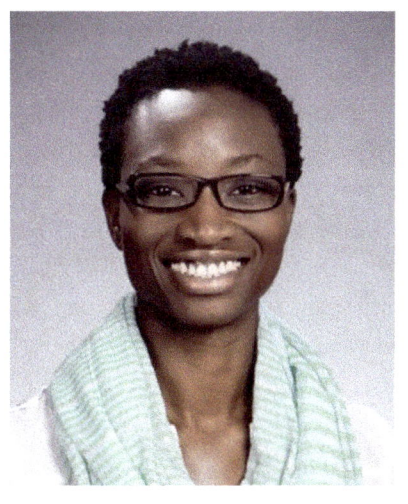

Dr. Kemi Doll is a gynecologic oncologist in the department of obstetrics and gynecology at the University of Washington in Seattle, Washington. She specializes in the surgical and medical treatment of uterine, ovarian, cervical, and vulvar cancers.

Dr. Doll earned her bachelor's degree at Duke University in Durham, North Carolina, and her medical degree at Columbia University in New York City. She traveled to Chicago, Illinois, to complete her residency in obstetrics and gynecology (OB/GYN) at Northwestern Memorial Hospital and returned to North Carolina to complete her fellowship training in gynecologic oncology at the University of North Carolina (UNC) Hospitals.

Her clinical interests include surgery, chemotherapy, and hormonal therapy for gynecologic cancers and minimally invasive and robotic surgery. She is honored to be part of a patient's cancer care team and believes every patient deserves honesty, respect, and compassion. Dr. Doll brings these values with her to work every day and is energized by the unique relationship she has with each patient and their family.

Dr. Doll grew up in a city outside of Atlanta, Georgia.

Her mother was a labor and delivery nurse, and this exposed her daughter to healthcare. She attended public school on the north side of Atlanta and grew up thinking, "I am going to school to be a doctor." Dr. Doll's mother is from Nigeria and instilled the importance of education in each of her children. Dr. Doll thought her options for a career were becoming a doctor, a lawyer, or an engineer. A doctor is what she liked. In college, she majored in biomedical engineering because she enjoyed biology but wanted to do something more interdisciplinary.

Dr. Doll attended Duke School of Engineering for her undergraduate studies. She received a quality education and learned a great deal, but the truth was she did not feel she had an enjoyable college experience. Her public school education made her feel poorly prepared for college. Because of this, she spent a great deal of time in the library. To be honest, she is not certain if it was that she was not prepared, or that she was intimidated. Due to many different factors, including a stressful home situation, she failed her sophomore year at Duke.

This was a difficult time but even after being academically suspended, she graduated as scheduled and was accepted into an Ivy League medical school, Columbia University in New York. The experience of going through failure and academic suspension and then needing to work extremely hard to stay on track to graduate on-time built tenacity and resilience in her.

Dr. Doll's medical school class was 25% underrepresented minorities and the Dean of Diversity was Dr. Hilda Hutchison who built a community of excellent students. All the students did well scholastically and had a great time together. Dr. Doll was the type of medical student who loved every rotation.

Initially, Dr. Doll was sure she would not pursue a career in OB/GYN. First, she rotated in general surgery and loved it. Then, she rotated in obstetrics and gynecology and, to her surprise, genuinely enjoyed it. In her third year in medical school, she chose to pursue a career in OB/GYN, a specialty she once thought she would never consider.

Dr. Doll feels navigating her path is her greatest

accomplishment. There were many times she felt she was stepping out on her own and trusting herself and developed the courage to navigate her own life and career.

In addition to being a gynecology oncologist, she is also a researcher and spends 75% of her time doing research. One to two days a week she sees clinic patients and performs surgery. Dr. Doll dedicates one day to administrative work. She completes paperwork regarding her various research projects including writing scientific papers and applying for grants to support her research.

Gynecologic oncology is a specialty where she sees a mixture of different cases. For instance, Dr. Doll may have a patient with ovarian cancer that requires debulking surgery, surgery to remove all the tumor that can be seen by the naked eye. Or, she may have a patient with cancer that has spread to the bowels and may benefit from the removal of that section of bowel.

She also counsels patients and teaches them about their diseases and the best treatment options and schedules surgery when indicated. Some patients who see her are in remission, meaning that their cancer is not present at that time.

Sadly, she also sees patients that are at the end of their lives and she considers all palliative care options, making patients as comfortable as possible. Because Dr. Doll practices in a tertiary center, she receives many patient referrals from doctors at smaller hospitals with complicated diseases and provides a second opinion.

Dr. Doll's proudest moment was being accepted into medical school after her difficult college experience because it taught her she could succeed despite prior failures!! It looked impossible for her to be accepted into the medical school she was accepted to and yet she was accepted despite the odds. This became a tremendous motivator for her in her career and in life. It let her know that just because something looks impossible does not mean it is. There is never harm in trying.

Dr. Doll remembers the many challenges as a black

female in training. She feels there is a double-edged sword of hyper-visibility. This means that everything you do is scrutinized. What she experienced was if you did well you were remembered because it was considered unusual for you to be in training at all and also because you are the only person who looks like you, so people remember. They remember you did well in that forceps delivery or gave a great morbidity and mortality (M&M) presentation.

On the other side of the double-edged sword is a very narrow margin for failure. Any little mistake you make is significantly amplified. People remember when you were late for a lecture, they remember when you did not deliver a great presentation in M&M, or that you missed a detail in sign out. (This is when healthcare providers hand off patients at the end of their shift to others taking over patient care.) Dr. Doll articulates these things well now that she has had time to reflect after training, but at the time she felt immense pressure to be perfect.

She saw a difference in what she perceived as relative freedom in her fellow residents or co-fellows. There were instances where after something happened, she said, "I could never do that." Whether it was not showing up to work, for a lecture, to M&M, or even in the types of emails that were sent to faculty and peers.

Despite all the challenges she faced, Dr. Doll did well and enjoyed the clinical work. She chose her residency program carefully and enjoyed what she was doing and where she was going. In fellowship, she focused on her clinical work and earning an advanced research degree.

The lessons Dr. Doll would like to share are, "In training, you must have a higher internal standard for yourself than anyone around you. You must learn early to set your own standard of excellence. It cannot be based on what everyone else is doing or what their expectations are because as black females we are either hold to 'too high' or 'too low' expectations. This is critical. I believe this was one of the things that helped me be where I am now. I had my own internal compass and knew exactly what I needed to do each step of my training. Sometimes the fire inside of us, our drive, can be misinterpreted by well-meaning mentors who want to protect us because they do not see things from our perspective and may worry that we are doing too much. But, if you have it in you girl, go for it. Go hard. Your standard must be high and your own. Also, deliberately cultivate a place of resilience outside your clinical or academic arena. A place where you remember what else you can do. Lean on your support people and have a place you can be 100% you and can recuperate. It takes a toll on everybody when you are this hyper-visible and you must have a place where you can relax and recuperate otherwise you will suffer from burnout early in your career. Take time out for self-care in your safe place where you can be your true self. And, lastly, you do not owe anyone your career, so it should be on your own terms. Trust yourself to know where you will thrive, whether this in residency or fellowship or your job as an attending."

After finishing medical school, Dr. Doll felt there was a great deal of outside input to her about where to apply for residency and this was the same for fellowship training. It was important for her to go where she felt she would grow as a professional.

She adds, "If you work hard and apply yourself, you can do anything, and doors will open for you. You are responsible for the quality of the career you will have. Do not allow others to make these choices for you."

"When I stand before God at the end of my life, I would hope that I would not have a single bit of talent left, and could say, 'I used everything you gave me.'" Erma Bombeck

Dr. Ebony Hoskins

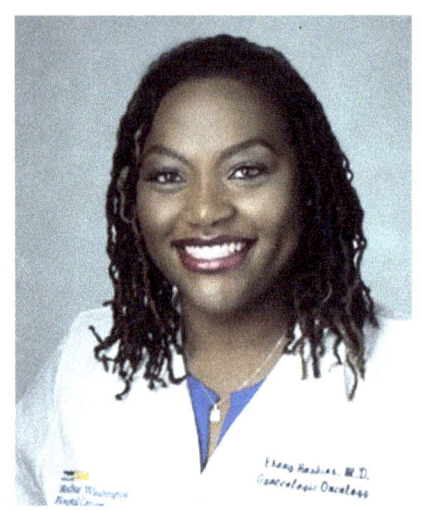

Dr. Ebony Hoskins is a board-certified gynecologic oncologist at MedStar Washington Hospital Center, Washington, D.C. She earned her medical degree at Wayne State University School of Medicine in her home state of Michigan. She developed excellent clinical skills during her obstetrics and gynecology residency at St. Joseph Mercy Hospital in Ann Arbor, Michigan, where she prepared for a clinical fellowship in gynecologic oncology at Magee Women's Hospital in Pittsburgh, Pennsylvania. She completed certified training in da Vinci robotic surgery techniques and qualifies patients for robotic surgery treatment of gynecologic malignancies (cancers). She has been practicing gynecologic oncology for nine years and continues refining her surgical skills.

Dr. Hoskins is a member of the Society of Gynecologic Oncology, the American Society of Clinical Oncology, and the American College of Obstetrics and Gynecology. She has been named a Washingtonian Top Doctor in 2016, 2017, and 2018 and has published various works including articles in peer-reviewed journals and abstracts.

She treats women with gynecological malignancies including endometrial, ovarian, vulvar, and cervical cancers. She sees women with complex gynecological surgical issues and considers minimally invasive surgical options for morbidly obese women.

Dr. Hoskins considers the use of robotic surgery because it offers patients many benefits including quicker recovery time, minimal hospital stays, and less postoperative pain compared to traditional open surgical techniques. She has completed more than 500 complex benign and malignant gynecologic surgeries using this robotic surgery technique. She also utilizes sentinel lymph node dissection for women diagnosed with endometrial cancer that may decrease surgical side effects associated with full lymph node dissection.

Her research interests include health disparity in women of African descent diagnosed with endometrial cancer and improving overall survival of women with ovarian cancer.

Dr. Hoskins grew up in Muskegon, Michigan. Growing up, she did not know anyone who was a doctor except the pediatrician she saw for check-ups and vaccines. She admired her pediatrician and in grade school, she decided she wanted to be a doctor. Dr. Hoskins remembers a time as a child she wanted to be a hairdresser, but her mother discouraged her from pursuing that career. After that, she never thought she could be anything other than a doctor.

A traditional student, Dr. Hoskins thought she was headed to a state school but was introduced to Xavier University in New Orleans, Louisiana. She loved the university and was accepted there for her undergraduate education. She attended medical school after finishing her bachelor's degree and followed the usual path, completing her residency and a research fellowship before completing her gynecology oncology fellowship.

As a third-year medical student, she was introduced to a program at Roswell Park in Buffalo, New York, where they were recruiting students to consider oncology. Dr. Hoskins completed a research project at Roswell Park, and this is how she was exposed to gynecology oncology surgery.

When she returned to complete her other rotations, she realized she did not love internal medicine and did not love obstetrics but enjoyed gynecological oncology. Dr. Hoskins was aware that to be accepted to an oncology fellowship she needed to be in a university-based program; preferably one that offered a gynecological oncology fellowship.

Dr. Hoskins did well in medical school despite not being

at the top of her class. She earned an average score on her USMLE Step 1 board exam but did exceptionally well on her USMLE Step 2 board exam. When she applied for her Ob/GYN residency, she was invited to interview for 10 residency programs. Some of these programs were university-based while others were community-based programs. In the end, she matched with a community program but at the time, wished she matched into a university program.

Looking back, being accepted into the community-based program was one of the greatest blessings of her training journey. Dr. Hoskins had a great experience and did not suffer from burnout because she was in a smaller program. Unlike university programs that focus on research, which helps match doctors into gynecological oncology fellowships, her program did not. The first time she applied for an oncology fellowship, she was not accepted. Instead, she was accepted to the National Institute of Health (NIH) for a two-year research fellowship. This was instrumental in helping her secure a position for a gynecological oncology fellowship when she applied again two years later.

Dr. Hoskins' journey was relatively smooth from her undergraduate studies to her residency. It was not until she started her fellowship training that she began feeling unsupported and wondered if her skin color had something to do with this lack of support. She felt she was treated unfairly by some staff. Dr. Hoskins had to dig deep within herself to find the strength to overcome these challenges. She had to believe in herself and have confidence in her abilities as a clinician. Her goal was to finish fellowship, so she persevered and kept going because complaining does not help. She just put her head down and worked hard.

To build confidence, she read a great deal. This helped knowing she had the answers when asked questions. She made certain she was well-prepared for cases and performed well in the operating room to the best of her abilities.

Like all doctors, Dr. Hoskins has learned to deal with

complications. She feels men and women process complications differently. She thinks men do not take complications as personally as women and are better able to compartmentalize. Men seem to better separate their emotions and are much more able to not take the complication personally.

Dr. Hoskins feels you must find a way to not let complications consume you. She does not expect perfection from herself because she knows no one is perfect except God. But she cannot relax until she has taken care of each patient and provided the best care she can. After complications occur, she wants to make certain the patient is better and is actively involved in her patient's care.

There are times when unexpected complications occur, and physicians need to know it is alright to seek therapy if these complications interfere with their ability to continue caring for patients. Sometimes there is no time to process these complications because many times when a complication occurs, the patient needs immediate care and you have other patients to care for as well.

Finding effective ways to deal with complications is imperative to prevent burnout and help your ability to care for the next patient confidently. You must remember all the great outcomes you have had and not focus on the negatives. You must separate the situation and remember that you are not a bad doctor and not let it paralyze you. Dr. Hoskins relies on God and the Bible for her strength and guidance, and she had a great co-fellow she frequently talked with. They supported each other.

On a lighter note, Dr. Hoskins' favorite surgery is a robotic hysterectomy with lymphadenectomy; taking out the uterus and the lymph nodes to remove cancer using small incisions and a robot. Patients do well, and it is an operation she enjoys doing.

She finds balance in life because her schedule is not as grueling as other disciplines and she enjoys reading as well. Currently, she is reading *The Purpose Driven Life: What on Earth Am I Here For?* by Rick Warren.

Some words of wisdom Dr. Hoskins shared are, "Apply to a program with mentorship because mentorship is important. Mentors help guide you and when you need an ally, you have one. Read. Reading develops confidence and when you are confident, others have confidence in you. When you do not know something, be honest about it. When there is a conflict, never try to resolve it alone. Make sure there is a third-party present. And, whatever you choose to do if your heart is in it, go for it!"

Dr. Hoskins' favorite quote is by author Leo F. Buscaglia, "The person who risks nothing, does nothing, has nothing, is nothing, and becomes nothing. He may avoid suffering and sorrow, but he simply cannot learn and feel and change and grow and love and live."

"A dream doesn't become reality through magic; it takes sweat, determination and hard work." – Colin Powell

CHAPTER FOURTEEN
Orthopedic Surgery

The scope of orthopedics includes the prevention, investigation, diagnosis, and treatment of disorders and injuries of the musculoskeletal system by nonsurgical and surgical methods. There are subspecialties as well, including: spine surgery, hand surgery, sports medicine, total joint replacement (hip and knee), pediatric orthopedics, foot and ankle, and orthopedic oncology.

Miss Samantha Z. Tross

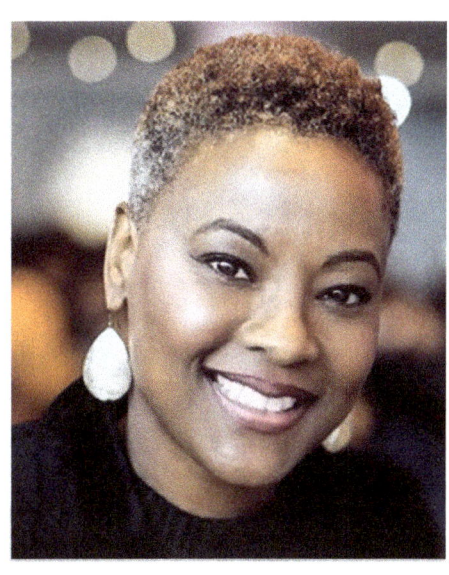

Miss Samantha Z. Tross is a consultant orthopedic surgeon in London specializing in conditions of the lower limb, specifically hip and knee preservation and replacement surgery. She is the first female consultant of Afro-Caribbean descent in the United Kingdom and one of 5% of the female orthopedic consultant surgeons practicing in the United Kingdom. She is a member of both the Royal College of Surgeons of England and Edinburgh.

Miss Tross earned her medical degree at University College London, England, before pursuing a career in surgery. She completed her surgical training at several London teaching hospitals including St. Georges, Guys, & St Thomas's and The Royal London. She also sought specialist training opportunities overseas at world-renowned centers in Toronto, Canada, and Sydney, Australia, where she gained additional experience in hip and knee surgery. She diagnoses and treats most orthopedic pathologies (bone diseases) and she utilizes minimally invasive surgical techniques whenever possible.

In addition to her clinical work, she is actively involved in medical education. She is an examiner for the Imperial College Medical School final examinations and an Associate Editor for the *Journal of Medical Case Reports*. She is an educational supervisor and mentors young surgeons, particularly female and ethnic minorities.

As a joint replacement surgeon in London, Miss Tross currently sees private patients at the BMI Clementine Churchill Hospital, BMI Syon clinic, BUPA Cromwell Hospital, and the Wellington Hospital. Her National Health Service (NHS) practice is at Ealing Hospital NHS Trust. NHS is the publicly funded healthcare system of the United Kingdom. The founding principles of the NHS are services should be comprehensive, universal, and free at the point of delivery.

Miss Tross has no idea what made her choose a career in medicine. She was seven years old when she announced she was going to be a surgeon when she grew up. Her mum was a nurse. Her grandmother and great aunt died at home. Miss Tross also had two friends that died when she was young – one from tetanus and the other in a traffic accident. Witnessing death at a young age had a huge impact on her. She was an avid reader and may have read something about medicine.

After being accepted to medical school Miss Tross knew early on she was going to be a surgeon. She chose orthopedics because the first female surgeon she ever saw was an orthopedic surgeon and she felt the orthopedic surgeons were the warmest and the friendliest. The specialty is nice because most surgery is done during daylight hours, and there is a diverse mixture of young, old, male, and female patients. Patients are generally in good health and recover quickly. This makes the results of her work quickly visible and appreciated. And, lastly, she has always been technically minded and enjoys working with her hands.

Miss Tross' greatest challenge has been overcoming self-doubt. When you are in an environment where there are few blacks and the system around you is filled with negative stereotypes, it is an uphill battle. She came to England from Guyana when she was 11 years old to go to boarding school. Her father's work kept her parents in Africa. Being away from her parents and culture made Miss Tross' journey difficult. The expectations others had for her were low because of the color of her skin. Her parents instilled self-confidence and belief in herself but without their presence, these were tested at times. Sexism is also an ongoing challenge. With more women entering the specialty, everyone is optimistic this will change with time.

Despite these challenges, Miss Tross has notable accomplishments. The first is becoming the first female orthopedic consultant in the United Kingdom of African-Caribbean descent. The second is being asked by one of her colleagues to perform knee replacement surgery for his mother, and another is being the first woman in Europe to perform robotic hip surgery.

A typical schedule for Miss Tross is starting her day attending a trauma meeting where the team discusses emergency admissions from the day before and plans care for their patients in the hospital.

Miss Tross is on duty one day a week and one in five weekends, but when she is not the admitting consultant on duty, she still attends the trauma meetings because she likes to have a consensus on treatment plans for the patients from all the team members. Then, she visits inpatients and evaluates their care and sees clinic patients with orthopedic concerns.

On her surgery days, she does not attend the trauma meeting. Miss Tross reviews pre-operative patients and then operates. She visits the patients after surgery to assess their status and order indicated care. She specializes in treating conditions of the hip and knee, so she performs knee arthroscopies where she evaluates and treats problems inside the knee with a small scope and camera. She also performs hip and knee replacement surgery. Lately, she has been doing robotic-assisted surgery.

Miss Tross is an educational supervisor for three surgical trainees (residents). This involves overseeing their career progression during the year they are assigned to her hospital. She meets with them throughout the day to catch-up on their progress. She also teaches medical students one day a week. She is also a faculty group tutor and oversees the educational needs of all the trainees in the orthopedic department during their four-month attachment.

With administrative duties, Miss Tross checks patient results, including labs and imaging tests. She replies to patient queries and reviews patient letters written by registrars (residents) before they are sent out. There is time during the week for personal reflection and keeping up to date with journals and courses. In addition to her NHS practice, she also works in private practice.

The best advice Miss Tross has received is, "There is no failure, only success and learning opportunities. Have a good support network and surround yourself with those on a similar path. Dream big!"

Miss Tross constantly searches for balance. This is a mindset and one you must work at she feels. Medicine tends to permeate all aspects of your life if you are not careful.

Her final words of encouragement are, "Believe in yourself. We spend a great deal of time worrying pointlessly. Believe that since you have been accepted to medical school, you are good enough to pursue any specialty. Give enough attention to your personal life. Plan to have your children if you so choose. Get involved in research and innovation, discovering new methods to treat diseases or inventing new and improved medical equipment."

"The future rewards those who press on. I don't have time to feel sorry for myself. I don't have time to complain. I'm going to press on." Barack Obama

Dr. Sonya Sloan

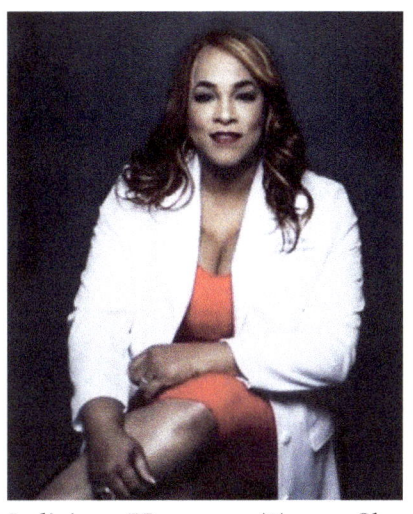

Dr. Sonya Sloan earned her undergraduate degree in chemistry at Texas Tech University, Lubbock, Texas, and her medical doctor degree from the University of Texas Medical Branch (UTMB) at Galveston. After graduating from UTMB, Dr. Sloan accepted a residency position in surgery at Baylor College of Medicine, Houston, Texas. She was the first African American female surgical resident in the history of Baylor College of Medicine. She completed several published research projects in orthopedic sports medicine and was involved in a joint venture with NASA Johnson Space Center researching exercise equipment for the International Space Station Intermittent Resistance Exercise Device.

Dr. Sloan's commitment to impacting lives reaches far beyond the hospital walls and is evident by her work in her community and internationally. She has established two specifically purposed non-profit organizations, ME&WE, Inc. (Motivating & Empowering Women to Excel), collectively reaching more than 5,000 women daily. The other is SLOAN STEM+Arts. This is a faith-based educational diversity initiative whose sole purpose is to increase the number of minority students in STEM careers through early exposure and mentoring, impacting financial stability for generations to come. In 2015, along with the Luke Church, she initiated the philanthropic efforts for an international medical clinic with the New Missions Organization in Haiti that now serves a community of more than 100,000 men, women, and children.

She currently serves on the Board of Trustees for the Institute of Spirituality and Health. Dr. Sloan is a consultant, blogger, and speaker for DairyMax, a national partner to the NFL and Fuel Up to Play 60 initiative, helping youth improve proper daily nutrition. She has been an adjunct professor at Concordia University with a focus on health care administration. As a partner in RoweDocs telemedicine, she launched her Virtual OrthoDoc venture as one of the first of its kind in telehealth for orthopedics.

In 2016, Dr. Sloan was chosen as one of the TEDMED Front Line Scholars. Additionally, she has been listed as one of the Top 25 Women in Houston and has been featured in magazines and several national publications.

In February 2019, Dr. Sloan's first book, *The Rules of Medicine: A Medical Professionals Guide to Success*, became an Amazon #1 Best Seller in medical education and training. Her work in medicine, as well as being a respected motivational thought leader, has positioned her as a highly sought-after public figure and speaker for health awareness, entrepreneurial mentoring, leadership development, and spiritual enrichment.

A proud member of the Alpha Kappa Alpha Sorority, Inc., she is the First Lady of the Luke Church in Humble, Texas, where her husband, Dr. Timothy W. Sloan, is the senior pastor. She is the founder of God's Women Rock, a nontraditional, international annual awards concert that honors spiritual women from all walks of life making a difference for a greater good. Her three greatest rewards in her life are her children.

This is Dr. Sloan's story in her words.

I have learned to appreciate the saying, "If you want to hear God laugh, then make a plan." When it came to my aspirations to become a doctor and a surgeon, God's sense of humor was in overdrive. No one looked like me in residency. No one had a background like me. But perhaps that was my saving grace, because no one had a drive like me to make it and be the first African American female orthopedic surgeon at a top residency in the United States.

I did not plan for it, but each step led me to whom I am today. I did, however, pray for it. And I do believe that blessings will sometimes chase you down from behind. But heed my warning, be careful what you ask the Almighty for. You will never be able to script each phase of your life or career. I think this makes the intrigue and the desire that keeps us going.

As women, we are fighters and are perhaps the 'never say give up chicks with medical degrees,' that just keep going. We have a tenacity that will not allow us to stop and a craving for success that cannot be curved. And more than anything, we know that we know we have a date with destiny that will not let us quit until we have achieved what we set out to accomplish.

So, what does a woman, physician, and/or surgeon do with drive, tenacity, and a date with destiny? She succeeds and then learns to pay it forward; the term that has changed the world since the movie *Pay it Forward* came to the big screen in 2000. Random acts of kindness and philanthropic endeavors have increased exponentially just with the idea of a heroic gesture with nothing expected in return. You have probably been part of this movement as a giver or a recipient whether you realized it or not.

Considering the current atmosphere we live in today, *Women's Movement, #METoo, Black Lives Matter*, all encourage everyone to believe they owe someone something. Make no mistake, you did not get to where you are because of your grades and good looks alone. There is always someone standing in the background, in your shadows, and in the recesses of decision-making board rooms. These people advocate for you. Not always because you deserve it or ask for it. These people are the ones who know that sometimes it takes a gentle push or strong nudge to usher your success in a positive direction.

Think of every man and woman who spoke life into you, encouraged you, and/or prayed for you. Recall every face who helped you to be who you are today. And do not forget those who wanted to see you fail. I call them the nay-sayers. At times, they can and will teach you more than others do.

So, I did not give you the most helpful hints for huge success as a female who wants to go into orthopedics, but you already know it. Work harder than anyone. Play the game to win.

You got this and I am here to remind you that you can do it. I did!

Lastly and most importantly, pay it forward. Do so because another young woman is looking to you for advice, support, mentorship, or just a hand up in a world where as women, we face unique challenges.

Dr. Pamela Samoyo

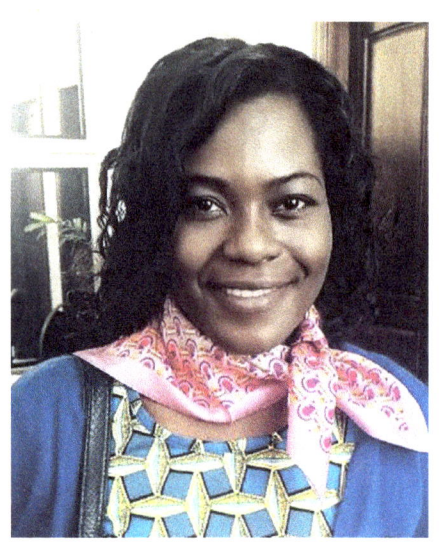

Dr. Pamela Samoyo is a specialist in orthopedics and trauma surgery. She earned her degree of doctor of medicine at the Ryazan State I. P. Pavlov Medical University, Russia (2010), degree of master of medicine in orthopedics and traumatology at the Kilimanjaro Christian Medical University College, Tanzania (2016). She completed an AO Alliance Foundation Trauma Fellowship (Kenya) and a COSECSA Oxford Orthopedic Link Pediatric Orthopedics Fellowship (Malawi).

She is an orthopedic surgery fellow of the College of Surgeons of East, Central and Southern Africa (COSECSA), Arusha, Tanzania. Currently, she is working as an orthopedic surgeon and serves as a pediatric orthopedic specialist at St. John Paul II Orthopedic Mission Hospital, Zambia. The hospital's main mission is conducting outreach programs and treatment for congenital orthopedic disorders free of charge to the needy and underserved community.

Dr. Samoyo is also involved in the treatment of adult trauma with interests in arthroplasty, surgical reconstruction or replacement of a joint, research, and teaching. She is a proud member of Women in Surgery Africa (WiSA) and has served as the treasurer for the organization since its launch in 2015. She advocates for gender equality in surgical training and leadership roles.

This is Dr. Samoyo's story in her words.

In high school, I enjoyed sports and participated in volleyball, tennis, softball, and other athletics. Growing up I wanted to train more aggressively in tennis and become a professional tennis player. Even though I considered becoming a tennis player, I was also passionate about and did well in science subjects, especially biology.

I balanced life between sports and school easily because I was passionate about both and had the support from my family that I could become anything in life without limits.

Because I loved science, I knew medicine was my field. This is a choice I have never regretted. Sports eventually faded from my life due to medical school demands, but nothing beats a good game of tennis.

My journey to becoming a doctor and an orthopedic surgeon has been difficult. After finishing A Level (advanced level) coursework in Zimbabwe (the equivalent of the first two years of college in the United States), I realized the country had one medical school that was not able to accommodate all interested students in the country. So, my family offered me an alternative to consider a different medical school at any university, provided the tuition fees were not excessive. I was accepted at Ryazan State I. P. Pavlov Medical University, Russia, in 2004 and my journey began.

The first few weeks after arriving in Russia were difficult. The racism I encountered on the street took time to become accustomed to. My brother, Dr. Brighton Samoyo, who was at the same university, encouraged me to keep focused on my goal of becoming a doctor no matter how difficult the studies and being away from home were.

After one month, I was able to brush-off the negativity and never looked back. Learning the Russian language was helpful because the communication barriers where what made the first few months so difficult.

In class, the professors spoke English, but knowing Russian made my stay more enjoyable. I enjoyed the six years I was in Russia and spent time site seeing, and I even learned to ski. I graduated in 2010 with my degree in medicine.

After finishing medical school, I began a new life in Tanzania. I do not regret this choice. I asked my mother for assistance with travel costs to relocate to Tanzania where I was accepted for internship training. She was in shock! How could I relocate to a country where we had no close family or relatives and where I did not know the language? She feared for my safety. All the same, I made my choice and was determined to get there.

Tanzania welcomed me and I broadened my medical knowledge during my internship at Kilimanjaro Christian Medical Centre (KCMC) (2010-2011) but above all, it gave me a platform to experience the different specialties in medicine. I loved both pediatrics and orthopedic surgery and was torn trying to choose between the two. Then my mentor, Dr. John Burrell from Utah, USA, came along. Dr. Burrell traveled to KCMC yearly as a volunteer lecturer with Health Volunteers Overseas (HVO). Dr. Burrell gave me career guidance and he and his family made an offer for me to stay with them for one month in the United States to observe at Davis Hospital and Medical Center, Utah, where Dr. Burrell worked.

This one month of observation in the United States opened my mind and cemented my thoughts. I wanted to become an adult and pediatric orthopedic surgeon. I am grateful to Dr. Burrell, Dr. Lyman, and Dr. Bean who were all instrumental in my education and career choices.

In 2012, I began my four-year residency in orthopedic surgery at Kilimanjaro Christian Medical University College (KCMUCo), Tanzania. My residency at KCMUCo was difficult mainly because I did not receive a salary, bursary, or stipend. I only had family support to rely on.

There were many barriers and lost opportunities because I was a Zimbabwean national and was unable to benefit from applying for jobs and/or sponsored external rotation/short course opportunities. These opportunities were reserved for the local students.

Kilimanjaro Christian Medical Centre declined three consecutive job applications and could not facilitate my application for a pediatric orthopedic surgery rotation in the Netherlands because these positions are reserved for nationals. I understood this and needed to find a plan 'B' for finances and placement for my pediatric orthopedic surgery training.

The Internet became my best friend. I searched for scholarships online for short courses and worked writing online articles for money. In 2013, I had a breakthrough. The Cosecsa Oxford Orthopedic Link (COOL) program offered me a fully sponsored position in Malawi for training in pediatric orthopedic surgery. It was a six-month fellowship at Beit Cure International Hospital, Blantyre. The Department of Orthopedic Surgery at KCMC was opposed to my going to Malawi because this took me away from my residency for six months. Malawi was intended as a sandwich program with the pediatric orthopedic fellowship lasting only a short time in between my training in Tanzania. I am grateful Dr. Rogers Temu advocated for me to train in Malawi and because of him, the University (KCMUCo) allowed me to complete the fellowship.

The pediatric orthopedic fellowship at Beit Cure International Hospital, Malawi was a dream. I took advantage of all they taught me and was able to maximize my learning. I wanted to learn everything I could.

The best advice I have received is from my mother when she told me to think outside the box! Which box? There never is a box, which means there are no limits to what you can do.

Now, my days are all different, but if I pick one day's activities to share, I pick Tuesdays. Tuesday, at 8:00 a.m., we drive out with the team to a local compound or clinic for outreach. At the outreach, we screen children with orthopedic disorders and give them appointments to come to our hospital for further examination, imaging, physiotherapy, orthotics, and/or surgery.

This usually takes until lunch time. Between 2-4 p.m., I see follow-up patients in the clinic for previously treated concerns.

My proudest moments are every time a child or patient with a previous disabling orthopedic condition returns to the clinic walking or smiling after surgical correction.

Balance can be difficult to find, but it is necessary. Balancing work, family, personal time, and rest avoids burnout. I try to find balance by daily prioritizing events like work, family and rest. It also helps to give everything you do your all, the first time and each time. I find this avoids unnecessary repeats. I also take time to read. Currently, I am reading *Born a Crime* by Trevor Noah.

I am grateful for all the Beit Cure Malawi staff. Between the years 2012-2016, I was fortunate to receive short-course training sponsorships that aided in advancing my career. I received sponsorships for the Cosecsa Oxford Orthopedic Link (COOL) program, the Institute for Global Orthopedics and Traumatology (IGOT) at the University of California, San Francisco, AO Alliance Foundation and SIGN. I am grateful for these. I graduated with a master's degree in Medicine in Orthopedic Surgery and traumatology in November 2016.

Currently in my career, I am completely in love with trauma surgery, pediatric orthopedic surgery, research, and teaching junior residents. At the same time, I felt I needed more hands-on experience, so I applied for a one-year trauma fellowship. The AO Alliance Foundation (AOAF) sponsored my one-year trauma fellowship in Kenya at Tenwek Hospital, Bomet and MOI Teaching Hospital, Eldoret. After completing my fellowship, I became a member of the College of Surgeons of East, Central and Southern Africa (COSECSA) after passing the exam in Maputo 2017.

Lessons I would like to share with the up-and-coming young female surgeons are build your confidence. Avoid apologizing unnecessarily. Do not allow others to make group decisions. Stop minimizing what you say and do not speak last. You are capable and your ideas are brilliant only if you tell the world. Learn to negotiate for better terms, for example, salary, flexible schedules, benefits, and more. Do not take criticism personally. Weigh criticism and make sure you understand what is being said, then use it to improve yourself or ignore it if it does not make sense.

The journey has been long. There have been many challenges. But, like a child in Africa who is brought up by the whole village, my career journey involved folks from all over the world. My career is a true definition of "I am because of who everyone was." I am grateful!

"All of us need a vision for our lives, and even as we work to achieve that vision, we must surrender to the power that is greater than we know. It's one of the defining principles of my life that I love to share: God can dream a bigger dream for you than you could ever dream for yourself."
– Oprah Winfrey

CHAPTER FIFTEEN
Cardio-thoracic Surgery

Cardio-thoracic surgeons operate on diseases affecting the chest, typically the heart and lungs but also the esophagus, diaphragm, and trachea. They operate on conditions that cannot be treated completely with medicine or interventional strategies. At times, surgery may be necessary for patients needing sampling of tissue from inside the chest to make a diagnosis, known as taking biopsy samples.

Dr. Ogadinma Mgbajah

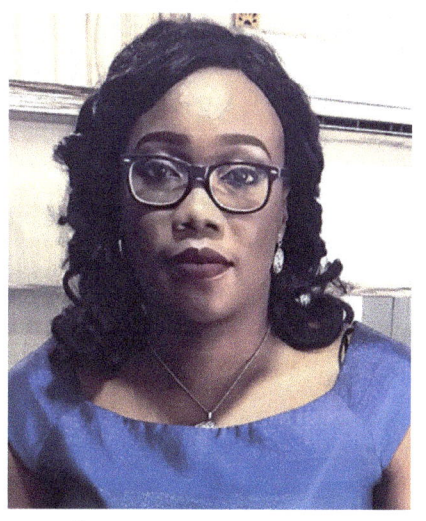

Dr. Ogadinma Mgbajah is a consultant cardio-thoracic surgeon at the Tristate Cardiovascular Institute at the Babcock University Teaching Hospital Ilishan-Remo, Ogun State Nigeria, Africa. She is the first woman cardio-thoracic surgeon in West Africa.

She earned her medical degree (MBBS) at the University of Ibadan in Nigeria. Following this, Dr. Mgbajah interned at the University College Hospital Ibadan. She completed her post-graduate surgical residency training in cardio-thoracic surgery and became a certified fellow of the West African College of Surgeons in 2016 and the first female cardio-thoracic surgeon in West Africa. Due to little availability of cardiac surgery in the country at the time, her residency training spread across India, the United Kingdom, and Ghana. In recognition of her achievements, she became the first recipient of the International travel fellowship award given by the Women in Thoracic Surgery (WTS) in collaboration with the American

Association of Thoracic Surgery (AATS) in 2017, aimed at fostering global collaborations in cardio-thoracic surgery.

Dr. Mgbajah's clinical interests include both adult and pediatric cardio-thoracic care. She is involved in efforts to build a completely indigenous team for cardiac surgery at the Tristate Cardiovascular Institute which has successfully performed more than 400 cardiac surgical operations in both the adult and pediatric population in the past four years. This is no small accomplishment because most of the cardiac surgical work in Nigeria is still heavily dependent on charity mission work.

Her research interests include sustainable cardiac surgery in a resource-poor environment, heart failure management and heart transplant, mitral valve repair, adult congenital cardiac surgery, and thoracic oncology. Dr. Mgbajah is presently seeking to attract global collaborations with larger and more established cardiac centers around the world to help build a sustainable cardiac surgery program in Nigeria. She is passionate about creating more opportunities and creating an environment to train more female cardiac surgeons.

Dr. Mgbajah does not remember why she chose medicine. Her mum says as far back as when she was a child, she always said she wanted to be a doctor. While her siblings considered various career options, she always gave the same answer whenever prodded!

She definitely knows why she chose surgery! As morbid as it sounds, Dr. Mgbajah looked forward to the cadaver sessions and, armed with a surgical blade, she dissected her heart out. No pun intended. Every other aspect of her pre-clinical studies seemed like a chore!

When she began her clinical rotations, her attraction to surgery became her passion. Dr. Mgbajah did not need to remember 25 possible causes of one ailment! With surgery, one or two possibilities for the causes of disease were enough!

Another consideration was she did not have to own patients for life. For example, if a heart valve needs replaced, she does so, and sends the patient on his or her jolly way. It is a practical specialty and she is a very practical person. So, it was love at first sight.

Dr. Mgbajah chose cardiac surgery because the heart made sense to her. All she had to do was draw a big box, divide it into four smaller boxes, put in gates (valves) and she was able to tell what happened if the gate refused to open or opened only slightly or if the gate flung wide open and refused to shut! She could tell what happens if there is an abnormal connection between the upper two or lower two boxes! Dr. Mgbajah was intrigued. She was hooked; it had to be cardiac surgery!

Dr. Mgbajah did not have challenges as a black surgeon because she trained in Nigeria where there are mostly blacks. But she did have numerous challenges as a female surgeon. Dr. Mgbajah had the support and backing of her family. It was an unofficial requirement for female residents, especially married ones like her. The question of having support always comes up in interviews! No one asked the male (married) colleagues if they had the support or the backing of their family!

She also had a few challenges with family. Most of the time, family does not have a full picture of what they are signing up for when they check the support box! Support in Nigerian culturally means being a wife, mother, and managing a home excellently (making meals, keeping the home) while being an excellent resident. The home cannot suffer because you have ambition! And culture requires you have a home (children and all) at a certain age. Dr. Mgbajah had three boys while training as a cardio-thoracic surgeon. It was an uphill task because she traveled to various countries to learn the skills she needed because cardio-thoracic surgery is still in its infant stages in Nigeria. Wherever she went, her family went.

It is bad enough Dr. Mgbajah dared to dream of becoming a surgeon as a female. Pediatric surgery was understandable, but she took her choices a notch higher and wanted to become a cardio-thoracic surgeon. Dr. Mgbajah dared to walk the paths trod exclusively by men! She endured the snide remarks, "Go and take care of your home!" "Can you saw open the sternum?" "Can you wire the sternum?"

Whenever she introduced herself as a resident in cardio-thoracic surgery, the reactions were predictable. No one paid attention! "She will change her mind." "How would she cope? Not going home for days?" were just a few of the common comments. Dr. Mgbajah was even rotated out of cases to favor male residents visiting from other hospitals, but she made her trainers and consultants believers, one after another!

Dr. Mgbajah was not always confident. She had timid moments and her, "I can't do this anymore" moments. She had her self-doubt moments and still does. A bit of self-doubt helps one grow. Dr. Mgbajah had moments when everything seemed to be going south, but thankfully, these times were transient, and confidence triumphed.

She feels there are many ways to build confidence. One way is knowledge. Dr. Mgbajah sought knowledge. She researched, read books and journals, and attended conferences. She made certain she knew her material! There is a level of confidence that comes with knowledge.

Another way to build confidence is practice. Dr. Mgbajah did things repetitively! She practiced suturing on cut pieces of foam! Those hand knots – she tied them over and over, frustrated at first and over time, it became second nature.

A third way to build confidence is mentors. The role of mentors cannot be overemphasized. In her case, it was friends. Dr. Mgbajah had two girlfriends training in general surgery and urology at the same time. They bounced ideas off each other, encouraged each other, picked up what was left of each other's confidence from time to time, and polished it till it shone!

A typical day in her part of the world as a cardio-thoracic surgeon in practice is anything but typical. They do not have work hours. Days easily roll into nights and nights into days, as they wear so many hats – surgeons, intensivists, respiratory therapists, and more. Dr. Mgbajah and her team rest when a surgical patient is discharged and there is often a break when there are no patients to operate on! Cardio-thoracic surgical practice in the most active center in a third-world country is an entirely different book of experiences.

Dr. Mgbajah's proudest moment was the day she received her degree and her award as the first female cardio-thoracic surgeon in Nigeria and West Africa, all with her husband and three sons by her side. This day she felt as though she had truly shattered the glass ceiling.

She gives heartfelt thanks to her husband, her sons and family, Mr. Bode Falase and Dr. Michael Sanusi (her primary trainers), and Dr. AGK Gokhale, Dr. Lauren Kane, Dr. Emily Farkas, Dr. O. C Nzewi (her secondary trainers). Seven years and three continents later, she became the first and only female cardio-thoracic surgeon in Nigeria and West Africa.

The best advice Dr. Mgbajah received is, *"You are responsible for how you turn out! Never delegate this all-important responsibility to any person, circumstance, or environment."* Her favorite quotes in residency were: "Every storm runs out of rain." (Maya Angelou) and *"And it came to pass." (The Bible).*

Dr. Mgbajah would like to share a few truths she has come to embrace in her journey, "Pace yourself. Run your race! Do not try to achieve another person's goal. Small victories add up and are easier to achieve! So, instead of wearing yourself out aiming for a huge dramatic win, aim for one small victory at a time. Trust me, the feeling is the same. Do not lose focus. Eventually, it will all add up. You are training to become a SURGEON, not a female surgeon! Notice our male colleagues do not refer to themselves as male surgeons. This is because the profession is surgery, your gender is your business! Don't accept lower standards, fewer calls, or less work because you are a female surgeon. Do not let anyone ask you if you need to scrub-out or if you want to rest a bit because you are a female surgeon. You are a surgeon, period! Show up. Put in the work and show out. Make certain your vision is clear and your motives are correct. Gather all the necessary information to make informed decisions, including options for places to train. When you have adequately counted the costs, get up and get it done. Pace yourself. Run your race. Set goals. Do not try to achieve goals set by others. It is a marathon and you've got this!"

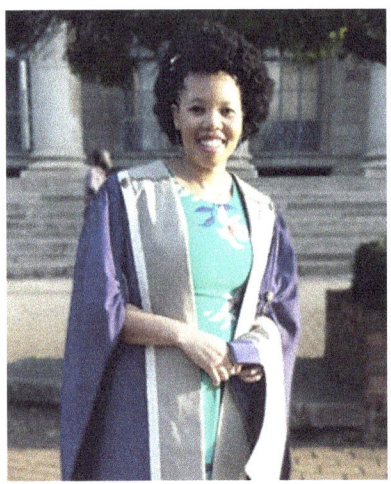

Dr. Lindiwe Sidali

Dr. Lindiwe Sidali is a cardio-thoracic surgeon at Inkosi Albert Luthuli Central Hospital, in Durban, South Africa. She received her medical degree from Facultad de Ciencias Medicas Sancti Spiritus, Cuba, and her training in cardio-thoracic surgery at Inkosi Albert Luthuli Central Hospital, Durban, Kwa-Zulu Natal.

Dr. Sidali's journey began a long time before she became an accomplished cardio-thoracic surgeon. She was born in a large family of eight in a small town called Dutywa, in the Eastern Cape, South Africa. Her father worked in the Wonderkop mine in Rusternburg, North West, so she lived between the two provinces.

She attended Rakgatla High School in Wonderkop and earned a bursary (scholarship) from the North West Department of Health to study medicine in Cuba. Dr. Sidali's parents were true feminists, so to speak. All the children in her family were treated equally in a culture that tends to have defined gender roles. Whether you were a girl or a boy, you were expected to cook, clean, and herd cattle and perform to the best of your abilities in school. Her parents taught Dr. Sidali and her siblings the value of hard work.

When she was in high school, Dr. Sidali volunteered at the Wonderkop clinic. The nurses there were wonderful and encouraged her to pursue medicine. Her family and teachers were also supportive and encouraging. While volunteering at the clinic, Dr. Sidali learned of the Southern African-Cuban scholarship to study medicine.

She applied and was accepted. She was interested in medicine because she has always wanted to serve her people and give back, not only by being a doctor but also by serving as a positive role model for every African child. Dr. Sidali wants to show them they can achieve anything they desire.

As for cardio-thoracic surgery, it happened by chance. During her rotations in medical school, she was interested in surgical disciplines but did not know which one to pursue. While rotating in general surgery, she was also a house officer completing her community service. In South Africa, physicians are required to do community service before they can complete official residency training. One day, a patient came to the hospital with a stab wound to the heart. The patient was taken to the operating room and, after experiencing a heart beating in her hands, she knew she wanted to become a cardio-thoracic surgeon.

Dr. Sidali does not think of her journey as a sacrifice. To her, it was time well-spent as she focused on her studies and advancing in her career. She has been fortunate to have many people supporting her and cheering her on along the way. She is grateful that her family has always been the cheerleaders of her life and her teachers too, the ones who expected the best from her.

She is grateful for her friends who were there for her through it all and everyone who saw potential in her and gave her a chance. From the Department of Health, North West, and to the Cuban community for their warm welcome and the knowledge they shared in medicine, they also taught Dr. Sidali to be proud of who she is and where she comes from.

She is also thankful to her mentors for the guidance and advice they generously gave, for believing in her and supporting her throughout her journey. She thanks the KZN Department of Health for its support. And, finally, she is grateful for the professors who taught her the art of surgery.

When she was asked what barriers she feels women face to achieve success in male-dominated fields, Dr. Sidali shared, "It is difficult to answer this question without sparking debate in other areas, but I suppose it is the same reason we still have not had a female president. These same barriers need to be broken. It is only when people see that one female can do it that they can give a chance to other females. It is uncharted territory for females, particularly African females because they are hardly ever given a chance. In my opinion, when women are given the same position as men, they are tested to the point of failure. This is where all intuitive direction points one to believe they cannot do it. So, the odds for African women are systematically, probably unintentionally, designed to drive us to not fight for more or to quit."

Dr. Sidali feels there is an increase in the number of female doctors in surgical disciplines overall. These disciplines have been famously known as the boy's club. However, African females have been given the least opportunities compared to their counterparts. They need opportunities and exposure. The most important thing that needs to change the future for all African children is the eradication of poverty. One way to do this is through education. This is how to truly liberate a person. But education requires money, which is the reason education needs to be free for those from disadvantaged backgrounds. There also to be more positive role models for young women. African girls need to see a girl who looks like them achieving success. This way they can see it can be done.

Dr. Sidali asserts her present position is just the beginning of a new dawn. She is excited to hit the ground running and sharpen her skills even more and teach and transfer her skills to the next generation of surgeons. She plans to pursue congenital cardiac surgery, a sub-specialty/super specialty in cardio-thoracic surgery dealing with structural problems of the heart present from birth. These structural defects range from a small hole between the heart chambers to complex abnormalities such as an abnormal spatial arrangement of the great blood vessels.

Dr. Sidali describes herself as aware. She is aware of herself, who she is and what she stands for, making it easier for others to be aware of her. She also describes herself as feminist, decisive, a dreamer, and dauntless.

She shares how she writes romantic fiction stories, but only for her friends, as she writes under a pseudo name. She intends to share her writing with the world someday, but no one will ever know it is her. Now that she has finished her exams, besides working hard, she is planning to practice more of her hobbies.

Dr. Sidali's final words are, "Everything in life is possible. Dream but create a plan of action in achieving those goals. Do not follow other people's paths. Create a new one for yourself and others."

"If the front side of the coin of success is the ability to set clear goals for yourself, then the flip side of the same coin is the ability to get yourself organized and work on your most valuable tasks, every minute of every day in order to achieve your goals. Your choices and decisions have combined to create your entire life to this moment. To change or improve your life in any way, you have to make new choices and new decisions that are more in alignment with who you really are and what you really want."
– Brian Tracy

CHAPTER SIXTEEN
Vascular Surgery

Vascular surgery is a surgical subspecialty in which diseases of the vascular system, or arteries, veins, and lymphatic circulation, are managed by medical therapy, minimally invasive catheter procedures, and surgical reconstruction. The vascular surgeon is trained in the diagnosis and management of diseases affecting all parts of the vascular system excluding the coronaries and intracranial vasculature.

Dr. Olamide Alabi

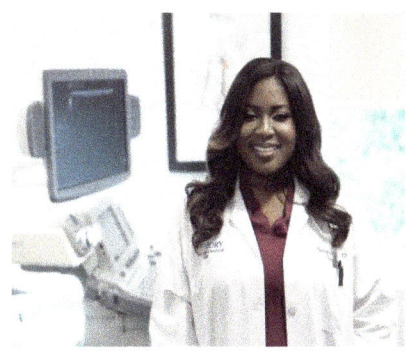

Dr. Olamide Alabi is a vascular surgeon at Emory University Hospital in Atlanta, Georgia. She received her medical degree from the University of Nebrask, College of Medicine, Omaha, Nebraska, trained in general surgery at Loma Linda University Medical Center in Loma Linda, California, and completed her fellowship in vascular surgery at Oregon Health and Science University, Portland, Oregon.

This is Dr. Alabi's story in her words.

When I was earning my undergraduate degree at the University of Nebraska, Omaha, I was interested in finding a scholarship for students who ere underrepresented minorities and from low-income families as well as first-generation college students.

At that time, I was not interested in medicine, but I did need a scholarship. As part of the program, we were required to go to the hospital, where I became interested in medicine. I stayed in the program and attended the medical school associated with the program, the University of Nebraska Medical School. Initially, I considered psychiatry, but felt this was depressing because I did not see tangible results.

During my first year in medical school, I accompanied a few primary-care physicians on a medical mission trip to Mexico. It was then that I realized I did not feel fulfilled treating medical conditions and returning to my life in the United States knowing there was no one in Mexico to follow up with the patients we cared for.

And, in my second year in medical school, I accompanied another team on a surgical mission trip to Haiti where we performed bread-and-butter surgeries like hernias, breast surgeries, and thyroidectomies. What impressed me most was the profound and immediate impact I saw on each surgical patient's life as opposed to medical patients who may have disease their entire lives. With surgery, a patient with an inguinal hernia that is large and debilitating can have surgery, and within a month be healed and again become the primary breadwinner for their family.

My life was changed. After this, the only question was what specialty of surgery would I choose? I did not have guidance and no one in my family worked in healthcare. I rotated through family medicine in rural Nebraska and had the privilege of working with a general surgeon who performed many different general surgeries including ruptured abdominal aortic aneurysms. This is a weakening of the wall of the major blood vessel that supplies organs in the abdomen and lower body that advances to the point where the blood vessel bursts causing blood to leak into the abdomen.

This experience is why I pursued general surgery but at this time, I was not aware vascular surgery was an option. To be honest, I wanted to complete my residency in a warm climate because I did not want to shovel snow early in the mornings as we did in Nebraska. I was accepted at the Loma Linda University Medical Center in Southern California for residency. This was the perfect place for me.

My residency was great. It felt like we were all a family and that I belonged to a community. This was perfect since I did not have family in California. When I began my residency training, I disliked vascular surgery because vascular patients are so ill and sometimes their conditions were severe enough for them to be in danger of losing a leg or losing their lives.

As a junior resident, vascular surgery is difficult to understand because the patients have complicated and complex problems. For instance, learning to read angiograms, pictures of blood vessels flowing to and nourishing areas of the body, to determine reasons a patient has abnormal blood flow to body areas is difficult at first. With time and experience, understanding vascular diseases and diagnostic and treatment modalities becomes easier. At Loma Linda, we rotated through vascular surgery each year during the first four years of residency.

When I was a second-year resident rotating in vascular surgery, I did not consider vascular surgery as a career until I replaced a senior resident who was unable to complete his commitment to vascular surgery for one month. This was my second rotation in vascular that year.

Initially, I thought I was being punished. Why would they put me on vascular surgery again? I was a second-year resident in the role of a senior resident. It turned out to be the best experience I ever had.

One night, a patient came into the hospital with a ruptured abdominal aortic aneurysm. I was on call with Dr. Sheela Patel. I called her and advised her of the patient's status and need for surgery. She replied, "Ok. Book it. Let's go." This meant for me to prepare the patient for surgery and make the necessary arrangements with the operating room.

I asked if she needed me to call a more senior resident or fellow and she asked, "Are you not going to be there?" I was shocked to learn she was comfortable doing the case with me. We performed the surgery together. I was in awe because typically this is a complicated case and the most senior resident is the person who assists the attending in this operation.

The next time I was on call, a patient presented with a type A dissection with associated limb ischemia. A bypass was indicated. A type A dissection occurs when a tear develops in the first part of the aorta, the largest vessel in the body, as it branches from the heart. In this case, occlusion (blockage) of the artery supplying blood to the arm occurred and needed repair.

The attending asked me to prep and drape and start dissecting the femoral artery and vein. I dissected and encircled the vessels the same way I saw my seniors do this and when I was finished, I asked if I should go to the other side. She looked up and said, "Wow, you are done? Yes, go to the other side." We worked well together, and I felt at home with the vascular team. They left a positive mark on me and I received so much support from them. One of the best technical surgeons I have ever worked with was our chief of vascular. Another surgeon, who was one of the most compassionate surgeons I knew and wanted to model my practice after, was there as well.

After these experiences, I wanted to train at the University of Oregon, Eugene, because this is where the chief trained, and he was amazing. I felt blessed when I matched in Oregon. My fellowship training was an amazing experience and again, I felt like I was part of the family. We did all we could for the patients as we worked well as a team.

One attending once said, "We may not agree on how to treat each individual case when we discuss them, but we do believe that whatever treatment we decide on is the best treatment for that patient. We don't cut corners or cut time, and no one is saying the patient is not a surgical candidate because we always do what is best for the patient." Of course, there were times patients would not benefit from surgery, but we made sure we exhausted all non-surgical options and provided the care that was in their best interest. I appreciated how the partners worked well and treated each other with respect where I trained.

I feel as a black female, there will always be challenges. There were no other black females in my program, but there were other females, and we had similar experiences. I remember being told to change my voice to make it softer and more pleasant. It seemed some felt my voice was harsh and I felt I was being criticized because I am female. I have always been concise and definitive, and this was not appreciated; the situation improved with time.

I remember one patient the urology service asked us to consult on. When I evaluated the patient, I determined they were ill enough to require intensive care unit (ICU) treatment. I transferred the patient to the surgical ICU and felt I acted in the patient's best interest by doing so.

Since I was unable to contact the chief resident, I spoke with another member of the urology team. When he discovered the patient was transferred to the SICU, he treated me meanly and told his attending what happened.

His attending discussed the situation with my attending, the chief of trauma. My attending reviewed the situation and realized I provided the proper care and made the right decision. He was objective and defended me. I was amazed when I heard this because this was an elderly white male physician who defended my actions. This does not happen very often. Having people advocating for you helps your career.

Confidence is an ongoing challenge for me, but I am becoming more confident as times passes. I never had the desire to be in academic surgery until my second year of fellowship training. Representation matters. We, as black females, do not have much representation. It is difficult to see where I am and where I wish to be because many times as black females, we must pave the way for ourselves and those coming after us. For instance, I never learned to write grants, but I am doing it. It is difficult, but I hear others agreeing it is difficult for them as well. I sometimes experience impostor syndrome and I combat these feelings by working hard, asking for help when I need it, and being humble. I tell myself, "Don't be afraid or feel ashamed to be yourself and you deserve to be there just as much as anybody else and maybe more."

As for my job, I spend half my time at the Veteran's Administration (VA) and the other half at the University Hospital because I am undecided about working full time for the VA or full time for the University Hospital.

I want to help VA patients because they are a vulnerable population. Veterans come to the VA for their care and I find it incredible to be able to serve those who served our country.

A typical week for me consists of two days seeing clinic patients and three days operating. This is split evenly between the VA and the University Hospital. We have residents and fellows in both programs. I enjoy teaching and mentoring students and surgical trainees.

My proudest moment is when I consider how we are trail-blazing for ourselves and those to come. Everything we do is a huge accomplishment and forges a path for others. My parents have advanced degrees, but neither felt their degrees were as important as my medical degree. I have a twin brother and when I graduated from medical school, he graduated with his master's degree the same day. I attended his graduation in Lincoln, Nebraska, early in the morning so I could see him walk across the stage, and he came to Omaha to watch me walk across the stage. I do not think my parents have ever been prouder!

In the middle of all my chaos, I am still searching for balance. Some weeks are better than others. You must be intentional about it. For my future downtime, I have five books that have been on my list to read for a few years. I am trying to make time for them when I can enjoy reading non-medical books once again.

There are several people I would like to have dinner and talk with and hear their stories. First would be a dinner party with my mother, father, and grandparents so I can listen to their stories. I wish my grandparents could see me now. I feel I am my ancestors' dreams fulfilled. I would love to sit with Vivien Thomas because I imagine he felt the way we feel, the feelings of not belonging and inadequacy. I would love to hear how he felt throughout the process and how he would feel knowing that his name is now included in the name of the shunt he helped create (The Blalock-Thomas-Taussig Shunt) for 'blue babies,' babies born with four heart defects. Also, I would like to talk to myself when I was 20 years old. I do not regret anything, and I do not regret my course. Maybe I could have convinced myself to complete a master's degree in public health. It would be interesting to hear who I thought I was at that time. And, I would love to talk to my 70-year-old me!

My final words to all are, "You have got to see it before you BE it!"

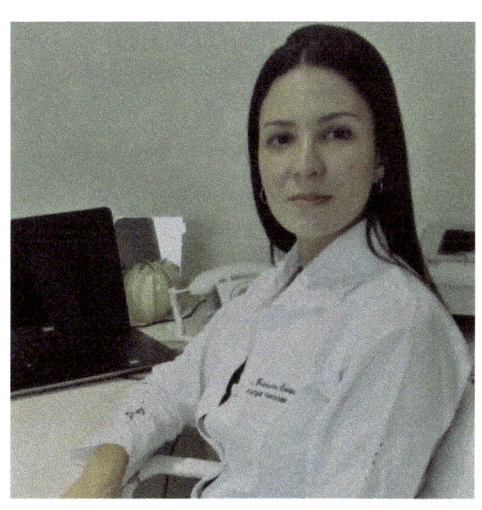

Dr. Fernanda Costa Sampaio Silva

Dr. Fernanda Costa Sampaio Silva is a vascular surgeon at the Centro Medico Hospital da Bahia, Department of Angiology and Vascular Surgery in Brazil, South America. She earned her medical degree from the Federal University of Bahia in Brazil and completed both general surgery and vascular surgery residencies at the Federal University of Bahia in Brazil and Ana Nery Hospital in Brazil. She is a member of the board of directors of the Brazilian Society of Angiology and Vascular Surgery (SBACV), regional Bahia and a member of the International Relations Committee, Society for Vascular Surgery (SVS).

Dr. Sampaio Silva is the daughter of a black father and a white mother. Unfortunately, in Brazil, there are still many remnants of the time of slavery. Racism is one of them. But she believes the greatest difficulty in being an Afro-descendant and wanting a medical career was economic limitation. In her country, she feels elementary and secondary education in public schools does not provide quality education. This makes it challenging for students applying to medical school. In the '80s and '90s, there was no quota policy at universities, so her parents had to work hard to pay for private education, otherwise, she would not have been able to fulfill her dreams of becoming a doctor.

Medicine is a prestigious profession in Brazil and difficult to achieve, which is why becoming a doctor was a great challenge. In Dr. Sampaio Silva's opinion, having professional freedom means not being afraid to deal with difficult situations. For this reason, she chose surgery, more specifically vascular surgery. She realized if she had the anatomical and technical knowledge about blood vessels, she would not be afraid to perform surgery on a human being.

Dr. Sampaio Silva has strong faith which maintains her confidence. She thinks becoming a doctor could only have been God's plan because looking at things in the natural realm, she would never have succeeded. When she investigated the paths her neighbors and childhood friends took, she realized they had different destinies than she. So, she is fully convinced that strength does not reside in her being, it comes from above.

At times along the way, Dr. Sampaio Silva struggled with impostor syndrome. It haunts her. Sometimes she feels she is in positions previously reached by rich, white people and grapples with thoughts that she does not belong where she is. Then, she takes a breath and remembers the reasons she is here. She asks herself, "Am I in leadership of any department?" And she answers, "Yes! And why did they choose me? Because I met all the requirements! Therefore, I am not an impostor!"

Dr. Sampaio Silva's greatest achievement so far was being selected as a committee member of a respected American society. No doctor in her specialty in her country has ever been selected for this position. And the best advice she ever received was, "No job, even if it is your dream, is worth your sanity." She had colleagues who committed suicide because they could not withstand the pressure of their own expectations.

To find balance, Dr. Sampaio Silva loves her husband and her son. Because she chose to have a husband and child, she makes sure she does not allow her career to absorb her. She constantly reviews her priorities, so she does not neglect them. And in her spare time, she is reading the article, *Leadership in American Surgery: Women are Rising to the Top*, recently published in the *Annals of Surgery* magazine.

Her father is the first of three people she would love to have dinner with and learn from. He died 10 years ago without seeing the results of his commitment to her career. He taught her to never give up. She would just like to say, "Thank you." Second is Rita Lobato Lopes, the first Brazilian female doctor. Dr. Sampaio Silva would like to hear what advice she would give her. And last would be Michael DeBakey, the pioneer in surgical procedures for treatment of defects and diseases of the cardiovascular system.

Words of wisdom Dr. Sampaio Silva would like to share with every reader are, "Do not let them judge you by appearance. Many may not call you doctor because you are black or have curly hair. But do not be ashamed to correct someone who confuses you with other professionals, such as a nurse or an assistant. Sometimes you will consider giving up. It is at this point you must rescue your roots and remember where you came from and how far you have come. Then keep walking. Have a life project beyond your career. Okay, you have become a surgeon and you have done a memorable job in society, but so what? Who are you outside the hospital? Do not lose your identity as a mother, wife, daughter, friend, and woman. It is to these places you will return when you feel overwhelmed and need to recharge your batteries to continue your career!"

CHAPTER SEVENTEEN
Ophthalmology Surgery

Ophthalmologists are physicians specializing in the comprehensive medical and surgical care of the eyes and vision. Ophthalmologists are the only practitioners medically trained to diagnose and treat all eye and visual problems including vision services (glasses and contacts) and provide treatment and prevention of medical disorders of the eye including surgery.

Dr. Sade Kosoko-Lasaki

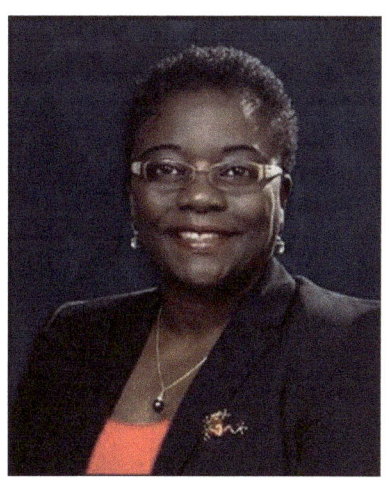

Dr. Sade Kosoko-Lasaki is associate vice provost of the Health Sciences Multicultural and Community Affairs (HS-MACA) Department at Creighton University in Omaha, Nebraska. She is also a tenured professor of ophthalmology surgery and preventive medicine and public health at the Creighton University School of Medicine. She is co-founder and co-director of the Center for Promoting Health & Health Equality.

Dr. Kosoko-Lasaki is a dynamite lady and has accomplished much in her 40-plus-year career. She is passionate about her work and, despite numerous obstacles along the way, she persisted and made a name for herself in her discipline. She completed her medical school in Nigeria and trained in ophthalmology at the University of Glasgow in Glasgow, Scotland.

She migrated to the United States and completed another residency at Howard University in Washington, D.C., and a subspecialty fellowship in glaucoma at Johns Hopkins University in Baltimore, Maryland.

She is a wife and mother of three, a stepmother of three, and a grandmother of three. She has been awarded multi-million-dollar grants for her research initiatives. She authored two major textbooks for ophthalmology and has authored multiple book chapters as well as numerous papers for publication. Her CV (resume) is 24 pages long. She is the epitome of an academic surgeon powerhouse.

Dr. Kosoko-Lasaki is passionate about eliminating health care disparities as well as minority health development and has won multiple national and international awards for her research in glaucoma, a disease of the eye resulting from increased pressure in the eye. Part of her research focuses on increasing minorities in the healthcare workforce. At Creighton University, she oversees the recruitment of disadvantaged students to the health sciences and mentors these students to retain them.

She lectures around the country and the world on cultural proficiency and health disparity issues. She focuses on the promotion of pipeline programs that prepare and support disadvantaged students from grade four through health professional schools so they may become successful health care providers.

She served as a consultant for the United Nations Children's Education Fund (UNICEF), the United States Agency for International Development (USAID), and Helen Keller International in West African countries, the Caribbean, and Asia. She expanded her outreach efforts to the Dominican Republic screening for glaucoma, performing eye surgeries, and combating childhood vitamin A deficiency.

Dr. Kosoko-Lasaki was instrumental in creating Glaucoma Initiative in the U.S. Virgin Islands, Nigeria, Rural Nebraska, Iowa, and Kansas screening of more than 20,000 individuals for glaucoma.

This is Dr. Kosoko-Lasaki's story in her words.

I was born in Sapele, Nigeria. My father, Dr. Babalola, was an optometrist, one of the first in Nigeria. He attended university in the United Kingdom and afterward returned to Nigeria where he opened his optometry practice. Before going to the United Kingdom, he was a pharmacist. Thus, I was exposed to medicine early in childhood.

When we were young, my sister and I went to our father's clinic and helped his patients select frames for glasses. I grew up loving optometry and told my father I wanted to be an optometrist like him. He told me if I wanted to practice with him someday it would be best if I was an ophthalmologist because I would be able to perform surgical procedures of the eye, which he was not able to do as an optometrist.

I was 13 years old and never knew there was such a field of medicine. I discovered that to become an ophthalmologist, I needed to attend medical school. I also realized I needed to work hard in school to earn excellent grades because this is a requirement for acceptance into medical school. At age 16, I was accepted into one of the premier medical schools at the University of Ibadan in Nigeria, Africa. I graduated from medical school at 22 years old.

After completing my national service at one of the largest hospitals for ophthalmology in Nigeria, an opportunity presented to apply for a scholarship to train in Scotland to specialize in ophthalmology. In some countries, doctors are required to complete one- or two-years work as a general practitioner in government hospitals after completing medical school. In 1979, I attended the University of Glasgow, Glasgow, Scotland, and completed my training in 1982. I planned to return to Nigeria to practice with my father.

I met my first husband when I was studying abroad in Scotland. He was from the United States. This is how my path took me to the United States after finishing my training in Scotland.

It was difficult for anyone from outside the United States to be accepted for a position to train in ophthalmology at that time. I started from the beginning in terms of residency training. It took me seven years to achieve my goal of becoming an ophthalmologist. While waiting for acceptance, I strengthened my application by earning a master's degree in public health. I worked as a consultant for the WHO, UNICEF through the Helen Keller Foundation. Through my research, we were awarded a USAID grant in St. Lucia in the Caribbean for research on glaucoma.

With a stronger application, I was accepted into Howard University, Washington D.C., for my residency in ophthalmology. After finishing residency, I was accepted to Johns Hopkins University, Baltimore, Maryland, for a fellowship in glaucoma.

I had two children before starting residency. My first child was born in 1983 and my second child was born in 1984. My youngest child was born in 1987. My children have always been my priority; even when I traveled internationally for research, I was able to take my children with me. I always made certain to ask for childcare as part of the package. Sometimes, I took my children to my parents in Nigeria for care because I became a single mother shortly after my third child was born. I have never used my children as an excuse for not getting my work done. I completed my work two to three days before due dates because I could never predict what could happen with the children. If they became ill, I was concerned this may cause me not to be able to complete my assignments or presentations.

I hired a live-in nanny to help during the week while I was in residency. I generally woke at 6 a.m. to prepare for the day. My day started with spending time with God. I took the train to work so I could read and complete my assignments. I worked moonlighting so I could afford to pay for a live-in nanny. This meant I had no days off because whenever I was not in residency training, I worked my moon-lighting shifts. My children were in bed by 8:30 p.m. every night so I was able to read and complete my assignments, which I usually worked on until 1 a.m.

When I finished my fellowship, I returned to Howard University in Washington, D.C., where I worked on faculty for 10 years before moving to Omaha, Nebraska, where I have been for 20 years.

Academic surgery does not pay as well as private practice,

so one must have a love and passion for it to choose this career path.

I recommend young women have specific goals to accomplish their career. For me, I knew I wanted to advance from assistant professor of surgery to associate professor of surgery within five years. The only way I would be able do this was by having scientific papers published in peer-review journals. I was disciplined. My day went from 8 a.m. to 5 p.m. each day, even on days I finished seeing clinic patients by 2 p.m. I used the extra time to do research, work on projects, and write papers. When you are ready to advance from associate professor to full professor, you need to add community service and committee memberships to your curriculum vitae.

A word of caution, you need to learn to say, "No," to committees and responsibilities that do not serve you well for advancement. It is easy to say, "Yes," to every committee you are asked to be a part of because you are happy you are being asked. But it is easy to become overwhelmed by too many responsibilities. I made a point to choose only three committees to be a member of at any given time.

Unlike many who pass-up opportunities because a job may not be in an ideal location or they do not want to be someplace where there is snow, I will go anywhere a great opportunity presents. I have never seen myself as a professional woman, but I am a professional. I learned early on that I am my own best advocate. I am my own champion and have learned to surround myself with people who champion me. For instance, my second husband has been a supportive partner who believes in me and wants me to be my best self.

My advice is to always be yourself because it does not matter what titles you have. At the end of the day, you are a physician and your calling is to serve patients. Your patients trust you to take care of them the best way you know how.

As I scrub my hands before each surgery, I pray for God's guidance. We are human and at times we become prideful of our abilities. I always ask God to help me remain humble and I know that God is in control in all situations. I have experienced complications, but the Lord always gives me the serenity to identify my complications and the humility to admit to them.

Part of my humility is that I know when to call for help or when to refer my patients to someone I feel will provide better care. I always tell my patients that if they have reservations about me as their surgeon, they should tell me, and I will find someone else to care for them. My mentor at Johns Hopkins taught me that I must remember every patient I operate on because they trusted me and took a chance on me. Another thing he said was to always, always be available to my patients such that when they call me, I take time to speak with them because they trust me.

When it came to finding balance, I took long walks with my children when they were young. I walked while they rode their bicycles. I do water aerobics two to three times a week and enjoy long walks to this day. I am extremely disciplined about what I eat. After turning 40, my metabolism slowed, so anything I put in my mouth I ask myself, "Is this food helping me or killing me?"

I visit my physician annually for health check-ups and make certain my cancer screening tests, my pap smear, mammogram, and colonoscopy, are up to date. I do not treat myself; I have my doctor who treats me. I make a point to keep my mind and emotions healthy and do not allow people or things around me that do not make me happy.

Currently, I am reading a book about military men who played a big role in the independence of Nigeria.

I have a mentoring group for undergraduate students on Facebook. I research articles and post them on Facebook for my group, so I read a great deal.

I also have another mentoring group for practicing physicians to help them avoid burnout, which has the added benefit of keeping me up to date with literature about burnout and physician wellness. Between these two groups, I read a great deal. I am busy, but I love the life I have.

CHAPTER EIGHTEEN
ENT Surgery

An otolaryngologist-head and neck surgeon is a physician who has been prepared by an accredited residency program to provide comprehensive medical and surgical care of patients with diseases and disorders that affect the ears, the respiratory and upper alimentary systems, and related structures of the head and neck.

Dr. Gina Jefferson

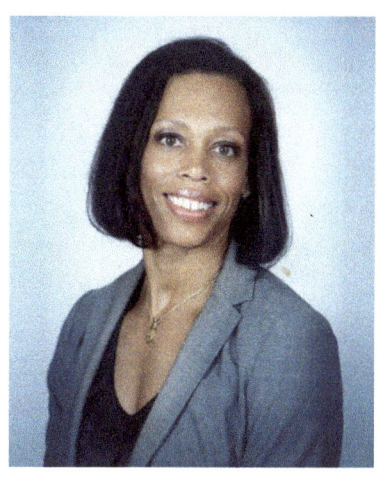

Dr. Gina Jefferson is an associate professor and chief of the division of head and neck oncologic and microvascular surgery, as well as vice-chair of education, in the Department of Otolaryngology and Communicative Sciences at the University of Mississippi Medical Center, Jackson, Mississippi.

She earned her medical degree from Case Western Reserve University School of Medicine, Cleveland, Ohio, and completed her residency in otolaryngology at Loma Linda University Medical Center, Loma Linda, California.

She continued to the department of otolaryngology, University of Miami, Miami, Florida, to complete her fellowship training in head and neck surgical oncology and microvascular reconstruction.

Dr. Jefferson is certified by the American Board of Otolaryngology. She specializes in head and neck surgical head and neck surgery oncology, microvascular reconstruction, and trans-oral robotic surgery. This includes the surgical management of adult oropharyngeal and supraglottic tumors and obstructive sleep apnea.

Her interests focus on research of head and neck cancers including patient outcomes, quality of life, and health care disparities among head and neck cancer patients. Dr. Jefferson has several articles in peer-reviewed publications and has presented at numerous national meetings including the American College of Surgeons, the American Academy of Otolaryngology, and the National Medical Association.

Dr. Jefferson grew up in Cleveland, Ohio. She and her sister were the first in their immediate family to attend college. Her sister has a Ph.D. Their parents encouraged them to be well-educated so Dr. Jefferson and her sister would enjoy a better life than they had. Dr. Jefferson had no aspirations of becoming a physician when she was a child but was proficient in math and science, and she participated in track. Because of her ability in track, she was granted a scholarship to Purdue University in Fort Wayne, Indiana, to study engineering. When she interacted with other athletes, she closely watched how they recovered after being injured. Their recovery was tremendous, and they were able to perform again despite their injuries. This fascinated her and she considered a career as a biomedical engineer.

As Dr. Jefferson worked toward her master's degree in biomedical engineering, she realized she is a people person and wanted to do something that allowed her to work with others on a team. Her first project was building a device that allowed children with cerebral palsy to swim. As she interacted with each child, she realized she really enjoyed working with children. This was when she decided she wanted to become a doctor. Initially, she thought her road would lead her to medical school to become an orthopedic surgeon.

During her third year in medical school, she considered gynecologic oncology but quickly changed her mind. Dr. Jefferson's mother was diagnosed with breast cancer when she was 37 years old. This made her consider breast surgical oncology, but she was not passionate about general surgery.

After medical school, she matched at Howard University in Washington, D.C., for her general surgery residency. It was during her residency that she was exposed to the ENT (ear/nose/and throat) specialty. As a first and second-year resident, she rotated on the endocrine surgery service. Dr. Jefferson enjoyed this her first year, but it was not until her second year of residency that she fell in love with ENT. She chose to complete a year doing research after the second year of general surgery residency and then matched with the Charles Drew Medical Center, Los Angeles, California for her residency in ENT.

During her second year of residency in ENT, her hospital (Charles Drew Medical Center) closed. Dr. Jefferson was forced to find another program. She was accepted at Loma Linda University Medical Center, Loma Linda, California, to finish her training.

Being the only female did not faze her; she was grateful for a program to train her. She was made chief resident in her chief year and her training was exceptional. Dr. Jefferson's residency at Howard prepared her for success in her current training and career because she worked with surgeons who looked like her and who were brilliant! They were great teachers and the residents, in turn, worked extremely hard and made sure they were prepared for rounds and operations.

Dr. Jefferson aspires to become a department chair because she wants to be able to give back and help others who look like her and are coming up the ranks. She wants young women thinking of a career in medicine to know mentoring and sponsorship are important for professional growth. And she thinks confidence comes in your own institution where you develop relationships with other doctors and specialties. It is important to be engaged in your own system. When you deliver presentations at meetings, the key is to be well-prepared. Always be well-prepared for cases, for rounds, for the clinic, for whatever it is you are doing. Preparation is key!

Dr. Jefferson is convinced that finding a mentor is

important. Find someone who is doing what you want to do. For those interested in pursuing a fellowship, she wants them to know they do not have to consider the specialty for which they are specifically trained. Fellowship training opens more doors and the ability to carve-out a personal niche, even in general practice. Fellowship allows the choice to do private practice or academic surgery.

Also, Dr. Jefferson advises her mentees to seek opportunities, shadow doctors, make early connections to familiarize yourself with medicine, always work hard because you never know what it is you will end up wanting to do, and do not be afraid to ask questions.

Dr. Jefferson credits her success to God. Her faith is important to her. For her, her time spent with God has evolved in a more structured way. Now that she has more control of her time, she makes a point to spend time with God in the morning before starting her day. She is grateful for her life and for the fact she is blessed to do what she loves to do. Dr. Jefferson works at a job she loves so much; not many people can say this. In residency, she had her Bible app on her phone and whenever she had time to read, she read and prayed, even in the car on her way to work or home. Finding time may be difficult, but it is important to try.

Now, in a typical work week, she spends three to four days in the operating room and one day, sometimes one-and-a-half days, seeing clinic patients. She spends half a day or one day doing administrative work.

If Dr. Jefferson could do one surgery, and only one surgery, every day for the rest of her life it would be micro-vascular free tissue transfers because it gives her the ability to reconstruct in many different ways. This procedure is when a block of skin, tissue, muscle, or bone is removed from a donor site and attached to the area in need of reconstruction. Dr. Jefferson must use a microscope to see and connect the tiny blood vessels in the free flap to the blood vessels at the recipient site. Very thin sutures (stitches) are used to join these tiny blood vessels.

In the operating room, Dr. Jefferson often plays "Black Eyed Peas" radio.

Three people Dr. Jefferson would want to have dinner with and learn from are Nelson Mandela, because of his perseverance and service to others; Oprah Winfrey, who wonderfully took advantage of the American dream and overcame some overwhelming odds and is the epitome of doing what you love and giving back to others; and Misty Copeland, because everyone told her she could not be a ballerina because she started so late. Not only is she a ballerina, but she is the best ballerina. She is the first African American woman promoted to principal dancer in the prestigious American Ballet Theater's 75-year history. She is pretty amazing.

Dr. Jefferson's final words of encouragement are, "You can do anything you set your mind to. Enjoy the process and do not forget to give back!"

Dr. Barbara Grandison

Dr. Barbara Grandison grew up in a family with many siblings in Spanish Town, Jamaica. She attended primary school in Spanish Town and then commuted every day to high school in Kingston, Jamaica. While in high school, she was in girl guides and rangers (girl scouts), and there was a program where the girls could be 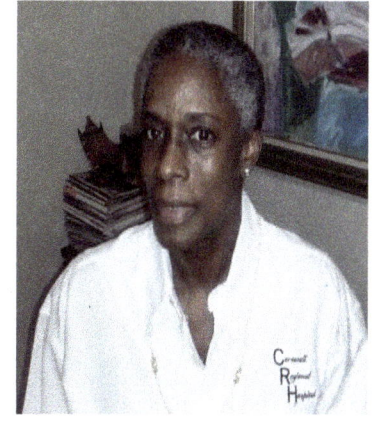 candy stripers at the hospital to help sick people. They also visited a home for mentally disabled children. There, they interacted with children with various congenital and mental disorders. It was at this time Dr. Grandison became interested in their care and decided she wanted to be a psychiatrist. When she discovered she needed to go to medical school to become a psychiatrist, she applied to the university with her friends because this made it fun and not stressful. Dr. Grandison was accepted to complete the preliminary courses at the university in preparation for medical school. She did well her first year and was accepted to medical school.

Dr. Grandison was not the best student in the class, but she worked hard and graduated from medical school. During medical school in her country, they were able do locums where they worked and were paid. Dr. Grandison did locums in the ENT (ear/nose/throat) department. This was when she realized she enjoyed this work and chose ENT as a specialty.

When Dr. Grandison graduated from medical school, she spent part of her internship training in ENT and the other time training in chest medicine. She began her ENT residency after her internship.

She was fortunate to have a great mentor during her residency at the University of West Indies, Jamaica, who helped her grow as a physician and surgeon. Dr. Grandison chose to work in public service, at a government hospital, in Montego Bay, Jamaica, where there were no ENT specialists and amazingly created a new ENT program. It was extremely challenging to start a program, so in the beginning she did everything on her own because there were no interns or residents. Dr. Grandison had a supportive anesthesiologist that made those first few years as the only ENT specialist more manageable.

It was great to watch the program grow. Now they have three consultant ENT surgeons and the program trains residents. Dr. Grandison also has a private practice she opened in 1987 at the same time she began working in public service. This is going well. If she could do one surgery for the rest of her career it would be tonsillectomies and thyroidectomies. Wait, this is two operations!

The challenges Dr. Grandison faced in the Caribbean were not due to being a female because women have been doing many male-dominated jobs for a long time. There are instances she passed on opportunities that could have advanced her career, but she chose to prioritize her family. Challenges were more institutional based, such as shortage of resources, manpower, and supplies, not discrimination or sexism.

To build confidence, Dr. Grandison advises new doctors to read about patients' conditions and treatments and about the operations and discuss everything with mentors. She felt empowered because her mentors empowered her and guided her. Dr. Grandison tells her residents there is no substitute for being well-prepared. Know everything about the patient. It is not about experiencing complications because complications will happen. It is about how you prepare for surgery, how you prepare your patients for surgery, and how you recognize complications and deal with them before they escalate.

She does not want her learning doctors to be afraid because something adverse may happen, but Dr. Grandison wants them to think about how to fix problems when they present. She welcomes suggestions. So, if she does something one way and someone shares how they find another way that works, she is willing to add to her armamentarium.

Dr. Grandison also coaches learning doctors to be willing to do what is required, sometimes more than what their job description is. Do whatever it takes to make things flow smoothly. The priority is the patients. It is important to be compassionate. Take time to talk and listen to patients. Dr. Grandison always treats her patients as she would her loved ones. She has a 33-year-old son.

Final words shared by Dr. Grandison are, "It is been a journey of learning and a journey of independence and dependence. Pave a way for others and after you finish your tour of duty you may end up being the patient. So it is important that what you leave behind will serve everyone so that even the least among us can receive great care."

"There is no passion to be found playing small — in settling for a life that is less than the one you are capable of living."
Nelson Mandela

Dr. Tonia Farmer

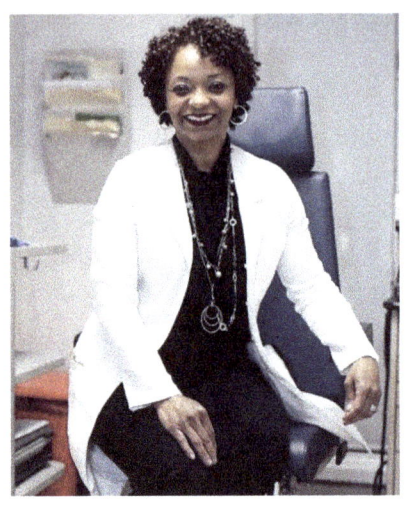

Dr. Tonia Farmer completed her medical school training at the Virginia Commonwealth University Medical College of Virginia in Richmond, Virginia, where she was inducted into the honor society, Alpha Omega Alpha. She remained there for her residency in Otolaryngology (ENT) and was the first female ever accepted into its residency program.

Otolaryngologist/Head and Neck Surgeon Dr. Farmer practices in Warren, Ohio. She owns the world-renowned Lippy Group for ear, nose, and throat care and the Lippy Surgery Center. In addition to her practice, she launched a company in 2018 called Salt Me! Her company specializes in Himalayan sea salt sinus and body care products, as well as provides easy to understand health and wellness education.

This is Dr. Farmer's story in her words.

The defining moment that made me choose medicine as a career was when my twin sister was diagnosed with osteosarcoma (bone cancer) when we were seven years old. My desire to become a doctor started with this experience and her being in and out of the hospital. How her doctors cared for her and our family impacted me greatly. I knew one day I wanted to be a doctor so I could do this for other people. Sonia died when we were nine years old. Though it has been a little more than 40 years since her passing, she has been the driving force behind my perseverance and success. I wanted to be a doctor for her, too.

One of the greatest challenges I faced during my journey was impostor syndrome. I did not know it had a name. I suffered from this when I was in residency and as a new attending. I battled feelings of not deserving my position because I was the first female and only black person in my residency program.

There were instances when I felt as if patients were looking past me because I was black. One example is when I was leading my team on rounds as a chief resident and a Caucasian patient refused to address me when speaking. This patient addressed their questions to the junior resident, a white male. The patient did this despite this junior resident redirecting him to me, the most experienced and senior member of the team. I experienced different feelings when I walked into a room with a Caucasian patient than I did entering a room with a black patient. I felt appreciated by people who looked like me.

There was an instance in training when a patient was blatantly racist. My attending removed me from this patient's care. He advocated for me so I would not be subjected to this type of treatment.

Another challenge I faced was my image was not accepted. I planned a vacation to a Caribbean island and had my hair specially braided. It is helpful for black women to keep our hair braided when we plan to be in water for long periods of time. When I returned from vacation, an attending told me my hair style was not professional because it was braided, even though my braids were professionally styled and neat.

The expectation was my hair be styled straight. This showed me I could not be myself and was forced to conform to society's idea of what is professional when it comes to black women's hair.

For the remainder of my training and into my early years as an attending, I wore my hair straight. Now, however, I wear my hair natural and am comfortable this way. It may seem like an insignificant topic, but for black women, these are some of the challenges we face.

Sometimes black women must conform and wear their hair straight or in weaves and wigs to be accepted into positions. Some have the courage to wear their hair natural once they are established in their jobs and can make their own decisions without it impacting their career trajectory.

In ENT, I felt my greatest challenge was being black rather

than being female. This field has many females, but a small number of blacks. I had excellent training and I did not feel I was treated differently from my male colleagues in terms of training opportunities. I feel ENT is a gentler surgical field to women compared to other surgical specialties.

A typical workday begins with making sure my children are ready for school in the morning before I go to the office. I need to be at work earlier on days I perform surgery. Those days my husband takes over the task of getting our children ready to go. We have our specific roles with the children. I take care of the clothes and hair for the girls and my husband makes them a hot breakfast every morning. I am usually home by 6 or 7 p.m. on days I have surgery and earlier when I see clinic patients.

I would say the secret sauce to my success in life is surrounding myself with mentors and a strong support system. While going through my schooling and training I learned I needed cheerleaders to help me along who were also experiencing what I was or who had experienced it already.

I have a woman named Betty Golden, who, along with her husband, were pivotal in mentoring my husband and me in our marriage. For us, it was important to have a Christian couple as mentors for a godly marriage. They have been such a blessing to us.

I am a member of Jack and Jill of America, Inc. This organization for mothers with children ages 2-19 is dedicated to nurturing future African American leaders by strengthening children through leadership development, volunteer services, philanthropic giving, and civic duty.

This organization provides a great support system and I have another mother who understands the struggles of parenting. Her support has helped greatly.

My family keeps me grounded. Growing up, my main pillars of support where my mother, grandmother, and aunt, and when I married, my husband became another major support person.

As I have grown older, my support system has grown. I

honestly believe in the African proverb that "It takes a village to raise a child." I am convinced it takes a village for a woman to become the best version of herself. Even though my twin sister is not with us, she is forever in my heart.

Finding balance is always a challenge. I work awfully hard because being in a private practice means I am a business owner. The work is never done. Gradually, I have learned to manage my time more efficiently and not feel guilty for not being able to do everything. I wear many hats in life. I am a wife, a mother of three girls, a daughter, and a doctor. I constantly check how I am doing in all these areas of my life. There is no way I will always have everything balanced.

In addition to my private practice, I started a company. Let me begin by saying that I love Himalayan sea salt! As you know, I am a board-certified otolaryngologist/head and neck surgeon (or ENT doctor) and I care for patients with sinus problems. Living in Ohio is good for my business because there are many patients with sinus problems here.

One of my patients introduced me to salt therapy (halotherapy) because she found it improved her chronic sinus symptoms. When I examined her sinuses with a scope, her sinus mucosa was healthy and appeared to be the healthiest I had ever seen it.

She shared how she began salt therapy sessions at Salt Sensations USA, LLC in Boardman, Ohio. I contacted the owner, Tracy Prizant, and visited her business. I experienced a salt therapy session with some of my staff members and was convinced that salt therapy was not only a growing spa treatment but also a beneficial, natural therapeutic option for my patients.

I spent hours securing and reviewing clinical research studies from Europe on the use of dry, aerosolized, inhaled Himalayan sea salt. These studies supported the benefit of salt therapy to improve respiratory and dermatological disorders.

I began recommending salt therapy to my patients as an adjunctive treatment to manage their upper and lower respiratory problems. I was interested to see how well salt therapy would work for my patients and how I could incorporate Himalayan sea salt into quality body and sinus care products that could be used at home. *Salt Me!* was born!

My love for entrepreneurship started early in life. During my surgical residency, I created a small business specializing in decorative, customized picture frames. It was a great DIY stress-reliever and allowed me to make a few extra dollars to help my tight budget. I have dabbled in other things along the way, including a party planning business I also do on the side. I really enjoy it, but I have not had much financial success from this because each job is usually a favor for my friends and family. But I must say, I do enjoy planning a great party and I am still considering making it an official business someday. In 2018, I launched Salt Me! This business has been doing well financially.

I enjoy success as an entrepreneur by co-owning the world-renowned Lippy Group for ENT and Lippy Surgery Center. The Lippy Surgery Center is a multi-specialty ambulatory surgery center established in 2008. We have delivered quality surgical and post-operative care to thousands of adults and children from around the world. Hearing-impaired clients have visited from all over the United States, Canada, and as far away as Israel for life-changing surgical procedures to improve and restore hearing.

Surgical specialties offered at The Lippy Surgery Center include procedures for eyes, ears, nose, and the throat as well as both functional and cosmetic plastic surgeries. Specialties related to ears include middle and inner-ear implants, bone anchored hearing aids, and cochlear implants. We regularly perform pediatric ear, nose, and throat procedures and maintain an outstanding safety record. We offer vocal and functional nasal surgeries as well as sinus procedures using high-tech CT guidance for optimal results.

Giving back by supporting small business owners is also important to me. They inspire me to keep growing. *Salt Me!* is a natural extension of my medical practice and allows me to put my desire to help others into action. It has become a family business because my three girls, Sonia, Simone, and Sanaa, as well as my husband Casey, provide the wind beneath my wings.

People I would like to have dinner with and learn from are first, Barack Obama. When I think of him, I think of grace under fire. Regardless of who he was dealing with, he was exemplary in the way he dealt with them. I want to know what made him walk with grace the eight years he was in office and dealt with racism and disrespect. I want to know how he managed to keep a level head and remain humble with all the accolades and praise. And, Harriet Tubman. When I think of her, I think of the phrase, "For such a time as this." She was born for the purpose of leading people out of slavery. Nothing deterred her from what she knew she had to do to bring freedom to others after she found freedom. She went back time and again. I would want to sit down and talk to her and glean small pieces of her strength and determination. Lastly, I would love to sit and have dinner with my twin sister, Sonia. When she was diagnosed with cancer, she knew she was going to die. My mother brought her home because the doctors told her there was nothing more they could do for her in the hospital. I remember that day. Sonia, who had her entire leg amputated and had multiple lung surgeries to remove cancer that spread there, was on home oxygen and could not breathe.

On the day she died, June 17, 1979, she said, "Mom call the ambulance because I can't breathe, and I am going to die tonight." She wrote a poem three months before she died. I have her poem on my wall, and I miniaturized it and laminated it and carry it in my wallet with me. She had the faith of a mustard seed. I want to sit and talk with her because at the time of her death, I did not understand her faith and what was going on. I want to know where her faith came from. How did it feel for her to know that she was leaving this earth and going to be with the Lord? I want her to see and know how much her life has meant to my life. I am who I am, and the doctor I am, for my patients because of her life. I want to be the kind of doctor who is loving and compassionate; the way her doctors were with her. Here is the poem:

February 29, 1979
<u>My prayer</u>
The Lord is our savior
We trust in Him. We love Him
You should pray to Him
He can see you and hear you
Everyone in the whole wide world loves Him
Some people do not love God and do not believe in Him
But I know I do
When you pray and ask God for something
You may not get it; God will wait until He sees you are ready for what you want
And sometimes you may not get it
But do not worry, God may think that you do not need it
Whoever does not believe in God
I will try to pray for you, for anyone
Sonia

My final words of encouragement are, "Do NOT accept other people's opinions about yourself. Always command YOUR future to achieve success. I believe in the 5 P's: Positioning can be Painful but is always Purposeful to Prepare you for your Place. This means that at times you must go through difficulties, but you must persevere because each difficult experience is preparing you for your success.

CHAPTER NINETEEN
Plastics and Reconstructive Surgery

Plastics and reconstructive surgery deals with the repair, reconstruction, or replacement of physical defects of form or function involving the skin, musculoskeletal system, cranio and maxillofacial structures, hand, extremities, breast and trunk, and external genitalia. It uses aesthetic surgical principles not only to improve undesirable qualities of normal structures but also in all reconstructive procedures as well.

Dr. Metasebia Worku Abebe

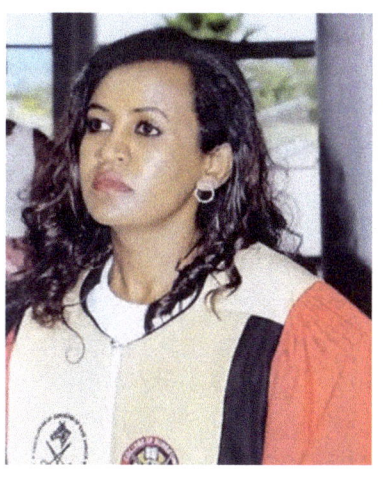

Dr. Metasebia Worku Abebe earned her medical degree at Addis Ababa University in Ethiopia, Africa. She completed her two years of national service required in Ethiopia after completing medical school as a general medical practitioner at Saint Paul Millennium Medical College in Addis Ababa, Ethiopia. She also earned a Master of Public Health (MPH) at Addis Continental Institute of Public Health in Addis Ababa, during the time she completed her national service. She was accepted for her general surgery internship and a plastics and reconstructive surgery residency at Addis Ababa University. She is currently a consultant plastic and reconstructive surgeon at Saint Paul Millennium Medical College in Addis Ababa, Ethiopia.

This is Dr. Metasebia Worku Abebe's story in her own words.

Persistence and hard work were my strongest steppingstones as a surgeon. As the younger of two daughters of hard-working middle-class parents who prioritized education, I had a wonderful support system at home. I went to an all-girls school where I competed with other hard-working girls striving to succeed. This produced unwavering confidence in myself. I have always known I can achieve anything I want to achieve if I put the necessary effort and time into it.

My journey in medical school, as anyone who has experienced any extremely competitive and demanding environment knows, was far from smooth. There will be times when you think you have given all it takes, but the results are not satisfactory. This requires even more determination and effort.

As with many higher-education programs, I feel medical school is a male-dominated field and surgery is even more so. You come across many personalities in your schooling as well as your workplace that will attribute your achievements to your gender rather than your commitment or hard work. It is important to push through all these hurdles and not lose sight of the goals you set for yourself.

I was one of the five female general surgery residents accepted into a program that accepted 30 residents per year. I knew surgery was my passion, but I also knew it would be demanding and I had to be focused, so this is what I did.

As a female in an environment not accustomed to having women around, I felt I needed to do twice as much work to balance my work and personal life, but it is possible, and I made it. I feel you will have role models you look up to, colleagues that lift you and support you, and there will be nay-sayers who will try to discourage you. If you put your focus, determination, and hard work towards your goals, you can and will achieve them.

What I have told myself from an early age is, "You are doing well, but there is always room for improvement. You can do it. Push through!"

Dr. Sharone' M. Jacobs

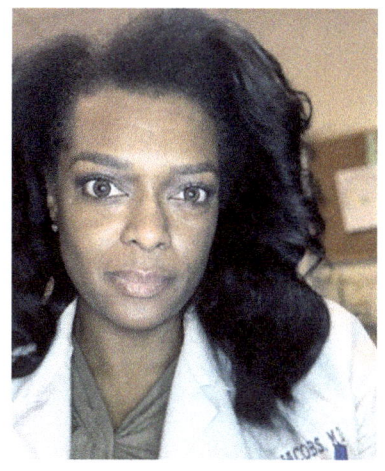

Dr. Sharone' M. Jacobs graduated from Duke University, Durham, North Carolina, earning a bachelor of science in biology and a minor in chemistry. She received her medical degree at the Louisiana State University School of Medicine in New Orleans, Louisiana. She completed her internship and residency in general surgery at New York-Presbyterian Queens hospital in Flushing, New York. She is an associate fellow of the American College of Surgeons.

Dr. Jacobs's story is a testament to the fact that your career may not go exactly as you imagined at times, but in the end, it is the best thing that ever happened to you.

This is Dr. Jacobs' story in her words.

I grew up in New Iberia, Louisiana, with a population of about 40,000 people. I had a good mixture of friends and experiences, which was much different than where I lived in New York for most of my adult life. I was enrolled in the honors program and did well in high school. I was a well-rounded student and involved in many extracurricular activities.

Initially, I aspired to become an attorney, so over one summer I had a job with a family friend who was an attorney in town. I worked at his office helping with faxing, filings, and occasionally researching cases at the courthouse. I loved it and thought I might enjoy practicing corporate law.

My first year in college, I studied biology with my boyfriend who was interested in medicine. Anatomy lab was love at first dissection! From there, I volunteered at hospitals over summer breaks in college. I was hooked from that point on and knew I wanted to be a physician.

Everything was easy initially. Undergraduate and medical

school were a breeze, relatively speaking. Reality hit in surgical residency. This is when I encountered obstacles. To be honest, the first two years as a junior resident were heaven. I loved everything about surgery and my training. The challenges were when I became a senior resident, when the weight of my clinical decisions was more imperative.

It took a while to build confidence. I feel confidence is built with time and comes when you realize you are good enough. I took two years off from clinical work to conduct research in a plastic surgery laboratory at Columbia. I was challenged when I returned to my surgical residency, and it took time to regain my confidence because my skills were rusty. I suffered from impostor syndrome after finishing residency and was working locum jobs where I was the only available surgeon. To conquer impostor syndrome, you must get out of your own way and keep believing in yourself. I knew I was trained to handle almost anything. It is helpful to learn to block out the self-doubt.

Then, amazingly enough, an opportunity presented in wound care. I worked with Vohra Wound Physicians initially, then went on to work at Montefiore Hospital in New York. I worked in the vascular surgery department. I managed the hyperbaric clinic and did administrative work for about four years before I received a flyer recruiting hair restoration surgeons. I usually discarded such solicitation, however, this one caught my interest because secretly, I wanted to have eyebrow restoration myself.

I responded and the rest is history! I started my hair restoration career in our Manhattan, New York, office before moving to Philadelphia to manage this office. I love what I do! Not only do I wake up excited (most days) about transforming someone's life, but my schedule also affords me time to spend with my daughter. Currently I arrive at work at 7:30 a.m. and typically perform 2-3 cases a day. I finish about 5 p.m.

I complete my cases in the morning and see consultations in the afternoon. Once we admit the patient, we take before photos. I draw where I will transfer the hairline to, then I get to work.

My job allows me to be creative because there is an element of finesse and design in the surgical planning. In addition, my job gives me autonomy, and a much better work-life balance.

But, to be honest, balance is still a work-in-progress. My current position makes everything easier because I arrive home at 7:30 p.m. or 8 p.m. Balance was easier when I had a live-in nanny. Now, my daughter is in daycare across from my office. This is convenient. I continue to work in a social life. When I figure out how to balance everything, I will let you know!

I feel my greatest accomplishment is my daughter. I never planned to have children. I was focused on my goals and establishing my career, so children were not a priority. I was 38 years old when I had my daughter, which is considered late, but she has been my greatest blessing.

Completing my surgical residency was another great accomplishment. Surgery training was difficult. There were times I wanted to give up, but I persisted. My father died when I was in medical school. His dying wish was to see me finish medical school and become a surgeon. Even though he was not here to see me through, I was still motivated to finish on his behalf. I could not let the sacrifices my family made (mom, I am looking at you), just fall by the wayside

As far as dealing with failure goes, I have a remarkable ability to block things out. I give myself a moment to mourn and be down about it and then I pick myself up and move on. I look at what caused my failure and make the necessary changes.

Lessons I would like to share with the up-and-coming young black woman who wants to be a physician are, it is especially important to read! Read all the time! It is important to take control of your education and development in surgical residency. Work hard to master your skills early on. It is important to have a strong support network, both at home and ideally someone at the hospital you can trust. Finding a mentor is key. I kept my mentors' phone numbers on speed-dial during my initial years as an attending. In medical school, don't take every student loan available just because you can, live simply. Try to live as simply as possible. Once in residency, start paying back the loans. Do this even if all you can afford is the interest-only payments. Learn about managing money early during residency. Protect your investment and find good disability insurance coverage early in your surgical training. Ideally you should do this before you develop any injuries or become pregnant because the premiums increase significantly for women thereafter.

My final words to all the ladies out there are, "I heard a wonderful quote by Suzy Kassem I love to recite to myself whenever I feel fear guiding my decisions. 'Doubt kills more dreams than failure ever will.' I hope this helps someone as much as it has helped me!"

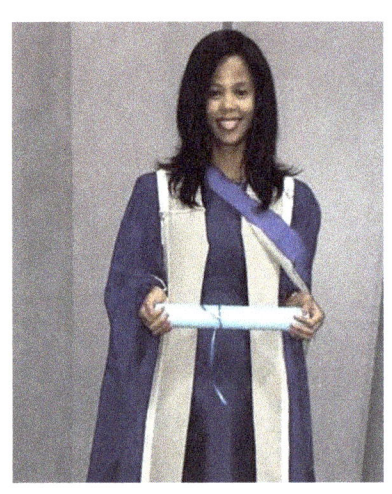

Dr. Elizabeth A. Xoagus-Makakole

Dr. Elizabeth A. Xoagus-Makakole is a consultant plastic and reconstructive surgeon at Inkosi Albert Luthuli Hospital in Durban, South Africa. She earned her medical degree at the University of Cape Town in Cape Town, South Africa. She returned to her home country, Namibia, and completed her internship as she worked as a medical officer in general surgery. She returned to South Africa for her plastic surgery fellowship and became Namibia's first black female plastic surgeon. She is a fellow of the college of plastic surgeons of South Africa.

Growing up, medicine is the only career Dr. Xoagus-Makakole dreamed of pursuing. As a child, she was motivated to pursue medicine when her mom was sick. Dr. Xoagus-Makakole felt helpless. Even when her mom was sick with a simple common cold it changed the atmosphere at home. Dr. Xoagus-

Makakole did not like this atmosphere or seeing her mom sick. She thinks this subconsciously made her pursue her dream to become a medical doctor as a way to help.

During her internship, her general surgery department head took it upon himself to convince her she should pursue a career in surgery. He believed she had the skills to do so. "You have good hands," he said. Dr. Xoagus-Makakole was the first female in a general surgery rotation performing general surgical procedures as a medical officer. This was not well received by many, including the nurses and some colleagues. Their reaction discouraged her from pursuing a career in surgery. She thanks God that her department head was insistent and pushed her to pursue surgery despite the opposition.

Dr. Xoagus-Makakole's first exposure to plastic surgery was when she was assigned to work with a group of visiting missionary plastic surgeons. There were no plastic surgery residents in her hospital at the time. During their two-week stay, the visiting team focused on reconstructive surgery. Dr. Xoagus-Makakole had the opportunity to observe a patient who was restored and regained lost function. This is why she fell in love with plastic surgery.

Her greatest challenge was facing and fighting discrimination. It was not easy, but she learned to be firm and knew what her rights were and are. She stood for what was right and is now well-respected in her field because she persevered.

Dr. Xoagus-Makakole attributes her strength and confidence to the fact that she is a born-again Christian. Her faith makes her confident because her confidence is in God and what He says about her in His Word. Her second source of confidence comes from her dearest mother who supported her and believed in her dream more than anyone else and who continues to encourage her. Dr. Xoagus-Makakole also draws support from the rest of her family and friends who believe in her and help keep her moving forward.

Dr. Xoagus-Makakole realized early on in her career path that she needed to prioritize things. Some things in life are of higher priority than others. Life requires one to be flexible and there are phases or periods where she prioritized some aspects of her life more than others.

It also means realizing and accepting she cannot do everything, and she must leave some things and defer others to another time. However, she feels it is crucial to remember that no important aspect of life should be neglected for too long.

Dr. Xoagus-Makakole considers her greatest accomplishments and proudest moments to be seeing her daughter following in her footsteps. Dr. Xoagus-Makakole does not mean her daughter talking about becoming a doctor but realizing she has set a good example for her daughter. Dr. Xoagus-Makakole sees her daughter dreaming big and believing in herself. This is reflected by her performance at school and her view and approach to academics.

When her daughter attended Dr. Xoagus-Makakole's master's graduation ceremony, she asked her mother what the highest qualification is that one could attain. When Dr. Xoagus-Makakole told her daughter, the highest qualification is a doctorate; her daughter promptly asked why she was not pursuing that! Dr. Xoagus-Makakole's daughter concluded her mother's not pursuing a doctorate was like dropping out of high school before completing her matriculation (final high school exams in southern Africa).

This was Dr. Xoagus-Makakole's proudest moment because she knows her daughter will achieve great things and she does not need to tell her daughter the importance of school, hard work, and striving for excellence. Her daughter knows these things. In other countries doctors have a master's degree as their highest degree and a doctorate is a PhD degree except for countries such as the USA and Philippines where a DO or MD degree is a doctorate.

On the flip side, Dr. Xoagus-Makakole finds how to deal with failure and complications a good question, but a difficult one. She does not think she will ever become immune to complications. She does not think anyone ever does! Dr. Xoagus-

Makakole thinks we are all able to handle minor complications well, but major complications are more challenging. They affect every surgeon, otherwise, we would not have hearts.

Dr. Xoagus-Makakole feels that the sooner she realizes and accepts the reality that complications are part of the profession, the better it is for her and her patients. She allows herself to mourn the failure, but she does not dwell on it. She similarly celebrates the successful cases quietly and with humility. The fact that the successful cases are more the norm than are failures/complications also helps to deal with the sentiments around the failure/complications quickly and keeps her moving forward.

A typical day for Dr. Xoagus-Makakole depends on whether it is a clinic day or a theater (operating room) day. She starts with ward rounds at 8 a.m. on a clinic day, which last about two hours, followed by outpatient consults in the clinic.

Dr. Xoagus-Makakole works in clinic as with her team, the registrars (residents), and medical officers. They usually complete their work before 4 p.m. and have an academic program starting at 4 p.m., with a presentation prepared by a registrar or medical officer. This is followed by a journal club presentation from 5 to 6 p.m. prepared by a consultant.

She usually arrives home at about 7 p.m. on clinic days. Dr. Xoagus-Makakole serves supper, cleans up, then she tucks her daughter into bed. She either does administrative work at 10 p.m. before she goes to bed or just goes to bed when she is too tired to work more. If she does not get to her administrative the night before, she wakes early to complete it.

A typical theater day starts at 8 a.m. and ends around 5 p.m. most days but can continue until 6 or 7 p.m. depending on the complexity of the surgery she is performing.

Finally, Dr. Xoagus-Makakole would like to add, "First, you have to believe in yourself, otherwise, no one else will. Secondly, know you are enough just the way you are! Do not seek external validation. Master your craft and shine. Lastly, choose your battles wisely. Not everything is worth a fight."

CHAPTER TWENTY
Surgical Oncology

Surgical oncology is the branch of surgery applied to oncology (cancer); it focuses on the surgical management of tumors, especially cancerous tumors.

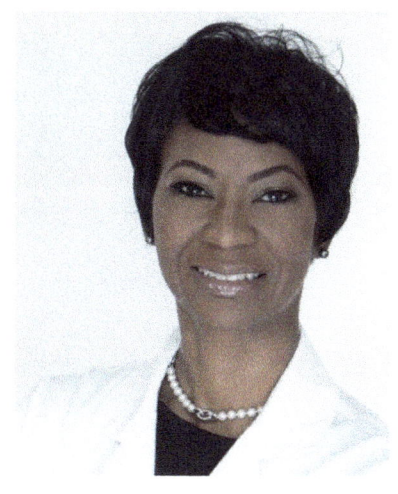

Dr. Lori Wilson

Dr. Lori Wilson is the division chief of surgical oncology at Howard University Hospital in Washington, D.C, and focuses on health disparities in underrepresented populations as well as breast, colorectal, and endocrine cancers.

She is also the program director of the general surgery residency at Howard University Hospital. As a graduate of Georgetown University School of Medicine in Washington, D.C., she completed her internship and residency in general surgery at Howard University Hospital. During this time, she was honored with the university's Chairman's Award, the Resident's Choice Award from the department of surgery, and was inducted into Alpha Omega Alpha, Gamma Chapter, Medical Honor Society, along with other honors.

She completed her research fellowship at the University of Cincinnati in Ohio, with advanced coursework in cellular biology, molecular genetics, and bioethics. She finished her surgical oncology fellowship at the John Wayne Cancer Institute in Santa Monica, California, where she was honored as a chief administrative surgical oncology fellow.

Dr. Wilson's personal struggle with breast cancer is

293

featured in the Ken Burns' PBS documentary, *Cancer: The Emperor of All Maladies,* based on the Pulitzer Prize-winning book by Dr. Siddhartha Mukherjee. She allowed cameras to film her surgery as she underwent a double mastectomy. She is a breast cancer survivor and works tirelessly to fight cancer daily.

This is Dr. Wilson's story.

My journey to become a surgeon began when I was seven years old. I always liked science and numbers in elementary school. I watched *MASH* and wanted to be like Hawkeye. He was the male surgeon who saved people and was good at what he did. It did not dawn on me that he did not look like me. I enjoyed watching the surgeons on *MASH* saving lives and using their abilities to help someone who was injured or sick. Even though this was fictitious, I loved how they immediately changed a patient's health.

When I was in elementary school. My parents purchased a set of encyclopedias that came with a medical encyclopedia as a bonus book. I liked the transparencies of the bones, muscles, and blood vessels. When I was in the 10th grade, I was selected to participate in a summer program focusing on cancer research. It was then that I decided I wanted to be a cancer surgeon.

My parents lived in the segregated south and waited until later in life to have me when more opportunities were available for black people. I was the first person in my family to finish college. My parents said if I worked hard, I could be whatever I wanted to be.

Now, I am a surgical oncologist, and I operate one or two days a week. I see patients in the clinic one or two days a week. I am also the program director for the general surgery residency managing 33 residents through their training. I also volunteer and provide more than 50 women with free mammography and clinical breast exams once a month.

My favorite part of my job is spending time with my patients and getting to know them as people. The operating room is my oasis. It is where I am most comfortable. Besides this, the best part of my job is knowing I have an impact.

My goal has always been making sure everyone has a fair and just opportunity and removing barriers that make outcomes different, whether these disadvantages are social, economic, or environmental. I spend my day partnering with women and men helping them understand the word cancer that has now become their diagnosis. I help them know what this diagnosis really means, what the treatment will do, and how they will look toward their future in a real and relevant way.

On a personal note, I was diagnosed with breast cancer in June 2013 when my son was 18 months old. After I stopped breastfeeding, one of my breasts did not decrease in size. This is abnormal, so I had a mammogram. I was devastated when I was told my diagnosis was breast cancer. I chose Johns Hopkins in Baltimore, Maryland, for treatment since I was well-known at Howard University Hospital where I worked. I just wanted to be a patient and Johns Hopkins was closer to my home.

On my first visit, I realized my medical oncologist was a woman I sat next to at a charity event months before. I was diagnosed with two types of invasive cancer in both breasts. One type of cancer was triple-negative, meaning the cancer cells did not have estrogen or progesterone receptors and did not make much of the protein called HER2.

HER2 cell receptors are special proteins found inside or on the surface of cells that receive signals from the bloodstream (hormones) that help the cells grow. So, this means triple-negative breast cancer does not respond to hormonal therapy medicine or medicines that target HER2 protein receptors because these hormone receptors are not present on the cells. This is the most aggressive breast cancer and has the worst prognosis for survival. I underwent 16 treatments of chemotherapy followed by a double mastectomy with immediate reconstruction. I also received 30 treatments of radiation to my chest wall and hormonal therapy. I am a survivor.

I think as a doctor I was a fairly good patient. During my last year of training as a surgical resident, my mother was diagnosed with lung cancer and I spent that year caring for her and experiencing cancer as a caregiver. My mother wanted to stay at home during the end of her life and this taught me about humility and letting go and allowing people to care for you.

I learned from her is that it is ok to let people who love and care about you take care of you when you really need it and are vulnerable. If I had not experienced this, I would probably not have been a good patient. But I was determined to let go and not direct my care.

I asked my doctors to treat me as they would any other patient and explain everything to me the way they would explain things to their regular patients. I was fortunate to have the resources I have. I had my surgery at Cedar Sinai in Los Angeles, California, by my mentor Dr. Armando Giuliano, who trained me thirteen years prior. Being a patient was a humbling experience.

Dr. Giuliano shared, "We all loved Lori when she was a surgical oncology fellow. She was very hardworking, very smart, fun to be with, completely reliable, and very inquisitive. She had a spark. I knew she would do something with her life and career!"

"You've got to follow your passion. You've got to figure out what it is you love—who you really are. And have the courage to do that. I believe that the only courage anybody ever needs is the courage to follow your own dreams."
Oprah Winfrey

CHAPTER TWENTY-ONE
Oral and Maxillofacial Surgery

Oral and maxillofacial surgeons are trained to recognize and treat a wide spectrum of diseases, injuries and defects in the head, neck, face, jaw, and the hard and soft tissues of the oral and maxillofacial region. They are also trained to administer anesthesia and provide care in an office setting. They treat problems such as the extraction of wisdom teeth, misaligned jaws, tumors and cysts of the jaw and mouth, and to perform dental implant surgery. Oral and maxillofacial surgery is a surgical specialty recognized by the American College of Surgeons and is one of nine dental specialties recognized by the American Dental Association, the Royal College of Dentists of Canada, and the Royal Australasian College of Dental Surgeons.

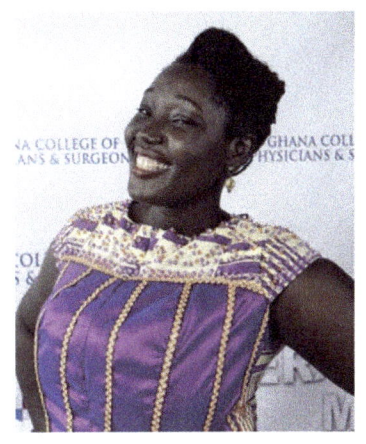

Dr. Sandra Oyakhilome

Dr. Sandra Oyakhilome is the head of dental and oral maxillofacial surgery (OMFS) at Cape Coast Teaching Hospital in Ghana, Africa. She completed her bachelor's degree in medical sciences at the University of Ghana in Africa. She earned a Bachelor of Dental Surgery (BDS) at the University of Ghana Dental School. She worked as a house-officer for two years at Korlebu Teaching Hospital & Ridge Regional Hospital, and as a medical officer at Cape Coast Teaching Hospital in Ghana.

Dr. Oyakhilome was admitted to the Ghana College of Physicians and Surgeons and completed her residency training in oral maxillofacial surgery at Komfo Anoyke Teaching Hospital in Ghana to become a member of the Ghana College of Surgeons.

She emerged as the first female Ghanaian-trained oral and maxillofacial surgeon in the country. She became the second female maxillofacial surgeon in the county, the first female maxillofacial surgeon was foreign-trained Professor Grace Parkins. She returned to Cape Coast Teaching Hospital after residency as a specialist. She is married with one child.

Dr. Oyakhilome chose dentistry because she loves to create things with her hands and put smiles on people's faces. Dentistry offers the ability to restore healthy smiles, OMFS because it extends beyond the mouth and also focuses on the face.

She practices in a government teaching hospital healthcare facility. This requires a great deal of mental and physical strength along with endless patience because of the doctor-to-patient ratio. Currently, there is one doctor to 4,000 people. There is a tremendous amount of skill required to work with limited resources and still save lives and have a life as a physician.

Currently, Dr. Oyakhilome is the acting head of her dental and OMFS department, so a typical day is a mixture of management duties as well as clinical and supervisory duties. She starts her day with her morning routine. She arrives on the patient wards to review patients admitted overnight.

She also sees patients in the accident and emergency department and discusses these patients with her team and colleagues. They make plans for patients to be discharged to home or be admitted to the ward.

Each day, Dr. Oyakhilome heads to the Dental/OMFS outpatient department (clinic) to evaluate patients. In clinic, she consults with patients and does minor surgeries. She trains and supervises doctors in training. Some days she is in the theater (operating room) doing major surgeries. At day's end, she passes through the wards to check on post-operative patients before heading home. Dr. Oyakhilome also attends meetings throughout the day. She frequently checks in with the emergency department to make sure there are no patients that need her attention before heading home, keeping her phone close in case of emergencies.

Dr. Oyakhilome considers her greatest accomplishment to be being the youngest first female Ghanaian-trained oral and maxillofacial surgeon to become a member of the Ghana College of Surgeons in 2018 and her proudest moment the day she became a mother.

When discussing balance, Dr. Oyakhilome claims that anyone working in a demanding profession, surgery or otherwise, who tells you that work-life balance is possible, is conning you. Life will never be in perfect balance. You must find a way to integrate all aspects of your life and make sure to constantly reevaluate, so you do not neglect an area in your life.

There is no such thing as a perfect parent, surgeon, or wife. You must be gentle with yourself and understand there is no such thing as balance.

She believes life is about sacrifice and the only things to balance are rest and recovery. The rest of the days you should be creating and focusing on your vision, passion, and goals. You should be growing. So, weekends are the days she spends resting and recovering. Dr. Oyakhilome shuffles between staying at home, going on outings with her family and friends, and fellowshipping with other Christians.

Dr. Oyakhilome feels that having lived in West Africa all her life, being black has never been an issue. She is blessed to be in an environment that supports women and respect is conferred once you are a doctor, whether male or female.

Her greatest challenge as a dentist is having people appreciate the importance of oral health as part of general health and not waiting until there is pain before they seek dental care. Public oral health education and access to oral healthcare services is a huge challenge.

Dr. Oyakhilome's encouraging and kind words for each reader are, "Have a long-term vision for your career and have faith in God to see you through. Take time to develop a career plan and set timelines. Be bold and just do it. Ask questions. Do not listen to people who have the, "It can't be done," mindset. Be persistent. Yes. We. Can.

CHAPTER TWENTY-TWO
Doctors in Surgical Training

Dr. Josephine Kusano

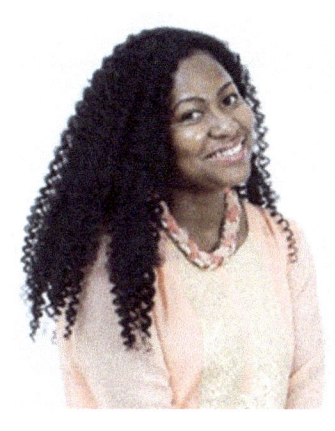

Dr. Josephine Kusano is a junior registrar (resident) in the department of urology at United Bulawayo Hospitals in Zimbabwe, Africa. She completed her medical school training at Wenzhou Medical College in Wenzhou, Zhejiang, China, and is completing her surgical training in Zimbabwe.

This is her journey from Ghana to China to Zimbabwe.

I was born and raised in Ghana, Africa. My passion to pursue medicine goes as far back as my primary school days in Ghana. I know most people think it is a cliché, but some doctors are inspired at a young age. I always thought of myself becoming a doctor when I grew up and I loved assisting our school nurse with wound care. I did not know what I was doing, but it made me feel good making my classmates think I could fix them. I made sure to work hard in school and I excelled scholastically. I told myself that one day I would be a doctor and all my classmates would come to me for care.

In junior high school, I attended a renowned private school in the capital city Accra in Ghana, Africa, and there were a few classmates who called me, "Miss Know-it-All." I remember my principal advised me to separate myself from these classmates to strengthen myself and excel.

These years were difficult because I had few friends and many enemies, but it never diminished my self-confidence. I told myself that if my parents, principal, and few friends saw something great in me, then I could be so much more than I could imagine.

When I was a senior in high school, I succumbed to a wave of peer pressure, a bit of truancy, and some regression in my academics. My mother threatened to pull me from the science program and move me to the home economics program. I cried and promised to do better. Luckily, my beloved father came to my rescue and gave me another chance to remain in the science program. He realized how much I loved learning science.

From then on, I worked extremely hard, but it was not enough to excel on my final national exams. Because I did not do as well as I needed to on my national exams, I decided to pursue law. I watched many television crime series and read legal thrillers, so I thought it would be a great career. I lost hope of being accepted into medical school because of my poor performance but thought I could excel as a lawyer.

My father never gave up on my going to medical school. He invited a friend who was a neurosurgeon to talk to me and encourage me to not give up. With this reassurance, I applied to medical school and was accepted into one of the medical universities in Ghana. I was excited but also afraid of the difficulties of a medical education. I heard stories about it being exceedingly difficult, and about some students succumbing to the pressures and committing suicide or quitting. I wondered if I was good enough to complete medical school.

As fate would have it, my mother decided she did not want me to complete my medical training in Ghana, where I would be exposed to my friends and peer pressure. She gave me the choice of applying to the University of Maryland in the U.S. to pursue a non-medical, non-legal undergraduate course of study or applying to the Wenzhou Medical University in China to pursue a medical degree. I chose China and this jump-started my journey to become a doctor.

Medical school was a roller coaster. I met my husband, a Zimbabwean young man also pursuing a medical degree. When we met, he became my best friend. We became each other's support system and helped one another stay focused on our studies. We joked that I was the medical physician and he was the surgeon in our study group.

I remember the dread I felt when I was the second assistant for a plastic surgery case. The patient was an adorable female toddler who needed her bilateral cleft lip repaired. A cleft lip is a birth defect that results in an opening or split in the upper lip and interferes with feeding.

When I started medical school, I considered medicine rather than surgery and intentionally avoided assisting in surgical procedures. However, this cleft lip operation was the turning point in my career.

Anxiously, I assisted by cutting the sutures at just the right length and exerting sufficient traction with the skin hooks. I avoided anything that might upset the surgeon operating because it could have resulted in a scolding. But, when I saw that child smile for the first time after we removed the bandages, I knew surgery was what I wanted to do for the rest of my life.

When I was an intern rotating in the surgical department at one of the main referral hospitals in Harare, the capital of Zimbabwe, I was stressed. After a traumatizing three months of general surgery, I was scared and petrified. I felt traumatized because general surgeons can be difficult to work with and training is intense. I spent long hours standing in the operating room dealing with distressing injuries and assisting with complicated surgeries.

I rotated on the maxillofacial surgery service and, even though they were more accommodating and patient than the general surgeons, I resisted the urge to develop an interest in surgery.

Interns are required to attend maxillofacial, dental, and plastic surgery clinics three times a week. I developed an interest in clinic patients because I was able to see post-operative patients. This was great because my consultant always took before photos, and when the patients came for their follow-up clinic visit, we took the after photos. The transformation was amazing.

Every day I told myself I would be the first doctor in my family when I returned home, work at the hospital of my dreams in Accra, and walk around wearing my white coat with a big smile. I imagined my mum looking at me, a successful doctor, and telling my dad how he had made the right decision allowing me to complete my science program in senior high school when she wanted me to switch to home economics.

I excelled in medical school until one month before my final exams. I was only weeks from graduation when my father died from bronchogenic carcinoma. I was devastated and I almost quit medical school out of anger and grief. I thought I was going to lose my mind. It was a dark time in my life. My husband and close friends rallied around me and helped me deal with my grief. I was able to study for my exams and passed. I wished my dad could have been here to see me become the great person he hoped me to be.

My husband and I moved to his home, Zimbabwe, and I began my internship at Harare Central Hospital. This was when I discovered my hidden love for surgery.

Everyone asked, "Why not pursue plastic surgery since this was the surgical discipline that originally captivated me?" After my internship, I accepted a job in Bulawayo as a hospital medical officer. This was the only available post (position) at the time. When I worked in the urology department, I developed a sudden interest in it. I found a great mentor who has been a great guide and helped me realize that even though urology is a male-dominated specialty in Zimbabwe, what matters most are my skills and not my gender. He said if I have a passion for urology, then I should do it.

Some days are challenging, and some are fulfilling. This is what keeps me going and makes me enjoy my career. With great support from my mother, my husband, and my children, I feel I can conquer all the obstacles I face. When I get home, I love turning some of my experiences at work into fictional bedtime stories. My children love my stories! I am glad to say I have motivated my two older children to aspire to be doctors in the future.

I have three children. My oldest is a 12-year-old girl. She

is my husband's biological child, but I have raised her since my husband and I met. She is mine. We also have two younger boys, a five-year-old and a seven-month-old. It has not been easy juggling work, family, and children. Sometimes I feel I am about to collapse from fatigue and exhaustion. I am someone who likes to put my whole heart and effort into accomplishing things I set my mind to do.

Urology training is difficult and terribly busy. I am training at a major referral hospital and there are many patients coming to our facility. Unfortunately, with the doctors in training strike, there are fewer of us to get the work done. Because of the strikes, my consult and I are on call every day. I rely on my support system, especially when I am working so many hours.

Sometimes, my children are disappointed when I leave them with their aunty who cares for them while I work. She is a wonderful lady and I am grateful for her help. On any free day, I make sure I cook our meals and bake with my daughter and sometimes take her for a girls' outing. Other times, my husband and I take all the children for a family outing or a short trip.

Luckily, my husband wants me to become a urologist as much as I do. He encourages me to fill my case logbook and to study urology. He asked one of his friends at the hospital records department to gather all the necessary data for my dissertation. My husband assists with some chores and sometimes visits me at work for lunch.

What keeps me going is knowing I make my family proud of me and also the sense of personal satisfaction when I see my patients grateful for the help I give them.

"You may not always have a comfortable life and you will not always be able to solve all of the world's problems at once but don't ever underestimate the importance you can have because history has shown us that courage can be contagious and hope can take on a life of its own."
Michelle Obama

Odinachi Moghalu Schulle

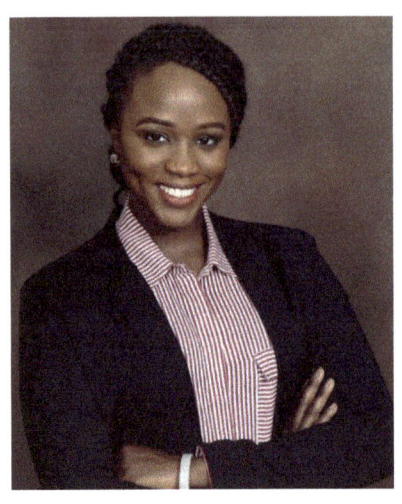

Dr. Odinachi Moghalu Schulle received her bachelor's degree in biomedical engineering from Baylor University in Waco, Texas. She has a master's in biomedical science from Touro College of Osteopathic Medicine, New York, New York, where she also received her Doctor of Osteopathic Medicine degree.

She completed an internship in general surgery at New York Presbyterian Queens Hospital in Flushing, New York. She is currently a post-doctoral research fellow at the University of Utah, School of Medicine in Salt Lake City, Utah, in the department of surgery, urology division.

Dr. Moghalu Schulle wanted to become a doctor since she was three years old. She does not recall any specific events that led her to this decision, however, after high school, she chose to pursue mathematics and physics. This led her to earn a degree in engineering.

Since she did not have a reason why she chose medicine, Dr. Moghalu Schulle wanted to make sure this decision was hers, not something her parents subconsciously instilled in her. So, rather than go straight into medical school after high school, how it is done in England where she lived at the time, she made the decision to pursue engineering. She chose biomedical engineering.

During her undergraduate studies, she realized she was interested in medicine, but at the same time, she did not want to let go of her engineering background. Dr. Moghalu Schulle's interest went from considering a career in medicine to finding how she would be able to merge her deep interest in engineering and human physiology.

During her third-year clinical rotation in medical school, she experienced the greatest joy during her surgery clinical rotations. When she was in the operating room (OR), in a place of controlled chaos, she had an overwhelming feeling of satisfaction. It was the most strenuous and tasking rotation, but it was the one rotation where she felt like she never wanted to leave the hospital.

Dr. Moghalu Schulle is currently a post-doctoral research fellow at the University of Utah in the department of surgery, urology division. She completed her general surgery internship.

A typical day as an intern was quite different from a typical day Dr. Moghalu Schulle now has as a research fellow. As an intern, her day started at 3:30 a.m. when her alarm went off and she prepared herself for work. She typically tried to be out of her apartment between 5:15 and 5:30 a.m. so she was at work no later than 5:45 a.m. On days she took sign-out (report to continue care) from the person who was on night float, she arrived by 5:30 a.m. to allow time to receive the sign-out, transfer the on-call phone, and not have to rush through the details.

General sign-out with the entire department usually started at 6 a.m., and they tried to be finished no later than 6:30 a.m. for team morning rounds. This is where they walked around and evaluated each patient on their list. Patients were in the emergency department, the patient units, and the intensive care unit.

Depending on the team she was on, Dr. Moghalu Schulle either headed to morning conference with the attending on call or could be found at her workstation at work on orders, notes, discharges, and patient care plans. When on day-call, she was not assigned OR cases or clinic time unless they were short-staffed on residents. If she was not on day-call, she headed to the operating room to learn to operate while assisting with cases.

Dr. Moghalu Schulle asserts graduating medical school, despite health issues that threatened her medical school journey, is the greatest accomplishment in her life so far. She is also proud of her determination and zeal.

Now, she is involved in an unpaid research position. This is difficult considering she could have stayed in general surgery, a specialty for which she has no deep passion. Dr. Moghalu Schulle made this difficult choice to take an unpaid research position hoping her portfolio will become stronger. This is so she can successfully apply to a specialty she is genuinely interested in, urology.

Dr. Moghalu Schulle feels her greatest challenge has been finding mentors who are black female urologists.

She has received so much good advice from people, but one bit of advice she finds herself going back to time and time again is, "You cannot be a doctor if you are dead." Her mum first said this to her when she was in high school. Her mum had been with her all her life, paying close attention to how zealously Dr. Moghalu Schulle extended herself to achieve success. Many times, this was to the detriment to her health. That day in high school, her mum finally had enough and insisted she drop everything and forced her to take time to rest.

Dr. Moghalu Schulle never took her mum seriously until she became extremely ill while in medical school and was almost forced to take a leave of absence. Her mum's words rang in her ears. They are true. Dr. Moghalu Schulle can only be a successful doctor if she is in the best health. She must prioritize her own health to best serve her patients.

Dr. Moghalu Schulle has had a few failures in her life, more like many, but has found that failure can either propel you or suffocate you. She finds when she experiences failure, she sits and cries. She cries out and expresses her feelings. She prays and then develops a strategy for how to get back up from that place. Dr. Moghalu Schulle looks at what she could have done differently and tries to separate things she can change from things she cannot change. For the things she can change, she works on these things to see how or where she can improve.

Dr. Moghalu Schulle considers herself an introvert and a recluse, so after a busy day or busy season, coming home and catching up on some of her favorite television shows or working out helps with stress. This for her is balance.

There are several lessons Dr. Moghalu Schulle would like to share. As a pre-medical student, she wishes someone had told her she did not have to rush to take the medical college admission test (MCAT) to fit a particular schedule.

She wishes the importance of seeking a mentor was emphasized. Dr. Moghalu Schulle also wishes she knew she could have taken time from medical school to pursue research in a specialty she was interested in. This is especially important since she had no research background before medical school.

Dr. Moghalu Schulle's lesson learned as an intern was people have more confidence in you if you have confidence in yourself. She is not talking about blind confidence or arrogance but walking into a room with the authority that earned her her place there. Being the only black female during her intern year, she felt like an impostor and several seniors took advantage of this. You must realize you earned that spot just like every other intern there, so act like it. Stay humble but be confident.

Dr. Weludo Ngwisanyi

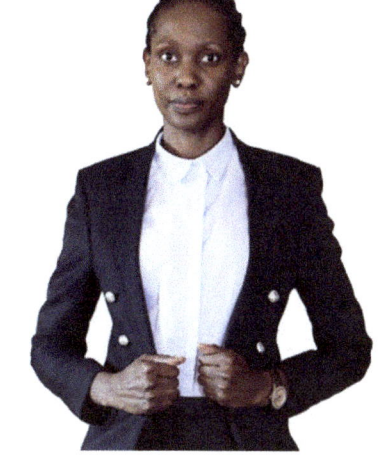

Dr. Weludo Ngwisanyi is a general surgery registrar (resident) at Chris Hani Baragwanath Hospital, University of the Witwatersrand, South Africa. She completed her medical school education at the University of West Indies in Kingston, Jamaica.

This is her journey from Botswana to Jamaica to South Africa.

On one Friday night, as I left the casualty area (emergency department), I heard my junior's voice echoing through the entire casualty area. "RESUS," she screamed. This means resuscitation. We walked quickly toward her. The nursing sisters (nurses) know what this means and came running with their resuscitation trolley. Everyone jumped into action and assumed their specific roles.

As a resident, I was the team leader when my consultant was not present. Our patient was a young lady stabbed in the chest during a robbery and she was being resuscitated. The team worked diligently to save her. They gave her blood transfusions, fluid drips, medications, oxygen, and as the team leader, I made the decision to operate. I felt this was necessary to save her life.

We ran through the hospital corridors to the theater (operating room) and moved her to the operating table within minutes. The amazing theater team understood the urgency and within minutes my consultant and I opened her chest. We found that her heart was stabbed. We took our time and carefully and skillfully repaired the injured tissue. She lived and was discharged to her home within a few days! On days like this, I realize how fragile life is, how every minute matters, and the importance of timely decision making. If you miss it or if you make wrong decisions, patients die.

I am a 31-year-old female medical doctor from Botswana, Africa. I completed my medical training in Jamaica in 2014 and after earning my medical degree, I returned to Botswana to work as a medical doctor.

In January 2018, I entered the University of the Witwatersrand, South Africa, as a self-sponsored trainee in general surgery. This is a five-year training program. I decided to be brave and sponsor myself because the government of Botswana did not have an allocated budget to sponsor doctors for post-graduate studies.

From a young age, I knew I wanted to be a medical doctor. I am the third of five children. We were raised by our single mother on a meager salary. To me, my mother remains a true reflection of the strength of a woman. Therefore, working hard has always been something our mother instilled in us. I partly attribute my mother's great qualities to her family, who would occasionally help her care for us.

My childhood was typical for where I grew up. In order to

attend junior secondary school, I walked 14 kilometers to and from school each day. Even after walking this distance, I was expected to help with daily chores in the house in addition to finishing my homework. My chores included cleaning the kitchen and looking after my baby brothers. I did not consider helping with chores work. I assumed this was part of the responsibilities of every girl child.

I spent my senior secondary school years at a boarding school. I left the only comfort I knew — my mother's house. When I met fellow students from wealthy families, I realized I was from a poor economic background.

A small group of us from poor families depended on the school for food, but the children from wealthy families had an abundant supply. After evening studies, our colleagues from rich families ate the food they brought from home while we poor students slipped under our blankets. We were ashamed and hoped our stomachs did not grumble. Despite these challenges, I was determined to become a doctor.

For me, it has always been about working hard and working smart. It never occurred to me I was intelligent. All I knew was I needed to work hard to pass exams. Like any other boarding school, the curfews were enforced, and I felt the evening study time was inadequate.

Against all odds, I successfully completed my senior secondary school with excellent grades and through my government sponsorship, I found myself in Jamaica at the University of West Indies.

You would believe it would have gotten better, but this is not so. Medical school was difficult, and it took more effort to keep good grades and learn. My secret strategy was being part of a study group. I do not believe one person can know everything. Sharing knowledge and teamwork were what helped me through the rivers and valleys. Being far from my family and missing home was one of the challenges I had to overcome daily, but I kept my eyes fixed on the prize. Time sure does fly when you are busy!

When I completed medical school five years later, I

returned home to Botswana. I was excited to be reunited with my family and serve the people of Mamaland. After studying medicine for five years, you would think this fully prepared me for the medical fraternity and all its challenges, but this was not true. I found myself saying, "I am not ready for this," half the time during my internship year.

One of the greatest challenges I faced, and still face, is having to deliver bad news to patients and families. This is even more difficult when a sudden or unexpected death occurs. Despite staring death in the face each day, it does not get easier. I guess this is because we are all still human at the end of the day.

Enduring long working hours, swollen feet, fighting sleep, and exhaustion, I finished my internship year. I progressed to junior medical officer. But, because Botswana, like other African countries, has challenges related to the shortage of doctors, especially specialists, this inspired me to focus on general surgery.

This is how I came to one of the busiest trauma centers in the world, the Chris Hani Baragwaneth Hospital in South Africa. On many occasions, I find myself and fellow doctors working late, running casualty (emergencies) alone or with only two doctors on busy days. Patients must wait long hours. Though this is exhausting, it is fulfilling work if you are passionate about serving people this way.

Currently, God willing, I will complete my surgery specialty training in three years and return to Mamaland (Botswana) to serve my people — as a qualified surgeon.

Surgery training in South Africa is one of the most intense programs. It is filled with a wide range of illnesses since it is one of the largest hospitals in Africa. Chris Hani Baragwanath Hospital has more than 3,000 beds. The trauma surgery department is such a busy place it makes you think there is a war underway. The experience has been amazing with a great deal of operating time and teaching. Currently, I am working on my research study, which I hope to have published in a year.

Training in general surgery is not without its challenges. I feel it is a male-dominated specialty. So, it goes with the territory that a young female must work extra hard to show she is capable. I find yourself on ward rounds with male surgeons I feel have huge egos.

As a resident, you are expected to know your patients thoroughly, operate on them, run the clinic, make academic presentations, and supervise and teach junior doctors as well as medical students. Additionally, I must work 24-hour call duty, which sometimes turns into 30-hour call duty, and work on my research. We have weekends off to recover and visit with family.

As an African woman, it is challenging to pursue a career and be a homemaker, find a partner, get married, and have children, as per societal expectations. You learn that even your family is not impressed with your choices when they feel other aspects of life are being delayed, because you are expected to focus on homemaking. When I think of the long working hours, the sacrifices, and the exhaustion, I know it will eventually pay off.

If there is any advice, I would give myself at each stage of life, it would be to remain focused and work hard. Also, never forget where you come from. The hardships in life make us who we are. We become strong young women because of where we come from. Always remember to stay grounded. Do not let anyone tell you what you can or cannot do. Never limit yourself. Spread your wings and fly like a butterfly, young girl. There are thousands of opportunities in the world, even beyond your current environment. Never be afraid to dream big dreams. Be ambitious and go all out. It is not easy, but it can be done. Remember everything happens for a reason. There is a God up there watching. You will overcome every obstacle. Never give up. Never quit! It is all worth it.

"The greatest problem of human life is fear. It is fear that robs us of happiness. It is fear that causes us to settle for far less than we are capable of. It is fear that is the root cause of negative emotions, unhappiness and problems in human relationships." Brian Tracy

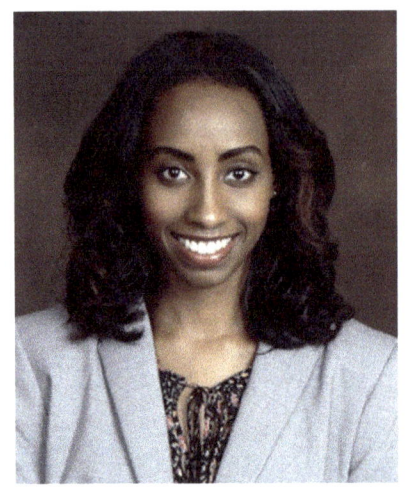

Dr. Ivy Godana

Dr. Ivy Godana is a general surgery resident at McLaren Greater Lansing, Michigan State University in East Lansing, Michigan. She earned her bachelor's degree from Baylor University in Waco, Texas, and a master's in clinical sciences from Boston University School of Medicine, Boston, Massachusetts. She completed her Doctor of Osteopathic Medicine from A.T. Still University of Health Sciences in Mesa, Arizona.

This is Dr. Ivy Godana's story in her words.

Mine has not been a straightforward journey. It seems many people know they want to be doctors from a young age. This was not so for me! I was born and raised in Kenya. I am half Kenyan and half Ethiopian.

We moved to Dallas, Texas, USA, when I was 10 years old. My parents were keen to make certain we understood the importance of education. My father said, "You are here to accomplish something, and you have to take advantage of the opportunity." Therefore, school was a priority for us.

When I was in high school, I realized I liked biology and I also liked health science classes. I loved English classes and read extensively, so my mom encouraged me to consider a career in medicine. I did not think I was smart enough or good enough to be a physician. However, I did have the courage to pursue the dream of medicine because I learned early on that courage is not the absence of fear but the doing despite the fear.

For me, high school was divided into two segments. During my first two years, I was not serious about school. I was satisfied with B's and did not push myself. My dad died when I was in the middle of high school. This was a difficult time, but it resulted in a huge shift in the way I approached life.

My dad wanted us to work hard and do well. He was an attorney and told my mom, my sisters, and me that education is the key to the future. Knowledge is power. This stuck with me, even till today. When I look back at my high school self, I would say, "You are having fun, but remember the important things in life. Keep going. You are doing well. You'll be fine."

When I took the SAT, I told God I wanted to go to Baylor for my undergraduate education and by God's grace, I did well on the SAT and was accepted into my number one choice, Baylor. My mother was excited for me. I was exposed to many things and had many opportunities there. I learned about global medicine and epidemiology. I had fantastic professors and it was a pre-medicine (pre-med) driven school. I became immersed in the pre-med world and knew for sure I wanted to be a physician.

I met one of my mentors in college, Dr. Baker. To my surprise, he coordinated an annual medical mission trip to Kenya, my own home country. The trip was to Western Kenya, so when I joined him it was as though I had come full circle. It was an amazing opportunity to see and feel what it is like to be a healthcare provider in my homeland.

I am proud of my heritage and because I grew up in Kenya, I am more familiar with this culture. Now, I am learning much more about my Ethiopian heritage. It was wonderful to be home and reconnect with everyone. I was grateful.

Being accepted to medical school was not easy because my MCAT score was not the best and my GPA was average compared to others applying. I knew I needed to do something to stand out. What followed was a life lesson in rejection. I applied to medical school after college and it was a resounding rejection from everywhere. I was extremely disappointed and sank into a depression.

I had this huge dream and I worked hard, but the doors kept closing in my face. You begin to think your dream is never going to happen. My mother encouraged me to keep believing and continue with my education, so I enrolled in a master's program at Boston University. After finishing my master's degree, I applied to medical school again. Guess what? Resounding rejection again!

Yes, it was difficult, but there is one thing I realized, in hindsight, I was usually a late applicant. This was a problem because most medical schools filled their seats by the time I applied. Just because there is a deadline does not mean you should wait until that deadline.

Be organized and get your application in early! I told myself, "You have to try again. There is no reason why you can't try again." I was more afraid of missing an opportunity than failing. So, I submitted my application early the next round.

I remember sitting in our living room and working hard on my secondary applications to medical school listing all the reasons I was good enough and would make a great physician. That cycle, I received many rejections, but guess what? I was granted one interview. One. One interview at A.T. Still in Arizona!

All I needed was one medical school to give me a chance. My first choice for medical school was the George Washington University because I wanted to live in Washington, D.C., and they had a well-known global medicine program. Later, by God's providence, an opportunity presented itself and I was able to complete my clinical years in Washington, D.C.

I cried tears of joy when I was accepted into medical school. I knew then that my dream was possible. I love reading. One of my favorite writers is Rumi. There is a quote where he asks, "Why have I received only this?" A voice replied, "Only this will lead you to that." I did not need a slew of choices. Sometimes God gives you exactly and only what you need. Revelation 3:7 says, "To the angel of the church in Philadelphia write: These are the words of Him Who is Holy and True, Who holds the key of David. What He opens, no one can shut, and what He shuts, no one can open."

When I sent my deposit to reserve my position, I felt this was something God had given me. It has not been an easy road.

I cried many times thinking it was over. Now, I marvel as I look back on my journey to becoming who I am today. I learned that your strength is in your perseverance. It is not in the things you have been successful in; it is in the many times where you fall and you decide, I'd rather get back up and fall again than not try at all. God is good!

It is because of all these experiences that I am better prepared for surgical residency. I didn't always realize it, but those moments when I had to pull every ounce of strength from within to get back up, were character building. One of the things that helps is this little poem by a little girl from Malawi. It says, "Little by little we go." A friend of mine sent it to me and I wrote it out. Training was difficult, the hours are long, and the stakes are extremely high. I am learning to take one step at a time, even if it is one little step every day until I achieve my goal.

When I look back and compare it with residency, medical school was not so bad. But at that moment, it seemed difficult. In medical school, you learn a great deal of information, but you also learn much about yourself. You learn how you deal with stress and how you respond to stress. I also learned much about time management. I learned about the importance of taking care of myself first. You must be strong in mind, body, and spirit to be productive, efficient, and successful.

I had great professors. If your mind and heart are open to receiving, you are going to receive the information. What worked for me was finding a study group and balancing studying with people and studying alone. Alone, because you are a physician alone. You are not going to be a physician with other people. You must determine what works for you because there is a great deal of information. The first two years are preparation for the next step. Learn to study well in college, so you develop the good study skills needed in medical school.

My clinical years were fun because I put what I was learning into practice. You are not writing real orders or doing real notes, but you are learning how the system works and the art of medicine.

I had an opportunity to rotate through Howard University in Washington, D.C, and it was so nice to be around people who looked like me. I developed relationships with other students and residents and was encouraged and inspired by many amazing residents and attendings. I had such a great time.

I would tell myself in those first few years, "Do not worry about the fun stuff. It will come later. Focus on the important things." In medical school, I would say, "Keep going. You are doing well. Everything is going to come together."

What I would like to leave every black girl or young lady with a dream of becoming a doctor is, "I want to say to those little girls to have huge dreams; no matter what your circumstances, you have a purpose. You belong here just as much as everyone else and you matter. Whatever dreams you have, it is like the valid words Lupita Nyong'o said, 'The world does not belong to a select few, it belongs to us all. Our greatest hindrances are our minds. If you say you are going to do something and you consistently put in the work and do your best, you will be rewarded."

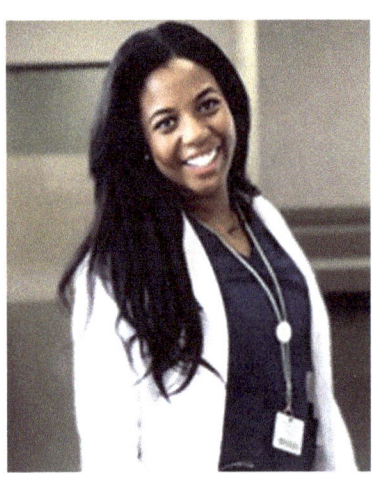

Dr. Amber Hardeman

Dr. Amber Hardeman is a surgical intern at the University of Mississippi Medical Center, Jackson, Mississippi. She earned her Bachelor of Arts degree in Spanish language and literature from Vanderbilt University in Nashville, Tennessee, and her master of public health from the University of Alabama in Birmingham. She earned a combined doctor of medicine and master of business administration from Tulane University School of Medicine and Tulane University A.A. Freeman School of Business, New Orleans, Louisiana.

318

This is Dr. Hardeman's story in her words.

I grew up as a military child. My parents were both in the Navy and, unlike most children, I moved from place to place. Moving was not an issue for me, but rather another adventure that optimized sharing experiences with others. I lived in many different states from California to Colorado to Texas, and other countries such as Japan and Australia. Every time I enrolled in a new school, I experienced a new culture, new friends, and new ideas. Another cornerstone growing up was golf. I was a member of the First Tee and not only played in the program, but I also participated as a mentor and eventual program director. I played in numerous tournaments on the Junior PGA tour, spoke at national PGA events, created PGA commercials, taught children to play golf, and eventually was recruited to play golf in college.

Growing up, I always knew I wanted to be a doctor because of my interest in science. As I became older, my passion for people solidified my career decision. I chose medicine because it empowers me to help people in a way that is not possible in any other field. Being a doctor is one of the most meaningful ways to positively contribute to society.

I chose surgery because there is a unique bond between a patient and a surgeon. The patient allows the surgeon to do something life-altering. The surgeon has the responsibility of someone's life in his or her hands. Complications are real, but positive outcomes and life satisfaction are exponential.

I believe healthcare is a right, not a privilege. I want to work in underserved communities as part of my mission to provide quality care. My desire to treat the patient rather than just the disease encouraged me to pursue an MD/MBA degree in addition to my MPH. I know that in addition to treating patients, medicine also involves understanding population-based health concerns, navigating the world of the healthcare business, and properly executing scientific knowledge to heal people.

As a bilingual black female, I have experienced firsthand treating patients who confide in me due to language and/or cultural barriers in care. I am dedicated to helping families have access to adequate healing support and diminishing disparities with adverse effects on public health.

My undergraduate experience was non-traditional. I was recruited for golf and accepted to Dartmouth College in Hanover, New Hampshire, in its early decision program. Over the course of the year, I realized I was not happy and searched for somewhere else to pursue my interests. I transferred to Vanderbilt University in Nashville, Tennessee, where I thrived.

I continued to play golf. I also dove deep into serving the Nashville community as a member of the student government Community Service Board. I became a Spanish interpreter at the Vanderbilt University Medical Center. After school hours, I worked at the Vanderbilt Childcare Center. Also, I was on the boards for other clubs including the Global Health Committee and the Vanderbilt chapter of the NAACP. My goals in college were to study hard but still have fun.

I studied in Spain while working on my Spanish honor's thesis. I also traveled abroad for community service projects in Costa Rica and Guatemala. I tried to make the best of my time, remain well rounded, yet also adequately prepare for the academic rigor waiting for me in medical school.

In medical school, I studied constantly. I studied all day, every day, almost nonstop. Some might think us type A personality medical students are studying this hard to get ahead. But the reality is that we do it just to keep up with the volume of material thrown at us and often we still feel behind.

At the same time, we are human beings, not robots. We also must sleep, eat, and enjoy laughter in our lives. On the weekends, I did try to attend local events, work out, see friends, travel, and grab some extra sleep. It is difficult and humbling to work so hard while feeling I have not mastered anything, with more and more work routinely piled on.

I became more efficient at managing my time. I learned to take breaks to maintain my sanity. No matter how difficult things became, I was grateful to be a medical student. This path is not easy, but I chose it for a reason. I love learning about medicine and would not have it any other way. Medical school taught me that success is a series of small wins. You must decide what your highest priorities are and have the courage to say "no" to things that do not always serve your purpose. I learned that the road to medicine is a slow process, but quitting will not speed it up.

I face challenges. I feel my greatest challenge is having colleagues who lack the historical context of what centuries of structurally racist ideas and practices are present within the medical community that leads to African American distrust of the system. I cringe when I hear colleagues complain about a patient when they have no idea of the cultural differences. I, however, do not always find it my place to correct them. I hope my colleagues join me in meeting the needs of our patients and I can constructively help them understand their own implicit biases.

Another challenge is having my position questioned every day. It appears I should only be a housekeeper, or in dietary, or a nurse as a black female, even when I introduce myself as a doctor and part of the surgical team.

I find myself being questioned by patients, "Are you actually my doctor?" I also find myself being doubted by colleagues. I strive to prove them wrong. I am daily reminded of the need to intensify the call to action for augmented diversity in medicine. I do believe racism exists in medicine and many African American physicians have their individual stories about being ostracized because of the color of their skin. I may be known to some as a black female first and as a black female who has worked to achieve the privileges afforded a medical doctor secondly. I will continue to try to break down these barriers, one person at a time.

I feel resilience is like a muscle. Difficult times are never fun, but they are what make us stronger. The days as an intern will be long and difficult, but I want to remain authentic. I try to keep my human touch and do my best to ameliorate the pain, suffering, and misery of my patients, even if all I can do is offer a friendly conversation.

A typical day for me involves seeing patients and making sure I keep things in order for the rest of the team. I typically wake up around 4:30 a.m. and arrive at work by 5:30 a.m. I check my patients' charts and review labs, imaging results, notes, and more before seeing them. I round with the team and am updated on things we are doing for each patient throughout the day.

Depending on the service, I spend the middle part of my day assisting with floor work or assisting in the operating room. At the end of the day, I round again and make sure daily tasks have been completed. I arrive home around 6 p.m. and eat dinner, sometimes exercise, study, and am in bed around 10 p.m.

My greatest accomplishment/greatest or proudest moment was competing as the only junior in a world golf championship at Pebble Beach — twice! And the last non-medical book I read was *Girl, Wash Your Face,* by Rachel Hollis. My dream vacation is laying on a private beach in Bora Bora while sipping a tropical fruity drink!

The best advice I received was, "Decide what kind of life you really want, then say no to everything that isn't that."

The pearls of wisdom I would like to share with others are, "Never stop challenging yourself. The day you do, you are falling behind. You inspire people who pretend to not even see you, trust me. Right now you might be in a situation you think you will not survive, but six months ago you were in a situation you did not think you would survive and two years ago you were in a situation you did not think you would survive. The point is, you will always surprise yourself and you will ALWAYS make it through. Just keep swimming."

"What could we accomplish if we knew we could not fail?" Eleanor Roosevelt

Dr. Rossana Chipalavela

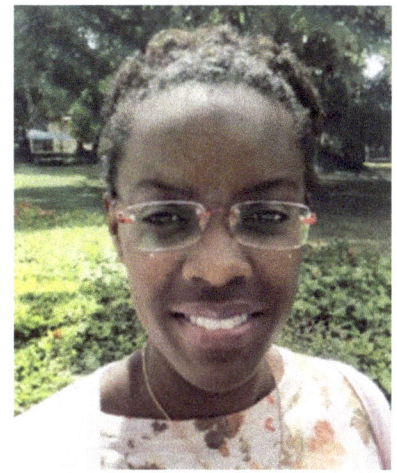

Dr. Rossana Chipalavela is a pediatric surgery registrar (resident) at the Hospital Pioneiro Zeca, Lubango, Angola, Africa. She is currently completing her training in Kenya, Africa.

This is Dr. Chipalavela's story.

When I was a child, I was always sick and spent a great deal of time in a pediatric hospital. I think the time I spent there created a deep passion inside of me to help others.

When I was in my third year in medical school, I went to the theater (operating room) for the first time to assist with a tracheostomy (creating a hole in the front of the throat of a patient) and this was the day I decided I wanted to become a surgeon. Since I love to work with children, I decided to pursue pediatric surgery.

On a typical day, I arrive at the hospital at 7 a.m. and time passes so quickly I realize patients are eating dinner and I have not had lunch yet! That is my typical day! We are busy taking care of patients in the unit and operating. The days go by ridiculously fast.

I find my greatest challenge is balancing personal life choices and career choices. This has been difficult. Also, I had to leave my country, Angola, and come to Kenya to pursue my dream. But the struggle is worth it when I see results.

I found an organization that works with cleft lip and palate defects and am able to work with them in my country. We perform free cleft surgery for both adults and children. When I watched a 52-year-old who spent her whole life with a bilateral cleft lip smile, it was one of the most amazing moments of my life. Currently, they are training me to do cleft surgery.

I build confidence by seeing examples of great brilliant women surgeons and what they have achieved. I always look at them and say to myself, "If they made it, I will also make it."

When failure or complications happen, I try to take the positive lessons I learn and apply them the next time I am in a similar situation.

I had a difficult time finding balance during my first year of residency and somehow this brought me closer to God. God is Who shows me how to balance.

Three people I would want to sit with and learn from are Jesus Christ. He is and will always be the greatest Doctor of all times. My mother. She is the most incredible woman I know. I don't know how she can do so much and never complains. She is my rock. And, Nelson Mandela. It is not easy to forgive people who hurt you, but it is even more difficult to still love someone who hurt you.

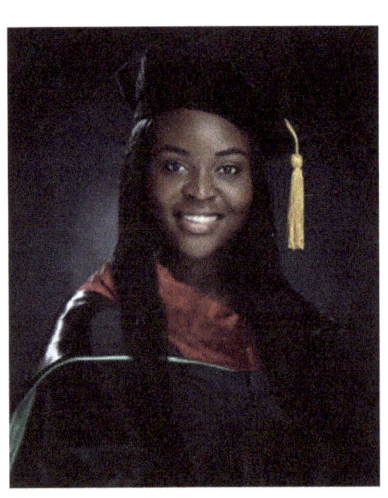

Dr. Sharon Cheryl Bonya

Dr. Sharon Cheryl Bonya is a surgical intern at Kamuzu Central Hospital, Lilongwe, Central Region, Malawi, Africa. She earned her bachelor's degree from Southwestern University in Cebu, Philippines and her medical degree from Emilio Aguinaldo College in Manila, Philippines.

This is Dr. Bonya's story. Perils of studying abroad.

"Where did you study?" she asked, giggling. One of the consults asked me this at the Kamuzu Central Hospital where I am completing my post-graduate internship. My colleague and I were doing morning ward rounds along with other doctors. Both of us studied medicine outside of Malawi.

We answered her with enthusiasm clearly stating where we studied. Her reply was rude and insulting. My colleague and I looked at each other, blankly, unsure of what she meant or why she was treating me this way. We had only been in the department for a few weeks when we met this consultant. Her insolent stereotypical statements did not infuriate me because I had endured such remarks from others.

At age 10, I moved from Malawi to the United States of America. Since I went to middle school and high school in America, I knew what diversity, prejudice, and racism meant. Being an African and a girl in such an environment was not easy, but I made it through.

I will fast forward to my years in medical school. I was a Malawian-born, American-raised woman, embarking on a journey in a new country in Asia, the Philippines, to pursue my medical degree. Things were not smooth here either.

The language barrier was one thing; colossal racism was another. I endured all of it. Often, I called my parents, who were thousands of miles away, to tell them I wanted to quit. All they could do is encourage me as any parent would.

In my final year of medical school, I rotated through the different medical and surgical services at the hospital daily and experienced patient care firsthand. Learning from my senior interns as well as residents and consultants was a great experience. But I felt lost because I was one of the five Africans in my class and the only Malawian.

Despite the discrimination I experienced from several colleagues as well as patients and their families, I did not give up. I still received a proper medical education that I will be able to use for the rest of my life. I would not trade this experience for anything because I learned to fix my eyes on my ultimate goal despite the challenges and obstacles I faced. I was even more motivated by the love and support I received from the senior interns, residents, and consultants who did believe in me.

I have not only become more proficient in my practical skills, but, because of my experiences, I have also become better at dealing with people as an intern medical officer at the Central Hospital in the capital city of Malawi.

Another encounter I had was with the consultant at Kamuzu Central Hospital. I do not know if it is the way I look or the way I speak, no one knows but her, but she also was rude to me. Sometimes others feel that since I am Malawian I lack medical knowledge and am, therefore, incompetent to diagnose and treat patients. Thus, I am labeled as such. I often find myself overworking to prove that I am as good as they are or, at times, even better.

In the end, however, it all depends on the environment in which you surround yourself. I choose positivity every day. I start my day with God to help me through challenges and obstacles each day, as well as end my day with Him. Always remember, you can build a solid foundation with the same bricks others use to throw at you.

What I would tell myself in grade school is, "Enjoy life. Make friends." What I would tell myself in middle school is, "Growing up is a trap, do not get too excited. Just kidding!" What I would tell myself in high school is, "Become the best version of yourself. Have fun, however, remember that your academic life is important." What I would tell myself in undergrad is, "Be present and avoid distractions. Life only gets tougher." What I would tell myself in medical school is, "You probably want to give up. Learning human anatomy and pathology is not easy, but you can and will do it." What I would tell myself before starting my internship is, "Ignore the mean seniors and patients. Learn and make mistakes while you are still under supervision."

"You gain strength, courage and confidence by every experience in which you really stop to look fear in the face. You are able to say to yourself, 'I have lived through this horror. I can take the next thing that comes along.' You must do the thing you think you cannot do."
Eleanor Roosevelt

Dr. Nadege Fackche

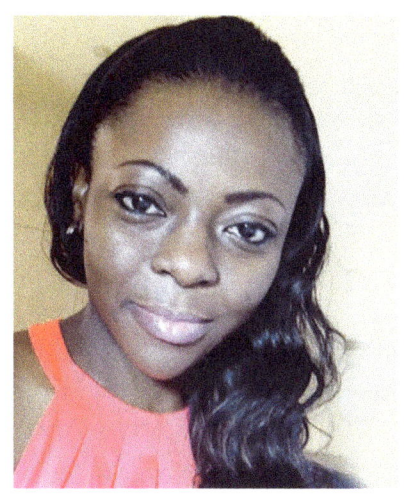

Dr. Nadege Fackche is a general surgery resident at Howard University Hospital in Washington, D.C. She completed her undergraduate degree in respiratory therapy at the University of South Dakota, Vermillion, and earned her medical degree at the University of South Carolina, School of Medicine, Columbia. She completed a two-year surgical oncology post-doctoral research fellowship at John Hopkins University in Baltimore, Maryland.

This is Dr. Fackche's story.

My father is a professor of math and was very intentional in letting me and my sisters know that it was important for us to be well-educated and self-sufficient and not rely on a man to provide for us. I have three sisters that are well-to-do and educated.

My grandmother was a non-compliant diabetic, meaning she did not follow doctors' directions to manage her high blood sugars. I accompanied her to doctors' appointments when I was a child and this exposure to the medical field influenced my decision to become a doctor when I was six years old.

When I was a young girl, I asked my father what the highest degree was that one can attain. He told me a doctorate was the highest degree. So, I knew from that young age I had to earn a doctorate. I started my medical school training in my home country, Cameroon, Africa, and one of my uncles who is an ophthalmologist in Virginia, wanted me to come and study in the United States. So, he and my parents made the decision for me to study in the States. I was not involved in the decision making. They made the arrangements for me to attend the University of

South Dakota.

I moved to the States in January and it was a huge adjustment. I found myself trying to figure things out as I completed my undergraduate training. It was different from how medical training is structured in Cameroon. My parents were not wealthy, so they could not pay for my tuition. My parents did not realize how expensive it is to attend school in the States. To this day, my father tells me that if he knew how difficult it would be financially and how expensive schooling is, he would not have made the arrangements for me to come to the States. I am glad he made the choices he did because everything worked out well.

I earned my undergraduate degree in respiratory therapy because this allowed me to work to support myself while pursuing my medical degree. I had a boyfriend when I was in Cameroon, but I did not think it was a serious relationship because I never saw myself as the marrying type or the kind of woman to have children. I imagined I would focus on my career as a doctor.

But God had other plans because our relationship became serious after I moved to South Dakota. We married and arranged for him to move to the States permanently. I worked for five years as a respiratory therapist and enjoyed my work while I prepared to apply to medical school and financial aid.

I considered a career in pulmonary critical care after completing medical school, but during my general surgery rotation, I fell in love with surgery. By the time I started medical school, I had two young children and wondered if I would be able to be a surgeon, a wife, and a mother. I realized after rotating through all the services in medicine, including OB/GYN and the emergency room, nothing made me as happy as surgery. My husband was instrumental in my decision to choose surgery because he noticed how much I loved being in surgery and how I felt about my other rotations. He promised he would be supportive and help me achieve my goal of becoming a surgeon.

I did my sub-internship (sub-I) in head and neck cancer surgery at Brigham and Women's Hospital in Boston,

Massachusetts, when I was seven months pregnant with our third baby. It was an amazing experience and I was nicely supported during this rotation. I worked hard and enjoyed every moment of my sub-I. I was at the forefront of cutting-edge surgical procedures and pushing the boundaries of science, medicine, and surgery. It was amazing for me.

We spent a great deal of time in the operating room doing ground-breaking surgery and I was in awe. While I was there, I realized I wanted to pursue surgical oncology. It is an exciting field and there is still much to learn in this area. My purpose is to improve cancer care for patients.

What drives me at this time is that there is an entire race of people, black people, which has not been studied in terms of cancer treatment and research. Different cancers affect black people differently from other races, and I want to contribute to how we can optimize treatment for this group of people.

To recap my education in a nutshell, I completed my undergraduate schooling at the University of South Dakota and my medical school training at the University of South Carolina, School of Medicine. I matched at Howard University Hospital, Washington, D.C., for my general surgery residency. I recently completed a two-year research fellowship at Johns Hopkins University in Baltimore, Maryland, between my second and third clinical years. I returned to Howard and am in my third year of clinical residency training.

When I was applying for residency, I was intentional about where I wanted to train. Howard University was my first choice because when I met Dr. Lori Wilson, the program director for the general surgery residency there, I knew she would support me and be a great mentor. She is a mother and wife as well as an excellent surgeon. It was important to have a great support system of other mothers who understand what you are going through because I suffered a great deal with mom guilt. My children are 12, 10, 7, and 5 years old. It has been a challenge to raise children while training to be a surgeon. This is where your village comes in, having a supportive partner and others to assist as needed and help with childcare when necessary.

As far as balance goes, I think there is no balance. There are times I need to focus on my school work and there are times I set my school work aside so I can focus on my family. There will never be balance for me, and that's alright with me. My greatest concern is to make certain to check in with my family frequently, especially my husband. Communication is important.

I love to cook and I often bake with my children, which is a great time to bond. During this season of life, my husband does most of the child-rearing. I make sure there are meals cooked days in advance to help lighten his load. We work well together to keep our home functioning well and thriving. I gave up the idea that I am in control of everything and this has helped to decrease the stress.

The best advice I received is, "You must own your story. Stop trying to make your story fit into other people's boxes. Be who you are and the people who matter will value you for being yourself. Do not try to be someone you are not so you can fit in or so you can be liked."

How I find strength is I pray a great deal of the time. When things are difficult, I give myself permission to cry. Then, I pray and move on. Having the complete support of my husband and children gives me strength each day. They are my reason for doing all that I do.

The lessons I would like to share with those coming up the ranks are, "Dream big. There will be obstacles, but you must fight hard to have the life you want. A support system is crucial to your success. You cannot live on an island. You need people who will encourage you along the journey. Networking is important. I used to believe hard work was enough to help you advance, but hard work alone is not enough. You need people who will open doors of opportunity for you."

Do your little bit of good where you are; it's those little bits of good put together that overwhelm the world." Desmond Tutu

Dr. Busi Mlambo (left)
Dr. Pamela Samoyo (right)

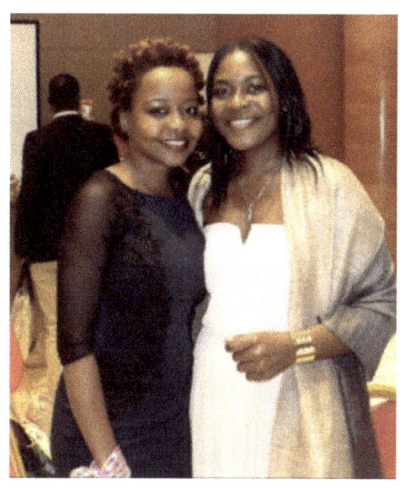

Dr. Busi Mlambo is a registrar (resident) in general surgery at the University of Zimbabwe in Zimbabwe, Africa. She earned a bachelor's degree in molecular biology, bioinformatics, biochemistry at the University of Maryland, College Park in the USA, and a bachelor of medicine and surgery from the University of Witwatersrand in Johannesburg, South Africa. She is a proud member of Women in Surgery Africa (WISA) and passionate about playing her part in empowering women in surgery.

Dr. Mlambo was born and raised in Bulawayo, Zimbabwe. She attended junior high and high school there. Her mom was a midwife when Dr. Mlambo was born, but her mother furthered her education in the medical field to attain additional qualifications in public health and adult education.

Her stepfather was a general practitioner. Dr. Mlambo feels our career paths are often guided by our areas of academic strength. However, when she reached her O-level training, she discovered she loved and excelled in both arts and crafts and sciences. As a result, the school referred her to a psychologist for career guidance counseling. The psychologist analyzed Dr. Mlambo and concluded she was suited for the medical field, particularly an area of medicine in which Dr. Mlambo would be able to use her hands.

The two recommendations highlighted were surgery and dentistry. Dr. Mlambo believes the combination of being raised by parents in the medical field and the results of this psychological evaluation set in place the first cobblestones on the path that led her to where she is today.

Dr. Mlambo chose surgery because she thinks surgery is the perfect balance between science and art. This is clearly where she belongs, somewhere in the middle of the two. Time flies when she is in the theater (operating room). Dr. Mlambo loses all sense of herself and is focused only on the task before her. She has a calm and rejuvenating feeling when she leaves the external pressures and stresses outside the theater and surrenders her mind and hands to the patient on the operating table.

Another reason she chose general surgery was her fear of regret. Dr. Mlambo worried she would regret not having followed her dreams had she chosen a different profession. One may ask, "Why should she have felt pressured to choose a different profession?" Because she knew surgery would not be a walk in the park for a married woman with children. She knew the demands of this career path and how the time commitment diverts time from family. Dr. Mlambo worried about the potential ramifications. She tried to investigate other less taxing careers.

She considered radiology, which has been dubbed an ideal specialty for women because it provides a rewarding lifestyle and the option of working from home. However, she found it unbearable to think she would not interact with patients.

Dr. Mlambo believes the close relationship between a surgeon and his or her patient begins the moment an initial history is taken and the patient is examined. She believes this relationship continues through ward rounds and clinic visits for follow-up care and is vital for the patient's well-being and holistic management of the patient. Dr. Mlambo feels this is vital for the surgeon as well. Her life would feel incomplete if her interaction with a patient began and ended in the theater or with the interpretation of their radiological imaging. She needs to know the person behind the images. She wants to know why they presented, why she made certain decisions about their treatment, how they progressed, and what their outcome was. Dr. Mlambo wants to know how she can build on the knowledge she gained to help other patients going forward.

When she accepted all these things about herself, she

knew her career had to be surgery. Dr. Mlambo explored traditionally female-friendly disciplines like ENT (ear/nose/throat), which she rotated through for six months hoping to fall in love with the specialty, but general surgery maintained its fierce grip on her heart.

Although she experienced some racism in her medical training in South Africa, Dr. Mlambo cannot say it scarred her for life. She quickly learned as a black female that if she stayed on top of her game, spoke out, and answered questions correctly and confidently, the color of her skin faded into the background. When the bedside tutorial seemed directed more towards her fairer-skinned colleagues, she engaged the lecturers with challenging questions or answered questioned in a manner impressive enough to re-focus the conversation. This resulted in her receiving the full benefit of the tutorial and future tutorials as well. Dr. Mlambo quickly learned that when the odds are not stacked in your favor, you have to stick your neck out much further to achieve an A in life, so this is exactly what she did and she succeeded.

Dr. Mlambo married a supportive husband who has backed her career choices since her final year in medical school. She had their firstborn son during her second year of internship, one and a half years before beginning surgical training. Internship in Zimbabwe varies from two to four years.

She had their second baby, a girl, during her third year of surgical training. Being a registrar (resident) in surgical training with two young children has been difficult because of the long hours she spends at the hospital. There is mom guilt associated with many working mothers, wondering if they spend enough time with their children?

Dr. Mlambo thinks comparison is the thief of joy. She tries not to dwell on this but at times she cannot help comparing herself to male colleagues because they have more time to read since their wives are at home caring for their children and homemaking. It is unrealistic to compare yourself to people who are different from you. For instance, one night she spent two hours trying to help the baby to sleep because she was fussy. Some nights her children needed to be breastfed several times during the night.

Also, there have been times one of her children was sick and she was up most of the night caring for them. Though she has support, when her children are sick, they want their mom. Finding balance has been challenging and she cannot say for sure she ever will find balance.

When she has difficult days in training, Dr. Mlambo finds the strength to keep going from colleagues at work. She feels everyone should know their team and not be afraid to call for help. She has mentors and keeps their numbers on speed dial. She needs someone to ask, "Did I do the right thing here? What would you have done? Should I have done anything differently?" She learns from experiences.

Dr. Mlambo keeps her family informed of when she will be home. She talks to her husband or her mom about challenging situations. And she remembers that through everything, it is important to maintain patient confidentiality and never provide information that could lead to the recognition or singling out of any patient.

She feels confidence relates to personality factors, and Dr. Mlambo is a type-A personality and an extrovert. So, confidence is not something she struggles with. As a matter of fact, confident is a word many people use to describe her, whether it is how she carries herself or how she answers questions. It is not something she focuses on or consciously puts on. She does think there are things anyone can do to make themselves feel more confident. These things are different for each person.

Dr. Mlambo feels dressing a certain way and presenting herself a certain way gives her confidence. So, on days she is not wearing scrubs, she dresses formally for her ward rounds and feels this boosts her confidence. Most importantly, she stays on top of her game. This means she knows her theory and she is operating well in the theater. This instills self-confidence, not only in herself but also in the consultants around her. This is vital in surgical training which is so mentorship-based.

If Dr. Mlambo had to choose one surgery to do and only one, she would have to say she would do a surgical oncology procedure because she makes meaningful and measurable differences in someone's life every day of her life. If she had to narrow it down even further, she would say surgical breast oncology, particularly the breast-conserving procedures where she rids women of their cancers while giving them the option of saving their breast. This translates into a preserved body image and beauty to many women.

She loves to play music in surgery. Yes, yes, and yes. She listens to anything and everything. Her theater playlist has a wide range of music ranging from artists such as Bob Marley to Maroon 5.

Dr. Mlambo will be the first to admit she has not done well finding balance. Most of the time, work comes first and everything else falls into place in whatever time is left over. Perhaps she should award herself with some protected time, be it an hour or two each day or a day of the week; time she commits to the people and activities that matter most to her outside work. It sounds close to impossible, especially for a surgeon in training; but it is possible. Dr. Mlambo loves to read but this is a difficult time to read for leisure because she has exams soon. The next book on her list is *This is Going to Hurt: The Secret Diaries of a Junior Doctor* by Adam Kay.

Lessons Dr. Mlambo shared are, "Manage time well. Everyone in the world has the same 24 hours a day you do. Apparently, there is a way to have it all as you maintain a balance between family and work, looking after yourself, exercising, and eating healthy food. When you figure this out, be sure to let me in on your secret! Keep your friends close and your family closer. You will need a social support system to get through surgical training. Get lots and lots and lots of help!! This may be in the form of help with childcare. Sometimes grandma's and grandpa's help with children. Keep your key people in the loop and informed about upcoming hurdles or challenges so they can anticipate any added stress you may be experiencing. For example, I told my husband ahead of time when my next rotation would be difficult. I informed him when I would be on call every weekend for six months and would be unable to do anything on weekends, including traveling. I informed him when I would only be home in the evenings. This helped him prepare for the difficult months, so he did not feel blind-sided and was able to deal with my absences and remain supportive. Ultimately, and most importantly, just do the best you can. Friends and family know they do not see me at family functions, and this is ok. Sometimes I miss my children's school events, and this is ok. I am not perfect, but I do the best I can! And finally, if you worry that a part of you will always be incomplete if you do not become a surgeon, then you must do this. The decision you must make here and now is to become a surgeon. As for the how, figure it out as you go. That is it!"

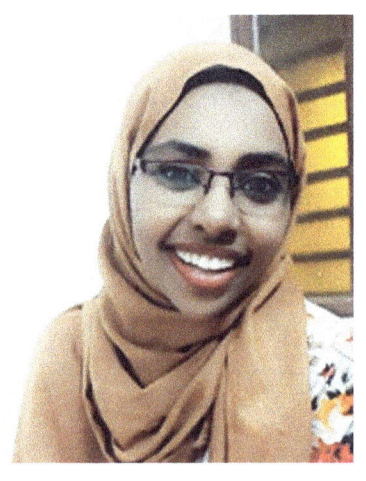

Dr. Eman Abdel Azim Elsadek Elhassan

Dr. Eman Abdel Azim Elsadek Elhassan is a fifth-year surgical resident from Sudan. She is a member of the Royal College of Surgeons, Edinburgh (MRCS-Ed). She received her medical degree from the Upper Nile University in South Sudan, Africa.

This is Dr. Adbel Azim Elsadek Elhassan's story.

I chose a career in medicine because my father is a doctor. I loved seeing him in a white coat with a stethoscope around his neck. During my medical school surgical rotation, I fell in love with surgery because of the fine motor skills necessary for surgery and the gentleness of surgery. Since it seems surgery is a male-dominated field and some women in my country of Sudan, for cultural and religious reasons, prefer a female surgeon, I feel I can offer them my expertise.

The challenges I face are working in a field with male predominance. Also, like other developing countries, we have a brain-drain where our highly trained professionals leave the country, and we are left without adequate staff. And, something that may be different for us is we do not have adequate call-rooms and healthy food making it challenging when working more than 24-hour shifts.

My greatest accomplishment and my greatest or proudest moments are when I see the junior doctors I teach excelling and doing well. This makes me enormously proud. Also, I was proud when I was admitted as a full member of the Royal College of Surgeons [MRCS] and received my certificate at the ceremony. I was so happy because I saw the pride on my parents' faces. My greatest achievement will be when I pass my final exam in a few months and officially become a surgeon.

The best advice I have received is "Read, read, and read as much as you can."

As far a finding balance goes, I am deeply convinced that God has a plan for my life, and He is in control of everything that happens. I remember when I was pregnant, I struggled due to the physiological changes of pregnancy. I waited for hours for public transportation to reach the hospital on time for my shift. I struggled with shortness of breath and fatigue. While standing for an hour or two doing a thyroidectomy or any other operation I experienced swelling in my legs. I remember the thirst I felt that drove me to drink three liters of water in one sitting. And then, my daughter decided it was time to be born when I was preparing to operate. Everything worked out well.

After she was born, I worked day and night, including weekends and holidays, to offer the best for my family. Now, I am studying for my final exam, holding my thesis in one hand and carrying my daughter with the other. It is not easy to find balance and I have accepted this. I am determined to be successful in all areas of my life. In my spare time I play the piano and write books.

Three people I would like to have dinner with and learn from are Benjamin Carson (American neurosurgeon), Maria Siemionow (Polish transplant female surgeon), and Reem Balilah (Sudanese hepatobiliary female surgeon).

Lessons I would like to share with the up-and-coming young black female surgeon are, "Being a surgeon is an amazing career. Do not shy away from it if it is what you desire to do. There will be people who do not support you along your journey to becoming a surgeon, but do not allow this to stop you. Let your personal life be parallel to your surgical career. There is no better time to get married, be a mother, and continue productive relationships with your friends and family. You will struggle much in your surgical career, but whenever you fall, you must find a way to get back up on your feet and keep going."

"Wherever you are in your journey, I hope you, too, will keep encountering challenges. It is a blessing to be able to survive them, to be able to keep putting one foot in front of the other—to be in a position to make the climb up life's mountain, knowing that the summit still lies ahead. And every experience is a valuable teacher." Oprah Winfrey

CHAPTER TWENTY-THREE
My Story

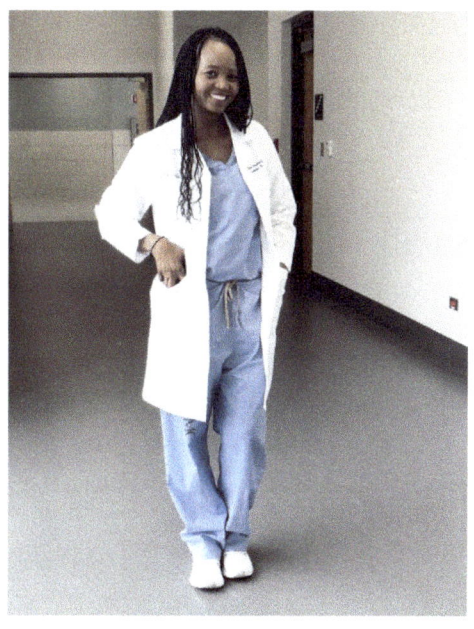

Dr. Praise Matemavi's story

For as long as I can remember, I wanted to be a doctor. When I was six years old, a medical team from Loma Linda University Medical Center, Loma Linda, California, came to my home country, Zimbabwe, to help start the open-heart surgery program at Parirenyatwa Hospital.

My father told me about this project and from this time on, my goal was to become a heart surgeon. We often drove by the hospital and I looked at the intimidating buildings that made-up one of the world's largest hospitals at that time, with more than 5000 beds. I imagined myself grown up, dressed in my white coat, and taking care of patients.

My parents encouraged my dream and in fifth grade one of my birthday gifts was the book *Gifted Hands* by Dr. Ben

Carson. I devoured the pages in one sitting. I was enthralled by the mysteries of medicine and surgery.

We moved to the United States of America when I was 14 years old. It was a cold and snowy day in mid-December when we landed at the O'Hare International Airport, Chicago, Illinois. I have always disliked cold and I never saw snow before but adapted quickly to our new home in Michigan on the campus of Andrews University where my father was studying for his master's in divinity.

Being a pastor's child, we moved many times. By the time we moved to Michigan, I had already attended six different schools, so it was an easy adjustment. Berrien Springs is a small village, population 1800. It is best known for being a Seventh - Day Adventist community. Muhammad Ali lived in our quiet, safe village that had two traffic lights and no Walmart. I loved the intimacy of my new community compared to the hustle and bustle of living in the outskirts of Harare, the capital city of Zimbabwe. I quickly made friends with other girls who lived on campus whose parents were also studying at Andrews University.

High school was fun and a breeze for me. I found the American education system much easier than the British education system I came from. American education was structured with study guides and multiple-choice questions and the British education system consisted of essay and problem-solving testing.

We did not have money for me to attend the university, but I had dreams and intelligence on my side. I enrolled in a community college where I was blessed with scholarships to cover my tuition. I planned to complete my prerequisites for a biology degree while working full-time to save money for university costs. As an international student, I was not eligible for student loans and the resources available to me were limited.

At age 18, I became pregnant. It was a devastating blow to me and my parents, who migrated to the United States so I could have the opportunities and resources necessary to follow my dreams of becoming a heart surgeon. This was the beginning of a difficult four-year period in my life.

I became a victim of domestic violence and later, a survivor. I felt alone despite having close family and friends who cared about me. I hid my pain. I was ashamed. During this time, I changed my course of study and completed my associate degree in nursing and was blessed with a second child.

By age 23, I was working full-time as a cardiac telemetry nurse and raising two beautiful children as a single mother. I was blessed to have the unwavering support of my parents and sister, however, my dream of medicine never died. Every time I encountered female physicians, it fueled my drive.

With sheer determination and hard work, I completed my prerequisites for medical school in two semesters. I took general chemistry, organic chemistry, biology, and physics at the same time I studied for the medical college admission test (MCAT).

By God's grace, I did well on the MCAT and applied to medical schools. I did not have an adviser. I researched and figured everything myself. I knew I needed a bachelor's degree to be accepted to medical school, so I enrolled in the university affiliated with our community college. I was able to complete the required 60 credits in one year! I was accepted to every medical school I applied to and chose my home-state medical school.

When I was 14 years old, shortly after arriving in the states, a family friend drove me and my sister to Michigan State University. It was a sunny Saturday afternoon and we saw the beautiful campus and toured East Lansing.

I am uncertain if our friend was considering attending Michigan State University or what her motivation was for taking the trip. We walked around the campus and when we arrived at the administration building with the big green S, my sister took a photo of me standing on the S. I wrote on the back of the photo, "This is where I will come for medical school someday." This was one of many instances in my life I had a vision of exactly what I wanted and years later, it happened.

When the time came to apply for residency training, I applied to both allopathic and osteopathic surgical residencies. At the time I was applying for residency, the osteopathic and allopathic matches were at different times. The osteopathic match (DO) was in February and the allopathic match (MD) was in March. For osteopathic medical students applying to both osteopathic and allopathic residency programs, we had the opportunity to take advantage of the allopathic match if we did not match into a residency in the osteopathic match. Though I interviewed for 12 osteopathic surgical residencies, I only wanted to train at Sinai Grace Hospital in Detroit, Michigan, and if I did not match there, then I would participate in the allopathic match. It was my heart's desire to train at Sinai Grace Hospital, Detroit Medical Center, Detroit, Michigan, and I matched at Sinai Grace and completed my internship year.

Three days after graduating from medical school, I married a wonderful man I met in medical school. He, however, matched in neurosurgery in New York. It was a difficult year for our marriage because we were both in demanding residencies. The following year I relocated to New York for general surgery training at New York Presbyterian Queens Hospital in Flushing, New York. This was one of the best decisions I made.

My surgical residency was difficult and during my third year of training, we divorced. It was another dark and difficult period in my life. I slowly drifted from God, though I continued to say my prayers. My relationship with God was at its lowest point. It was during this dark time I rebuilt my relationship with my Creator. I needed His strength to get out of bed and make it through the difficult days.

I put a smile on my face and continued to work hard, learning how to be the best surgeon I could be. I had a 10-minute walk to work and used this time to talk to God and listen to uplifting Christian music. Eventually, I began to heal and rebuild my life as a single mother again. God has shown me time and again that His grace is sufficient for me. I forged through the fourth year of surgical residency without many incidences. This is a year you have the opportunity to operate a great deal and it was amazing.

In the second half of my fourth year I applied for a transplant surgery fellowship. I traveled the country, interviewing at phenomenal programs. Through all the travels and interviews, my heart set on a fellowship at the University of Nebraska Medical Center in Omaha, Nebraska. This was my last interview.

When I was a second-year medical student at Michigan State University, a professor once saw me reading a book about a pediatric cardio-thoracic surgeon called, *Walk on Water: The Miracle of Saving Children's Lives* by Michael Ruhlman. This professor said that to him, the only other surgery that was technically challenging and beautiful in its own right, was a pediatric liver transplant surgery. He knew a surgeon who did this named Dr. Alan Langnas in Nebraska.

That day, I researched all I could about liver transplants and decided that I would work hard so that I could go to Nebraska to train to become a transplant surgeon under Dr. Langnas' tutelage. You can imagine how excited I was to open my email that June afternoon eight years later as I sat in Central Park to find out that I was matched with Nebraska for my fellowship training. This was by far one of the best days of my life!

I breezed through the first half of my chief resident year, my last year of residency, but three months before my graduation, I faced another dark period. My beautiful mother, who was my prayer warrior and the president of my fan club, was diagnosed with extremely aggressive triple-negative breast cancer. She died within one month of her diagnosis.

I was devastated and had many regrets because I did not realize her time on this earth was this short. I regretted not spending time with her at the end of her life. I took one week off after her funeral and returned to work, business as usual. I dug deep within myself to find the strength to continue each day even though all I wanted to do was cry.

Each time I saw a patient on a ventilator, it brought back memories of her last few hours before we disconnected the ventilator and made sure she was comfortable. During this painful time, I developed a deep respect and appreciation for palliative care physicians. God saw me through, and I graduated from residency and relocated to Nebraska for the ride of a lifetime.

Fellowship was a beast. Nothing prepared me for the long surgeries and even longer days. Also, the flights in private jets to various hospitals around the country, often arriving in the middle of the night, leaving with precious lifesaving and life-altering organs for our patients, was something new to me.

I worked with the most amazing team and grew professionally and personally more than I ever thought possible. Even with the long hours and busyness, I managed to meet the love of my life. He has been a great support and friend. Often, I look back at my journey and marvel at how God led me each step of the way. Even in my darkest days, He was there.

It has been an amazing journey and I see the hand of God in every step, especially during my darkest moments. I have had the opportunity to meet many amazing people along the way, men and women who believed in me and opened doors for me.

In this season in my life, I am exactly where I am supposed to be. I feel extremely blessed to have incredible partners in my practice who support me and have made my transition as an attending smooth. I am grateful for all the trials and tribulations, for they too have shaped the woman I am today. I would not be where I am today was it not for my family and friends who have been through thick-and-thin with me, always encouraging me to keep going. It truly took a village to produce the first Zimbabwean multi-visceral transplant surgeon.

A note about some of the women in this book.

Along the way, I found friend after friend. Now, I am sincerely grateful to each and every one of them for helping me tell my story and theirs.

It was a pleasure and amazing opportunity to talk with Mr. and Mrs. Gordon about their daughter, Dr. Sherilyn Gordon-Burroughs. Dr. Sherilyn died three months before I graduated from my surgical residency and began my multi-organ transplant surgery fellowship. I never met her, but I knew about her because there were only six black female transplant surgeons practicing in the United States at that time. She was the third trained in abdominal transplant surgery. Being such a small group of black female surgeons, everyone knows one another. As I write this book, there are 10 practicing black female transplant surgeons. I hope there will be many more in the years to come! I believe anyone with a dream can have it come true. I want Dr. Sherilyn Gordon-Burroughs to be remembered for the amazing and strong woman she was and thank her for her inspiration.

Dr. Sherilyn Gordon-Burroughs and I share our experiences with domestic violence. I want to share her story in this collection to ensure she is not forgotten. I am also a victim of domestic violence and in my journey to healing, I met some incredible women who share this with us.

Another beautiful woman I have had the pleasure of meeting is Dr. Arika Hoffman. I first met her when I interviewed for my transplant surgery fellowship at the University of Nebraska Medical Center in Omaha. We had many things in common and quickly became close friends. We are both from Michigan and discovered we knew many of the same people. This made talking easy and we naturally found something to talk about all the time.

Also, both our mothers died the same year and we understood each other's grief. When I needed to go home to California in an emergency, she quickly booked a plane ticket for me to leave that day. She has been a mentor, sponsor, confidant, and, most of all, a friend.

And another of my favorite women is Dr. Velma Scantlebury. The first time I met Dr. Scantlebury was at the society of black academic surgeons meeting in Birmingham, Alabama, in 2018. I knew she would be attending and was looking forward to meeting her. I had been corresponding with her for four years via email prior to our meeting.

When I was a third-year general surgery resident, I emailed her telling her I wanted to be a transplant surgeon and asked for advice. She emailed back that same day and from then on mentored me through residency and fellowship and now as a new attending. She is always so well-dressed and put together. I love shoes and can always tell a fellow shoe-lover. I can only imagine what her shoe closet looks like! She is the first black female transplant surgeon in the United States of America. She is a wonderful mentor and my hero!

I researched everything about Dr. Scantlebury when I was a medical student, watched every interview, and read every interview. I also read her autobiography in one day when I was on vacation. I feel I know her life story. I know she wanted to be a doctor since she was seven years old and moved to the United States when she was 15 years old from Barbados. I always wondered what this was like.

Dr. Scantlebury was trained by Dr. Starzl, who is considered the father of liver transplant surgery. I read his memoir, *The Puzzle People* multiple times. I was sad when he retired before I was ready to train in transplant surgery. Because I trained at the University of Nebraska Medical Center, I feel I have a little piece of him since he trained Dr. Bud Shaw who trained Dr. Alan Langnas, who trained me. I consider Dr. Langnas my father of transplant surgery.

Another phenomenal surgeon I admire is Dr. Patricia Turner. I first met her when I was a second-year surgical resident. One of my mentors, Dr. Armando Castro, introduced us at an American College of Surgeons Leadership and Advocacy Summit. There were no surgeons who looked like me in my home institution and he made it a point to connect me with her. She does not know this, but throughout my training, she was a surgical idol of mine.

I followed her rising career with enthusiasm and excitement to see a beautiful black woman surgeon accomplishing so much, giving me hope for what I could accomplish in my career.

I remember leaning in and listening to her intently each time she spoke, whether it was in a large conference room or at the networking dinners. She is the epitome of black girl magic. I love how humble she is and how hard she works to make sure that underrepresented minorities' voices are heard. I could sit and talk with her all day and bask in her wisdom. I was pleased when I told her I was writing a book as a tribute to Dr. Sherilyn Gordon Burroughs and she was happy to be a contributor.

Dr. Iyore James is also dear to me. When I prepared for my general surgery oral boards, I told her how nervous I was to take this difficult exam since I had been in transplant surgery training for two years and not done general surgery and trauma surgery for that long, which was what would be asked. She took time out of her schedule to coach me and review cases two days before the exam. She is a great friend and mentor.

My first time at the Society of Black Academic Surgeons Scientific Session in 2018 which was held at University of Alabama in Birmingham, Alabama, I had never seen so many black female surgeons in one room before. I thought to myself, "Wow, these amazing, beautiful black women are excelling in this male-dominated field." I stood at the edge of the room with my mentor and friend, Dr. Arika Hoffman, because I wanted to take it all in. I trained at an institution where I was the only black categorical surgical resident in the six years I was there and there was only one male African American surgeon who was in private practice. So, one can imagine how excited I was to be in the same room with women in my field who looked like me.

As I stood there in awe of my colleagues, Dr. Zaria Murrell walked into the room. She had an energy about her I admired. I leaned over to my friend and said, "I have to know who that woman is."

I watched this woman who was the epitome of grace, style, elegance, and unmistakably a powerhouse. I learned she was a pediatric surgeon and I was slightly intimidated. Pediatric surgery is one of the most competitive surgical fellowships one can be accepted into and to me, they are the true general surgeons because they cover such a wide breadth of surgical disease processes. Their range is anything from thoracic (lung) surgeries to abdominal surgeries to the skin and soft tissue surgeries. I worked up the courage to approach her and ask to interview her for my book. She was warm and gracious to me. I enjoyed chatting with her and by the end of the interview, I was blown away by her tenacity, authenticity, and just how extraordinary she was.

Dr. Miriam Mutebi is a great friend and supporter. When I told her I was writing this book and including stories and interviews of black female surgeons, she was the first one on board with the project. She helped me contact the women in the Pan African Women Association of Surgeons. She is a powerhouse: the epitome of a triple achiever; a surgeon, a scientist, and an educator. She also has an amazing fashion sense and we share a love for beautiful shoes.

I was introduced to Dr. Portia Siwawa by a friend of mine Dr. Tobe Momah. Dr. Momah is a physician at the same hospital where I work. He was the first to welcome me to Jackson, Mississippi, and he and his wife have been a great resource for me and my family. When I mentioned I was creating a book about black female surgeons, he told me a friend he met during his residency was a surgeon from Botswana and helped me contact her. It was great to talk to my neighbor (Zimbabwe and Botswana are neighbors) who was an African girl-child who also survived surgical training in the Big Apple!

Dr. Violet Onkoba is one of my best friends. It is funny how we met. I was a fourth-year medical student applying for my general surgery residency. I wanted to train at Sinai Grace in Detroit, so I decided to make an appointment with Dr. William Anderson, a nationally known general surgeon and civil rights leader who, at the time, was the Vice President of Academic Affairs in Osteopathic Medical Education at Sinai Grace Hospital. I was given an hour of his time and went intending to consider the different osteopathic general surgery residencies and deciding which ones I would interview for. I had been granted interviews at more than 20 osteopathic surgical residencies and needed to narrow my list to 12.

After talking for a short time, he paged Dr. Onkoba to come to his office so I could meet her because he said to me, "You cannot be what you cannot see." I never met a black female general surgeon or resident, so what he did for me was not only tell me that it is possible, but he also showed me it is possible. I matched at Sinai Grace for general surgery training. We discovered we had much in common and became close over time. She is one-of-a-kind and I am grateful to call her my sister and my friend!

I cannot remember how I discovered Dr. Omofolasade Kosoko-Lasaki on the internet during my first year as a fellow in Nebraska, but I am glad I did. I emailed her asking to meet with her at her office. She responded graciously. She was not working in the same institution I was, so I drove downtown to her office at the Creighton University in Omaha, Nebraska, where she is the associate vice provost of the Health Sciences Multicultural and Community Affairs (HS-MACA) Department.

As we talked, I wanted to absorb everything she said. She taught me many lessons in the hour I spent with her. I could go on and on listing her accomplishments. She is an amazing woman and I am proud to call her my mentor. When I was an avid blogger, she is the one who inspired me to turn my blog posts into a book someday. Well, this is that book!

And I do not want to miss the opportunity to thank Dr. Lori Wilson. As I watched her documentary, I cried because I lost my mother to triple negative breast cancer. Her story hit very close to home. I thank her for sharing her pain, suffering, uncertainty and eventual triumph; for being vulnerable and giving us all a glimpse into her journey.

These and all the wonderful women in this book mean everything to me and I am so grateful for their participation in this book and as my friends. My world is wonderful and beautiful because of them. Thank you from the bottom of my heart, ladies.

ACKNOWLEDGMENTS

This book has been a labor of love which has come to life because of so many wonderful and amazing people. Without their generosity, grace and support, this publication would not have been possible. It took a village of many people to help me achieve my dream of becoming a transplant surgeon. I wanted to mention a few people, there are so many more I am grateful for, they fill a book on their own.

Thank you, Terrie Sizemore, my editor and publisher, visionary and writing partner, for seeing this book as a reality from that first phone call. Thank you for recognizing the importance of our voices. You have a vision for this book that was even better than the vision I have for this book. You put your soul and energy into every word and every story. Editing and reediting until it was perfect. You took time to revise and refine more than 125,000 words until it is a masterpiece. You provided critical and insightful feedback without taking away from my originality. You painstakingly fixed every error and polished this piece and now it shines! Your love and patience are invaluable.

Thank you, Brenda Carter de Treville, for copyediting, proofreading, wordsmithing, layout, and for your insight and constructive criticism. You took time out of your busy schedule to make this dream of mine a reality. I am grateful for all the handwork you put into making this book great!

To the 74 other women who agreed to be featured in this book, thank you for believing in my vision as a place for our voices to be shared. Thank you for willing to share your stories and experiences so that others who are following behind us may benefit from them. You are ALL so inspiring and phenomenal women. I am grateful for the friendships I have developed with each and every one of you during the compiling of this book. To Mr. and Mrs. Gordon, thank you for sharing a little piece of Sherilyn with me. I am so glad to know you.

Dr. Barbra Ross-Lee, thank you for reading every word of the book and for your insight and constructive criticism in how to make the book flow better without losing the reader. Thank you for supporting me with this book. When I was a medical student at Michigan State University College of Osteopathic Medicine, I often stood in the hallway in Fee Hall and gazed at your photo on the wall among a sea of white men. You were a trail blazer and you showed me that anything I dreamt was possible. You overcame barriers during a time when African American women physicians were not common. You went through medical school as a single mother of two children and I was motivated also as a single mother of two to succeed. You worked hard and shattered glass ceilings time and again, becoming the first black female dean of a medical school. A pioneer and legend. Thank you for showing me and others what is possible!

I am indebted to the following individuals who agreed to review the manuscript and write blurbs for me despite their own impossibly busy schedules.

- Dr. Pringl Miller
- Dr. Roberta Gebhard
- Dr. Ainhoa Costas
- Dr. Felicitas Koller
- Dr. Wendy Grant

To my wonderful and amazing work family within the surgery department at the University of Mississippi Medical Center: Dr. Christopher Anderson, Dr. Mark Earl, Dr. James Wynn, Dr. Shannon Orr, and my work sister and BFF Dr. Felicitas Koller. I am so grateful for being part of this family. I know that God brought me here for a reason and I am grateful for the support and growth during this first year of my attending life. You all have guided me and have been patient and made it a smooth transition from trainee to attending.

I need to acknowledge a few surgeons who have made the greatest impact in my training. I am grateful to each of you that has had a hand in my development as a physician and surgeon beginning in medical school. Dr. Shirley Harding, for believing I could achieve my dream of becoming a surgeon; Dr. Susan

Seman for being an example of a phenomenal clinician and surgeon early on in my training; Dr. Sample for being a great mentor to me throughout my residency, for believing in my abilities; Dr. Satterfield for being gracious to me and allowing me to have a safe place to voice my concerns when I felt I was not seen or heard; Dr. Armando Castro, for giving me a chance, without you my career would have turned out very differently; Dr. Tiszenkel, during the difficult days when I doubted and wondered if I was good enough, I went back to the words you spoke upon me as a brand new intern doing an inguinal hernia with you. You said to me, "Doctor, there are very few people I have come across in all my more than 25 years as a surgeon who have what you have; you are destined for greatness!" To this day I don't know if this is something you told every intern, but this was exactly what I needed to know that I belonged – to work hard, and excel. Ms. Donna DeChirico, thank you for your dedication to the surgeons who pass through your doors. I am grateful for all you did for me.

To my transplant surgery family, I am grateful for all the surgeons who took the time to teach me to be a transplant surgeon. Your patience, guidance, and support throughout my two years at Nebraska Medicine is what made the long days' worth it. To my transplant father, Dr. Alan Langnas, thank you for being a great teacher, not only of the art of surgery, but also of how to talk to patients. Dr. Wendy Grant, you believed in me from the first time I met you and because of you, I am. I hear your voice the most when operating. Thank you for always being there to support me and to mold me and direct me. For all the coaching and counseling, not only for me but also for my dear transplant surgery best girlfriends, I am so grateful. I love you very much and my life is better for knowing you! Dr. Shaheed Merani, you taught me so much my first few months of fellowship; you made my transition smooth and almost easy. Thank you for taking the time to coach me a day before my general surgery boards and preparing me for the exam. Dr. Blaire Anderson, I don't have words to describe what you mean to me.

Thank you for being the best litter mate. You made fellowship enjoyable. Dr. Alexander Maskin, Dr. Luciano Vargas and Dr. David Mercer, thank you for educating me and molding me into a well-rounded surgeon.

To my patients — each and every one of you that I have served and will serve — thank you for entrusting me with your care. Because of you, we are able to fulfill our life purposes of relieving pain and suffering. To the medical students, interns and residents I have worked with and work with who have taught me invaluable lessons about medicine and life, thank you.

Thank you, Sonal Johal, for helping me identify women who could contribute to the project and helping me with transcription of two of the most difficult interviews.

To my father, my late mother and my sister, Faith, I am one lucky girl to be part of this family. I appreciate your love and support through everything. Dad, thank you for reading through the first draft and for your constructive criticism. To my stepmother, I am grateful for your encouragement and input. My husband, Ryan Tiemeyer, thank you for letting me be me and for spoiling me every single day. My Shantelle and Noel, you have been through so much with me and are my constant companions and supporters. Jacob, Trent, and Daniel, Tatenda, Branden, Tiwirai, Habakuk and Hope, I am blessed to be in your lives. You all bring me so much joy. Mufaro, you light up my life. I am grateful to have a best friend like you. Shorai Ndoro-Maswela and family, I am grateful for you. Pat Burnham, Mrs. Tsikirai, Ms. Chandra, and Mama Paulina Abbey, thank you for being my prayer warriors. Dr. Shannon Davis, I appreciate you!

Over the years, mostly in retrospect, I learned a variety of lessons, and one of the most important is this: You can't hit a target you can't see. You can't accomplish wonderful things with your life if you have no idea of what they are. You must first become absolutely clear about what you want if you are serious about unlocking the extraordinary power that lies within you. Brian Tracy

CPSIA information can be obtained
at www.ICGtesting.com
Printed in the USA
BVHW021912160620
581684BV00017B/959